# PRINCIPLES OF VENOUS HEMODYNAMICS

# PRINCIPLES OF VENOUS HEMODYNAMICS

CLAUDE FRANCESCHI

AND

PAOLO ZAMBONI

**Nova Biomedical Books**

*New York*

For permission to use material from this book please contact us:
Telephone 631-231-7269; Fax 631-231-8175
Web Site: http://www.novapublishers.com



**LIBRARY OF CONGRESS CATALOGING-IN-PUBLICATION DATA**

Principles of venous hemodynamics / editors, Paolo Zamboni and Claude Franceschi.
p. ; cm.
Includes index.
ISBN 978-1-60692-485-3 (hardcover)
1. Hemodynamics. 2. Veins--Physiology. 3. Veins--Diseases--Treatment. I. Zamboni, Paolo. II. Franceschi, Claude.
[DNLM: 1. Varicose Veins--therapy. 2. Hemodynamics. 3. Veins--physiology. 4. Venous Insufficiency--therapy. WG 620 P957 2009]
QP105.P75 2009
612.1'34--dc22

2008047100

*Published by Nova Science Publishers, Inc. ✦ New York*

# CONTENTS

# FOREWORD

## AN INTERNATIONAL PRESENTATION

Dear Colleagues,

Treatment of varicose veins based on hemodynamic considerations and especially the CHIVA concept have influenced phlebology for more than a decade. These ideas are not historical but are also a part of new treatment concepts including sclerotherapy and modified surgical procedures. Pre-treatment duplex investigation has become the gold standard.

Today, more than ever before, there is a lively discussion and a lot of controversies on how to treat varicose veins best. In the moment there is no definite answer to this question based on published prospective comparative studies. Many questions still remain open and hopefully may be answered in the near future.

In these discussions hemodynamic based treatment is always an issue although many of us are not sufficiently familiar with the basics and the nomenclature of the CHIVA concept.

It is the merit of Claude Franceschi and Paolo Zamboni, two of the CHIVA mentors, to give us all the information we need for a better understanding and recognition of these thoughts. The chapters of this book are not only well illustrated with excellent colour pictures but also based on the actual literature.

This book is a mandatory reading for every phlebologist, may she or he be performing CHIVA treatment or not. It is the basis for a better understanding of this concept and for fruitful discussions on the best way of treating varicose veins in the future.

With kind regards

Professor Eberhard Rabe,
University of Bonn, Germany
President Union International de Phlebologie

## An American Presentation

It is with great pleasure and honor that I introduce this book to the reader. Some may be quite familiar with the concepts proposed by Claude Franceschi in his first book on the subject, Conservative Haemodynamic Cure of Incompetent and Varicose Veins in Ambulatory Patients published in 1988. Certainly there has been an evolution of these concepts over the past two decades, resulting in the present work by Profs. Franceschi and Paolo Zamboni.

I must admit that on this side of the Atlantic, very little attention has been paid to the fundamental notions of venous hemodynamics, whether in the basic understanding of the concepts of valvular function, or the application of these concepts as they relate to treatment of chronic venous disease. While our academic colleagues in the U.S. may have a greater understanding of basic venous hemodynamics, the great majority of clinical work involving superficial venous disease has resided not in the world of academia, but in the realm of private practitioners who evaluate and treat large numbers of such patients on a daily basis. And sadly, as one such private practitioner myself, understanding of the basic principles of venous hemodynamics and their application to therapeutic maneuvers is severely lacking for most of us.

I believe that the greater our depth of knowledge of these important principles, the better the outcome we can expect for our patients. Acquisition and application of this knowledge for better outcomes in the treatment of patients with chronic venous insufficiency will present a challenge for many. This work by Franceschi and Zamboni should greatly lessen that challenge.

I expect this book to help begin to bridge the gap that separates Phlebology as it is understood and practiced in the U.S. from that of Europe and other parts of the world. I also expect the book to stimulate vigorous discussion regarding basic principles of venous hemodynamics and valvular function as they are presented in this work, and the application of those principles to various treatment options. And ultimately I look forward to facilitating the presentation of these discussions to phlebologic symposia and congresses here in America.

Nick Morrison, MD
Morrison Vein Institute
Scottsdale, Arizona, USA
Nick Morrison, MD
The Vein Institute, Scottsdale, AZ

# PREFACE

## A FRENCH PREFACE

This book represents the updated English version 20 years later my first CHIVA book, that was entirely hand written.

Venous Hemodynamics was not properly studied before the Duplex scan era because invasive investigations were not appropriate enough, due to their static nature. The second reason is that people interested in venous superficial disease where mostly oriented towards dermatology and cosmetics, which doesn't require physics and hemodynamics. So, varices were more or less considered as "tumours" to take away, due to histological wall changes , and their recurrences were assigned to a biological hereditary status.

I was working in arterial pathology and developed Doppler signal interpretation from 1975. I have been interested in varicose veins in order to spare the draft material for arterial by-pass; so I tried to understand the pathophysiology of venous disease. In the medical literature I didn't find any convincing response. My previous knowledge in haemodynamics gave me the keys for understanding more. I was happy to find a coherent model. I didn't foresee that many would perform pseudo "CHIVA" without any knowledge of it and would be "disappointed" not by themselves but by the method "theoretically fascinating" but "practically inefficient". So, some tenors of Phlebology sang around the world that CHIVA didn't work. But it works!

Claude Franceschi

## AN ITALIAN PREFACE

The development of the original haemodynamic concept of Claude Franceschi, along the last 20 years, gives me the opportunity to remark how several recognized cornerstones in duplex evaluation were originally described by CHIVA authors. The original sin in spreading novel concepts was certainly the French language, and my impression is that a lot of phlebologists around the world are still unaware of the contribution of CHIVA studies in the development of modern venous duplex investigation. Duplex anatomy is the necessary premise of a correct duplex mapping. CHIVA studies introduced the followings:

- the standing position for duplex investigation of CVD cases
- the introduction of different manoeuvres for eliciting reflux, providing a coherent interpretation of their significance.
- the use of transverse duplex access and the saphenous eye sign
- the alignment sign for localization of the AASV
- the concept of the duplex saphenous compartment and the tributaries layer.
- the end of the concept of varicose saphenous vein

This is well apparent by comparing the consensus conference on duplex venous anatomy published on EJVES in 2006 with the chapter of Mark Bailly published in 1993 on the Encyclopedie Medico-Chirurgicale. The Bailly's chapter contains more than 80% of what was approved 13 years later by the Consensus Conference in San Diego.

The haemodynamic inseparability of the reflux phenomenon from the re-entry one, is the key for understanding the concept of the vicious circles defined as venous shunt. The duplex individuation of the venous shunt provides a coherent model to achieve the target of Doppler guided surgery of CVD. If someone should reflect on the different models of venous shunt herein described, and on their infinite variations in our patients, it will appear very clear the impossibility to correct the disease always with the same conceptual approach: the saphenous vein destruction.

This book shows how this approach is incoherent in the majority of cases, including the presence of a competent terminal valve (more than 40% of cases), the presence of pelvic shunt (around 10% of cases in female), the presence of a saphenous trunk completely or almost completely competent, etc. Preoperative duplex assessment gives us the possibility to tailor surgery achieving the goal of reflux suppression while maintaining the drainage function. It is a fantastic opportunity for introducing in vascular surgery the concept of venous restorative surgery because a surgeon, by learning venous haemodynamics, can redirect venous flow exactly where he wants, without destroying the saphenous vein.

Paolo Zamboni, MD

*Chapter 1*

# PHYSICAL PRINCIPLES OF VENOUS HAEMODYNAMICS

***Paolo Zamboni***
University of Ferrara, Italy

## 1. BASIC HAEMODYNAMICS

### 1.1. Fluid-Static: Correlation between Pressure and Energy

The venous system functions under two conditions: fluid stasis and fluid dynamics. It is necessary to review some principles of physics in order to define and correctly interpret the phenomena described below [68].

First we will examine the principles that govern the behaviour of venous blood under conditions of stasis. There is a widespread opinion that fluid motion within a conduit is produced by the pressure difference or gradient between the two ends. If this were true, then if we stood a closed-end cylinder vertically and filled it with a fluid, we should expect upward motion in the fluid, from the bottom, where the pressure on the cylinder walls is greater, to the top where the pressure on the cylinder walls is less. But this does not happen (Figure 1.1)

In reality, pressure on the cylinder walls (defined as static or lateral pressure) represents only one part of the total energy of this system; another part is gravitational potential energy linked to the height level that the fluid occupies (hydrostatic pressure). Since static or lateral pressure, greater at the bottom and less at the top, is perfectly offset by gravitational or hydrostatic pressure, greater at the top, less at the bottom, then total energy is absolutely identical in all parts of the system.

Analogous to the zero principle of thermodynamics, which states that no exchange of energy can occur between systems or between points within a system at the same energy level, we find no fluid motion (and therefore no exchange of energy) within a cylinder between points that have the same total energy level [53,54,257].

## 1.2. Fluid-Dynamics: Definition of Potential, Pressure and Gravitational Energies

Now let us imagine two cylinders placed vertically, connected to each other through a conduit with a removable rigid diaphragm installed internally at the level of the base of the cylinders. If the height of the fluid within the cylinder on the right is greater than the height of the same fluid in the left cylinder, then an energy gradient exists between these two systems. Both lateral and hydrostatic pressure are greater in the right than in the left cylinder because the fluid on the right is at a higher level. The energy gradient in this case is totally independent of the absolute heights of the fluid; instead, it depends solely on the inequality of the levels within the two cylinders.

The second principle of thermodynamics states that energy is spontaneously transmitted from a system at a higher energy level to a system at a lower energy level and not vice-versa. Therefore, it is logical to expect fluid motion (i.e., work) and thereby an exchange of energy from the right cylinder to the left cylinder whenever the rigid diaphragm that separates the two systems is removed; this is something that regularly occurs by reason of the **principle of communicating vessels** (Figure 1.1).

To sum up, we believe it is more correct to regard fluid motion within a conduit as the result of an energy gradient instead of a pressure gradient.

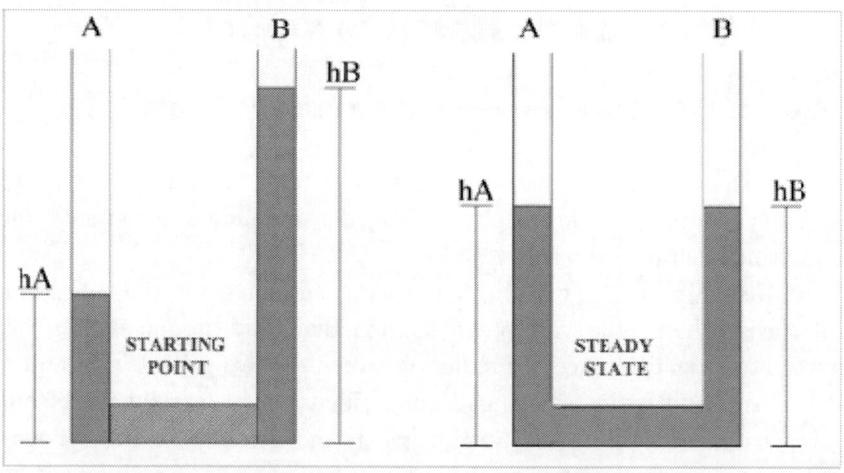


Figure 1.1. The principle of communicating vessels and its application in the superficial and deep venous system physiology, characterized by different height columns (Fig. 2.5).

# 2. Re-Entry Gradients

## 2.1. Required Elements for Flow Determination

If, however, we apply energy in the form of pressure to one end of a rigid conduit filled with fluid, while the other end is closed, we do not produce any fluid motion within the conduit. In this situation, the total energy of the system increases in response to the increase in pressure, but pressure at the distal end of the conduit increases immediately, and any pressure gradient between the two ends is also immediately eliminated.

Therefore, the application of energy in the form of pressure to one end of a conduit clearly represents a necessary element, but insufficient in itself, for producing a gradient that endures for the time required to overcome the inertia of the system and to produce fluid motion within the conduit [68].

Another element, also necessary and insufficient in itself, is represented by the capacity of the conduit, and/or of systems connected to it, to receive the volume of fluid in motion in such a way that the exit velocity of the pressure at the end of the conduit (opposite the entry point where energy is applied in the form of pressure) does not exhaust the gradient prematurely [257].

## 2.2. Compliance

This capability to receive fluid in the conduit and to maintain the gradient over time is expressed in physics as the 'compliance' of the system. It depends on the elasticity/rigidity, the length and (to a lesser extent) the radius of the conduit and also on the degree of filling. For example in the venous system there is a different behaviour when the vein is filled and distended by the blood (Figure 1.2) [10-12,73-75,261-262,275-277].

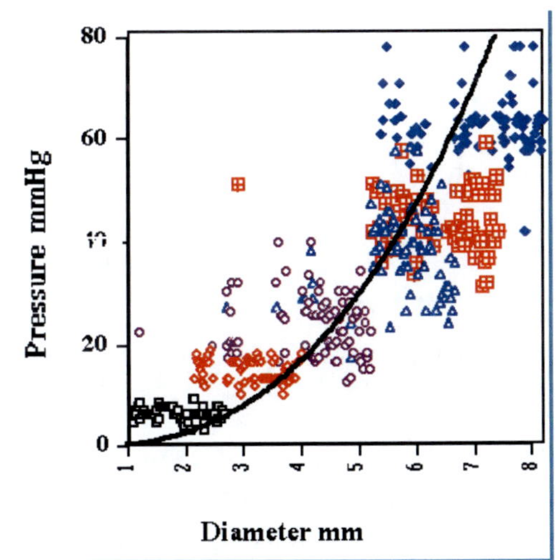


Figure 1.2. The pressure-diameter curve demonstrates during the filling phase greater increasing in diameter with no correspondent increasing in pressure(fig B). The linearity of the relationship starts after the completion of the vein filling. In the GSV this happens at a pressure around 20 mmHg.

We know from classical physiology that the relationship between vein volume and pressure is characterized by a significant increase in volume with little change in pressure during the filling phase [93,231-233], in which the vein is distended by the increase in blood volume. In other words, during this first phase the pressure/volume relationship is not linear. Instead, during the distension phase following the filling phase, further increases in volume are proportionally reflected by pressure increases, so that linearity of the volume/pressure relationship in veins can be demonstrated starting from pressure values around 20 mmHg. On the other hand, after completion of the filling phase, vein diameter is geometrically related to vein volume (provided that vessel length is constant). This may explain the finding of a linear pressure/diameter relationship in the saphenous vein at the thigh, starting from 20 mmHg [261].

Compliance (c) is a characteristic of every hollow system. Volumetric increase (dV) of the content is correlated with pressure increase (dP) inside the container (the equation is c= dV/dP); compliance therefore represents the slope of the volume/pressure curve within a system [1,10-12,75 –76,275-277].

If a system has high compliance, it can receive a significant volume of fluid with a small increase in pressure; the curve will not be very steep.

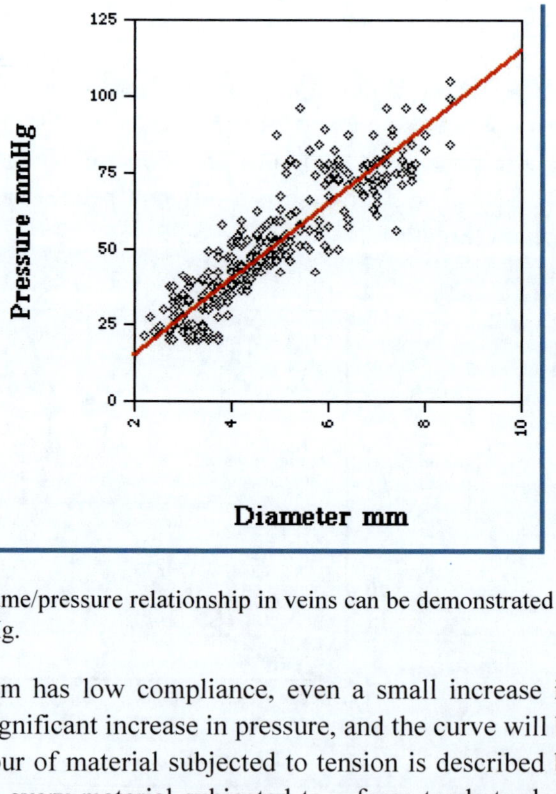


Figure 1.3. Linearity of the volume/pressure relationship in veins can be demonstrated starting from pressure values around 20 mmHg.

Conversely, if the system has low compliance, even a small increase in fluid volume within the system causes a significant increase in pressure, and the curve will be steeper.

The mechanical behaviour of material subjected to tension is described by Hooke's law (F= E.dL), which states that every material subjected to a force tends to develop a reactive force (F) proportional to the elongation produced (dL), in a linear ratio through a constant (E) (the Young modulus) which is characteristic of any material and represents the slope of the line (E= dL/F) [68].

Biological materials, however, do not obey this law and demonstrate a ratio between applied force (or developed force) and produced elongation that is curvilinear in form. The slope, called a tangential modulus, varies from point to point on the curve in proportion to the produced length and therefore is not a constant like the Young modulus.

By analogy with the tangential modulus of the force/elongation curve, compliance in biological systems (i.e., the slope of the pressure/volume curve) also varies from point to point in relation to the filling volume of the system.

The shape of the compliance curve is determined, therefore, by the physical characteristics of the material involved [10-12] in the system, as well as by the volumetric extension of the system and its geometric configuration. It is evident that the greater the volume of a container, the greater its capacity to receive the volume of the contents with a small increase in internal pressure. It is also evident that in a hollow spherical system the extension of the system is correlated solely with the radius, while in a hollow tubular system it is correlated principally with the length of the system and only to a small degree with the radius or diameter.

The actual value of compliance is, instead, correlated, as we mentioned, with the filling volume of the system [186,231,262]; this in turn is determined by the kind of system in question. In a hydrostatic system, with the fluid in stasis, the degree of filling in the system is influenced only by the initial volume; but in a hydrodynamic system, with the fluid in motion, the degree of filling in the system is influenced not only by the initial volume but also by the relation between input rate and output rate.

## 2.3. Flow: Castelli's Law, Bernoulli's Principle, Venturi Effect

Whenever energy in the form of pressure is applied to a high-compliance system, the gradient is capable of enduring for the time required to overcome inertia and produce fluid motion, or flow, inside a conduit [68,261].

Under normal conditions, that is, during the time in which the flow is continuous and constant, **Castelli's law** (a development of the equation of continuity, or the Leonardo law) states that flow velocity is inversely proportional to the area of the conduit sections. This means that if the area of a conduit section is reduced, flow velocity increases and conversely, if the area of a conduit section is increased, flow velocity decreases. In addition, if the conduit divides into several branches and the sum of the area of the sections in the different branches is greater than the area of the section in the main conduit, then flow velocity will decrease; conversely, if several branches unite to form one conduit and the sum of the area of the sections in the different branches is greater than the area of the section in the main conduit, then flow velocity increases.

Whenever flow is produced in a conduit, the total energy of the system is represented at each point not only by the sum of the pressure potential energy and gravitational potential energy, as in the case of a closed-end cylinder in a vertical position, but also by the kinetic energy produced by fluid motion.

According to **Bernoulli's principle** for fluids in an ideal state, the sum of potential energy (lateral and gravitational pressure) and kinetic energy is constant at any point. This means that in a hydrostatic system (one with the fluid in stasis and velocity at zero) the sum of potential energy is at its maximum, while in a hydrodynamic system (with the fluid in motion) the sum of potential energy is decreased proportionately to the **velocity of the fluid**. In other words, the lateral pressure exercised on the conduit walls by a fluid in motion is less than that exercised by the same fluid in conditions of stasis, and the greater the velocity reached by the fluid, the more marked the reduction in pressure.

If we have two equal and parallel communicating conduits and the fluid in one of them moves at a greater velocity, then by Bernouilli's principle the lateral pressure there is lower. In this way a gradient is created between the conduit in which the fluid moves at a lower velocity and the one in which it moves at greater velocity. The latter thereby causes an "aspiration" effect upon the former; this phenomenon is known as the **Venturi principle**.

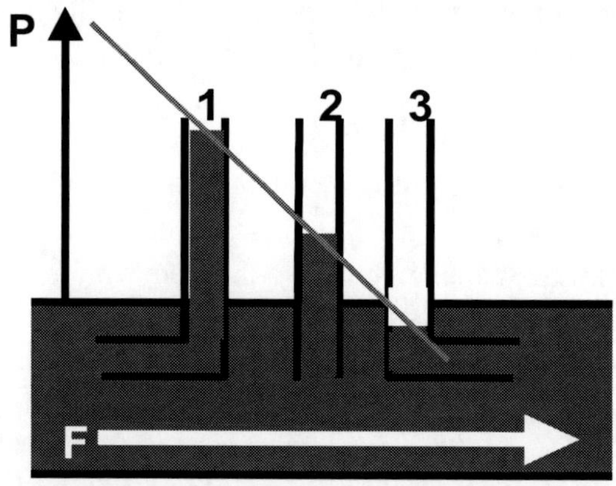


Figure 1.4. Classic experience of the tube of Pitot, demonstrating the aspiration of fluid thanks to the Venturi effect in collateral tubes with different lateral pressure gradients.

We have spoken generally in the preceding paragraphs of a "fluid" and a "conduit" in an ideal state, that is a fluid free of internal friction and a conduit with walls that produce no friction during contact with the fluid moving past them.

In the biological environment, however, blood possesses complex visco-elastic flow properties, and vessel walls produce friction through contact with circulating blood.

An extension of the second principle of thermodynamics, called the law of entropy, states that in the case of real fluid circulation and real conduits, part of the energy is dissipated in the form of heat and increases the share of energy no longer available for doing work (system entropy).

Therefore, while Bernouilli's principle remains basically valid even for real fluids, it could be "corrected" by adding entropy to the two forms of equilibrated energy, potential and kinetic.

Nature has already performed a similar "correction": the thermodynamic purpose of the series of pumps placed along the cardiovascular system is, in fact, to restore vascular system energy dissipated in the form of heat due to friction.

## 2.4. Turbulent Flow

The characteristics of blood viscosity and vascular wall friction also affect kinematics, that is, the geometry of fluid motion.

Blood flow within the vascular system is, for the most part, laminar, which means it behaves as though it were composed of very fine, concentric, cylindrical layers that slide over one another. The layer in immediate contact with the vessel wall is practically static; proceeding toward the center of the vessel, the individual layers move with increasing velocity up to a certain distance from the wall; from there on, the velocity is practically constant.

Under certain circumstances, flow can become turbulent, or completely irregular; particles of fluid stream toward the center continually and form vortices. Turbulent flow is characterized by a huge expenditure of energy because the kinetic energy vector that normally points straight along the vascular trunk breaks up into a very high number of vectors pointing chaotically in all directions. Whenever this type of haemodynamic condition occurs, for example, in the saphenous trunk, it is accompanied by development over time of dilation of the trunk [69,94-95,268].

The transition from laminar to turbulent flow depends on fluid density and viscosity, conduit diameter and flow velocity [68,69].

All of these variables have been united in a nondimensional parameter, the Reynolds number, which, if higher than 2,000, is predictive of turbulent flow.

Turbulence is one of the major causes of vein wall dilatation and is significantly associated to segmental dilation of the GSV (figure 1.5). Turbulence plays a major role in veins walls dilation respect to pressure [95,268]. This explains why when you replace with the saphenous conduit an artery, in bypass surgery, the GSV does not appear dilated in the outcome despite the increased blood pressure. Therefore, blood pressure in a laminar flow system does not produce vein walls dilation and varicose veins. In contrast, wasting forces applied to the vein wall along time determine varicosity and dilation.

Oscillatory flow, in upward direction during muscular systole, and in downward during diastole, is considered one of the major stimuli to vein wall inflammation and valve remodelling and injury [23].

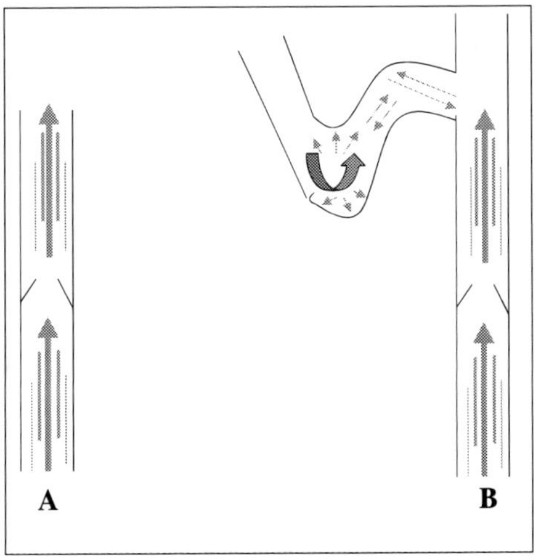


Figure 1.5. A: Laminar flow characterized by higher velocity in the middle of the vessel and decreased velocities towards the walls. B Mechanic effects of turbulent flow: reflux with flow conflict and turbulence in a collateral vein of the GSV with dilation.

*Chapter 2*

# BASIC ULTRASONIC ANATOMY OF THE LOWER LIMBS VENOUS SYSTEM

***Paolo Zamboni***
University of Ferrara, Italy.

## 1. INFORMATION FROM VASCULAR ULTRASOUND DEVICES

EchoDoppler and color-echoDoppler diagnostic systems are able to furnish at least three levels of information. The first level is the B-mode image, which offers morphological information [57,61]. This is of extraordinary importance since it allows us to integrate successive information with reference to a perfectly localized and anatomically catalogued vessel segment. Historically, this information brought about improved diagnostic accuracy with respect to CW Doppler systems that only allowed for "blind" hemodynamic analyses. In certain sectors of the venous tree, as for example in the popliteal fossa, the pocket/CW Doppler does not permit differentiation of the signals that come from the veins in that area, possibly leading to numerous errors [72,107,109,121,130,163,169,179,181,184,234,245].

The second level of information is that of the velocity-meter Doppler. Thanks to the B-mode image, the small cursor of the Doppler volume sample can be precisely sampled inside the venous segment being analyzed, generally with a 60° angle, bringing to the center of the preselected vessel [61]. In this way, information can be obtained about the direction and velocity of blood in the veins of the lower limbs in muscular systole and diastole, respectively. This information can be represented as waves reflecting the echoes of the red blood cells moving inside the veins. These tracings, the significance of which we will learn to identify, are characteristic of echoDoppler devices. Color echoDoppler represents the different flow velocities and directions with color coding visible inside of the vessel lumen. Practically speaking, it does not provide additional information, but rather the same information as the Doppler tracing, presented in a different form. Nevertheless, color coding allows for the sampling of a number of vessels contemporaneously, thus providing integrated information simultaneously and more rapidly. In addition, it facilitates the identification of veins in areas difficult to explore.

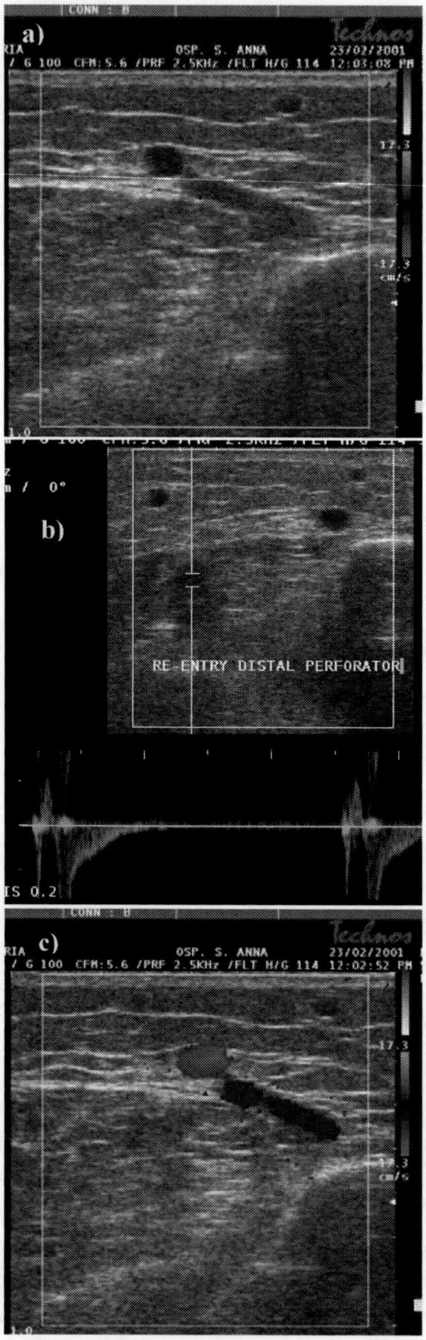


Figure 2.1. a) B mode imagine providing morphological information of saphenous vein connected with a perforating vein. b) The velocity-meter and flow direction Doppler information thanks to the Doppler sample of a duplex system placed into the perforating vein. c) The coloured-Doppler integrated information shows flow direction in both saphenous and perforating vein.

The third level of information is represented by the Doppler sound of the unsonorized vessel. This allows us to identify quickly, for example, flow phases in a venous area when they should be physiologically absent, as during the Valsalva maneuver or during muscle relaxation.

## 2. Functional Anatomy of the Veins of the Lower Limbs

The B-mode level of information is fundamental to avoid gross diagnostic errors for those who analyze lower limb veins using an echoDoppler system. It is absolutely indispensable to orient oneself through recognizing anatomic markers constantly present in the sections or scanning that is carried out during the course of the examination.

In an anatomic section of a lower limb, we need to know how to recognize the inter-tegumentary layers (cutaneous and subcutaneous), the superficial and muscular fascia.

As shown in Figure 2.2, the layer of imbrication of the superficial fascia and of the deep fascia contains the saphenous axes, and anatomists now consider it a compartment; in fact, it is called the saphenous compartment [7,19,35-41,49,158,230,252-253,255,257,258-260,268].

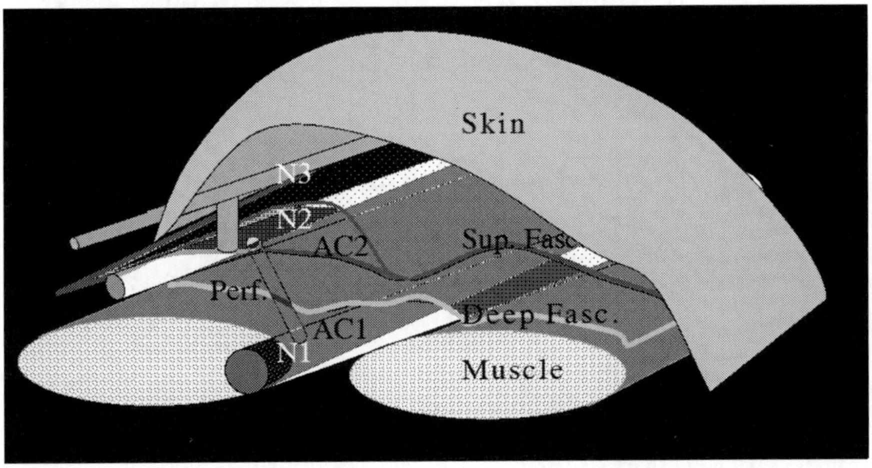


Figure 2.2. Anatomo-functional subdivision of lower limb veins.

All of the veins above this layer are intertegumentary veins that represent the superficial venous system and are tributaries of the saphenous axes. Analogously, all of the veins below this layer represent the deep venous system. Finally, all of the veins that perforate the imbrication layer of the fascia, joining the deep venous system with the superficial one or with the saphenous axes represent the perforating veins [6-9, 35-41, 53, 57, 61, 105, 124, 145, 148, 158, 200, 252, 260, 262, 268].

On the basis of these anatomic premises, by using an echographic probe at extremely high frequencies, it is possible to differentiate three venous compartments that are characterized by precise anatomic markers (Figure 2.2-2.3):

a) Compartment AC1, containing the deep venous system (DVS): represented by the venous structures situated beneath the deep fascia (femoral, popliteal, tibial, peroneal, gastrocnemius and soleal); network 1 (N1)
b) Compartment AC2, saphenous compartment, network 2 (N2): represented by the venous structures contained in the layer between the superficial fascia and the deep fascia (constantly the great saphenous vein (GSV), the accessory anterior saphenous vein (AASV), the short saphenous vein (SSV), and the vein of Giacomini (GIAC); inconstantly, the tributary paratibial antero-lateral (T vein). The echographic finding in transversal scanning of the saphenous trunk on the inside of the division of the superficial fascia is reported in the literature as "saphenous eye".
c) Compartment AC3, superficial venous system (SVS), network 3 (N3): represented by the collaterals and saphenous tributaries, situated above the superficial fascia;

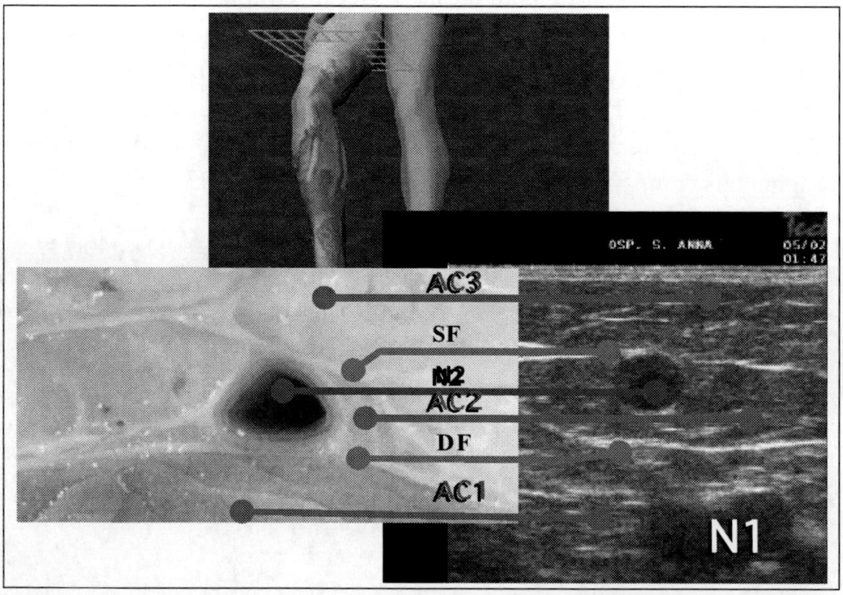


Figure 2.3. Anatomical and ultrasonographic transverse access of the medial aspect of the thigh. Legenda: AC 1, 2, 3 = ANATOMICAL COMPARTMENT 1, 2, 3. N 1, 2 = venous NETWORK 1, 2 SF = SUPERFICIAL FASCIA; DF= DEEP FASCIA.

When the veins of the SVS connect different segments of the saphenous compartment, entering and exiting from the superficial fascia, they are defined in the literature as N4 networks. These veins, being situated above the superficial fascia, belong to compartment AC3 and functionally represent intersaphenous branches, between the same saphenous axis (N4 longitudinal) or between different saphenous axes (N4 transversals) (Figure 2.4).

The veins of the deep venous system, that is, the N1 compartment, consists of two subsystems:

a) the intermuscular veins, situated between one muscle group and another, or between a muscle group and a fascial structure, are represented by the following veins: superficial femoral, deep femoral, popliteal, anterior tibial, posterior tibial, and peroneal. These veins, which are "comites" veins in the homonymous arteries, are generally bifurcated, but the two branches are not necessarily equally developed. Valvular density is at its greatest at the level of the leg and decreases progressively towards the base of the limb (Figure 2.5).

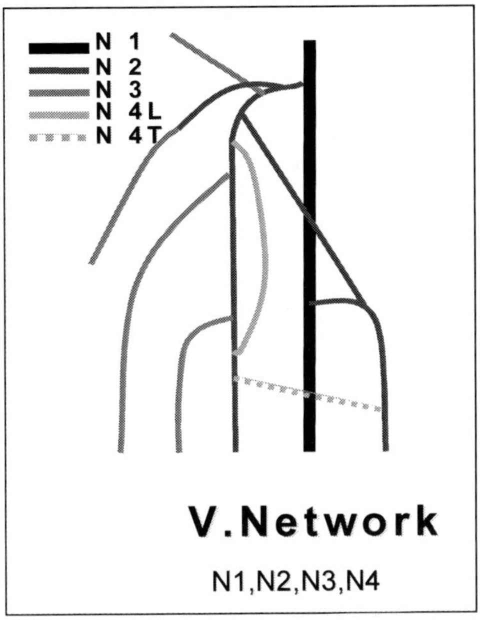


Figure 2.4. Different compartments of the lower limb venous drainage.

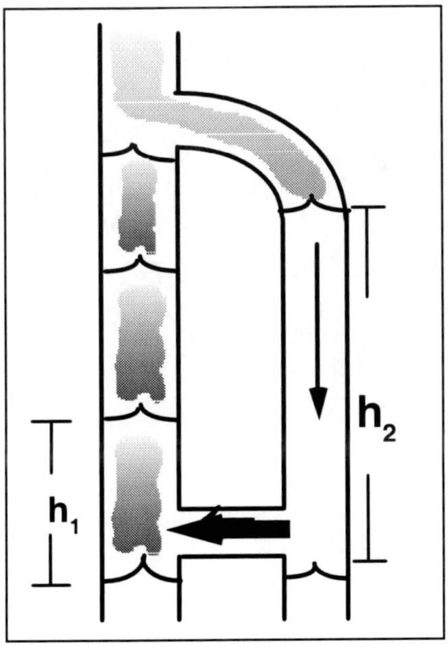


Figure 2.5. Decreasing valves density in the N1 compartment from the leg to the thigh (see Fig. 1.1).

b) the intramuscular veins, situated inside the muscular structure, are represented by the gastrocnemial and solear veins, the latter being, it is known, lacking in valvular apparatus.

At the level of the leg, all of the venous groups, both intermuscular and intramuscular, are profusely anastomosed among themselves sometimes forming a sort of plexum as, for example, at the level of the posterior tibials (sural plexus).

In addition, at the level of the leg, both types of veins are surrounded by very rigid structures (deep fasciae, dissepiments of the muscular cavities, interosseal membranes and flat bones), which render particularly efficacious the energy transfer caused by the increase in the transverse diameter of the muscles during contraction and, at the same time, perform a retention role with respect to the veins.

Compartment AC2, which forms the true saphenous systems, recognizes in its own anatomical marker (that is, in the fact of being contained in the imbrication of the fasciae) the principal physiopathological characteristic, that of being the retention-providing component in the superficial venous system.

If we observe the veins in the saphenous compartment in transversal scanning, we see the characteristic construction of the "eye" image, related to the combination of the round black circle of the transversally sectioned vein and the hyperechogenic fascial "eyelids" that surround it (Figure 2.2).

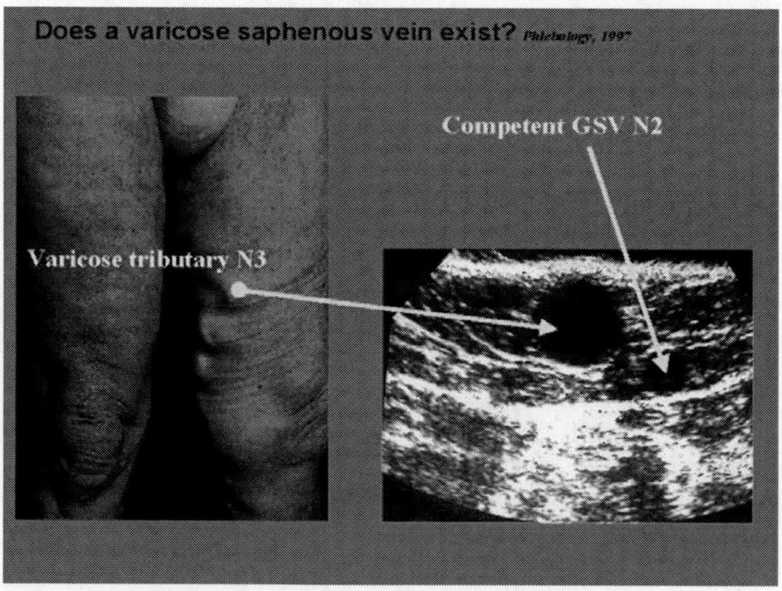


Figure 2.6. Classic misdiagnosis of varicose GSV in a frequent case presenting with a visible and palpable longitudinal vein trunk of the internal thigh . US imaging reveals that the varicose vein is a vein located above the superficial fascia in the AC 3, network N3. The cited study demonstrated in 101/103 limbs, 98%, that a varicose trunk visible at the internal side of the thigh is a saphenous tributary, always lying more superficially as compared to the GSV. Unfortunately, still today the misdiagnosis of varicose GSV represent the best indication to surgical avulsion.

This constant and characteristic image allows us to recognize and localize the saphenous axes precisely and to differentiate them from other veins. This enables us to eliminate gross diagnostic errors. One of the most common errors is to diagnose the GSV as being varicose. Figure 2.6 shows a large chordal varix running longitudinally along the medial surface of the thigh. The B-mode image of reference shows, based on the displayed criteria, a GSV recognizable by the undilated and nonvaricosed "eye," while a collateral vein in compartment AC3 is varicosed. This latter vein runs a few mm more superficially but outside of the superficial fascia.

If, instead, we insonate the veins in compartment AC2 with longitudinal scanning, they will be recognizable as lying on the muscular fascia and being covered by a reinforcement (this, too, hyperechogenous) of the superficial fascia.

The transversal image of the eye requires additional knowledge of the echographic anatomy at the level of the thigh in order to differentiate and recognize quickly the GSV from the AASV, both of which are marked as already stated, by the eye image. The alignment sign is particularly useful for this purpose, precisely where the two veins run parallel, or, in the superior and middle third of the medial face of the thigh [8,57] (Figure 2.7).

At this level, the eye of the anterior saphena, in contrast to the internal one, appears to be aligned with the deep veins, the artery and the superficial femoral vein. These appear perpendicularly beneath the single anterior saphena, situated more deeply than the layer of imbrication of the fasciae, between the muscle heads of the quadriceps and the adductors [8] (Figure 2.7).

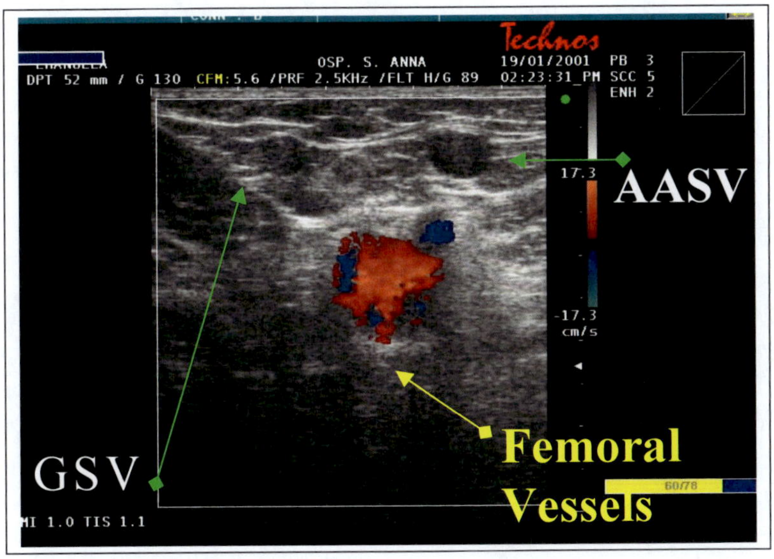


Figure 2.7. The aligment sign between the anterior saphena and the deep veins.

The superficial fascia is a rigid structure and, as such, is able to perform two important functions: 1) to allow the transfer of energy brought by an increase in the transverse diameter of the muscles during contraction (even though the interposed layer of reticular adipose tissue tends to damp the phenomenon), and 2) to carry out a retention role for the veins contained therein.

In order to improve even further the transfer of muscular energy to the saphena, the saphenous compartment is furnished with a ligament, called the saphenous ligament, that facilitates the pincers-like squeezing action that the imbricated fasciae perform on the saphenous axis (Figure 2.2).

The anatomical organization, in light of the physical principles set forth in Chapter 1, enable us to understand the reasons behind the physiology of the venous system of the lower limbs. If it is true that the energy propulsor, the so-called peripheral heart of the venous system of the limbs, is the surrounding muscular mechanism, it is evident that the transfer of energy from contraction will be maximal in the deep layer and gradually less intense as we move towards the superficial layers. In pratice, the kinetic energy of moving blood will be higher in the deep venous system, high enough but certainly lower in the saphenous system, and very low in the veins belonging to compartment AC3. Therefore, applying Bernoulli's theorem (Chap.1), we can conclude that the lateral pressure will be lower in the deep venous system, which permits, based on the gradient, a moving of blood in systole from the saphenous and AC3 compartments to the deep system through the perforating veins, and from the AC3 compartment to the saphenous system. The latter becomes, in short, the polarizer of the superficial venous flow due to the high kinetic energy transferred to it from the fascial and ligamental structures of the saphenous compartment, with respect to the other veins of the SVS (Figure 2.2).

Unlike in the deep venous system, the valvular density in the saphenous systems is minimal at the level of the leg and increases progressively towards the saphenous junction, though always remaining lower than that in the deep veins.

The AC3 compartment includes all of the other superficial veins, and among these even the so-called posterior saphenous arch, or Leonardo's vein, and the so-called accessory saphenas, which, not being contained in the division of the superficial fascia, are not saphenous systems.

Even in this case, the anatomical marker (i.e., the fact of being situated above the superficial fascia and immersed in the subcutaneous tissue) constitutes for the compartments in question the principle physiopathological characteristic. In fact, the subcutaneous tissue, in addition to damping to an even greater degree the transfer of energy caused by an increase in the transverse diameter of the muscles during contraction, is unable to carry out any retention role for the veins contained in it. For this reason, the veins in compartment AC3 represent the retention-lacking component in the superficial venous system.

The functional differences between compartment AC2, on the one hand, and compartment AC3, on the other, are also confirmed by the histological structure of the venous walls. The saphenous trunks present, in fact, a double layer of muscle fibers that are circular internally and longitudinal externally, in the media coat much more developed, and a layer of longitudinal muscle fibers at the subintimal level, completely lacking in the collateral veins.

These observations explain why findings of "tortuous and varicose" saphenas are extremely rare, while such collateral veins are often reported (Figure 2.3).

Besides the venous compartments described are the connections between the superficial network and the deep venous axes, represented by the perforating veins [15,16,18,27,29,49,70,79,106,107,113,137,150,173,177,185,209,212,221,230,278]. The latter can be made up of a single trunk (mono-trunk perforating veins) or several trunks (multi-trunk perforating veins).

The connection, which can be a short or long passage, can be direct, that is, without muscular veins as intermediaries (direct or intermuscular perforating) or indirect, that is, with muscular veins as intermediaries (indirect or intramuscular perforating).

There are also mixed perforating veins, that is, multi-trunk perforating veins in which one or more trunks reach the deep venous circle as direct perforating, while other trunks reach the deep venous circle as indirect perforating.

Perforating veins present a variable number of valvular mechanisms, usually three (of which one is on the deep side, one on the superficial side, and one in the intermediate section), which oppose the reflux of blood from the depths towards the surface.

Their place of entrance, at both superficial and deep venous levels, is always in the commissural area [243], that is, in the area in which, based on the kinetics of the valvular opening, the flow velocity is greatest, and the consequent drop in lateral pressure is maximal, during muscle contraction. Nevertheless, many anatomic studies indicate that very often the valvular mechanisms, especially in the smallest perforating veins, are absent or rudimentary, and in some cases oriented in the anti-physiological direction. This enables us to understand how their flow direction is almost exclusively owing to the hemodynamic laws set forth in Chapter 1, rather than being regulated by the valvular mechanisms.

Because their walls have no external sustaining structure, the perforating veins represent a retentionless component of the venous system. Due to this structural characteristic, they are more or less dilated according to their flow volume. Analogously, their mechanical and parietal compliance characteristics enable them to reduce their diameter, thereby decreasing the hemodynamic overload.

At the level of the saphenous trunks the perforating veins are particularly numerous, even if often they are invisible echographically because of their small caliber.

The primary function of the perforating veins is to allow for a rapid emptying of the superficial network, especially of the saphenous trunks, into the deep venous axes.

In addition, Boersma has demonstrated that the perforating veins also carry out the drainage of muscular branches and subfascial structures [32].

The saphenous junction, which represent the transfascial connections between the superficial venous circle (in the case in point the AC2 compartment) and the deep venous circle, must be considered for all effects as perforating [31].

*Chapter 3*

# VENOUS COMPARTMENTS AND THEIR HIERARCHICAL ORDER OF EMPTYING

***Paolo Zamboni***

University of Ferrara, Italy.

Venous drainage of the lower limbs occurs in two directions [14,17,19,23,26,30,78,102-105,183-185,193,234,242]:

a) from the distal area towards the heart, therefore in the antegrade, dromic, upward or centripetal direction; and
b) from the superficial area towards the deep area, therefore in the "cutifugal", inward direction.

There are, however, two exceptions to this general pattern. The first is a portion (about 10%) of the blood contained in the venous sole of the foot, which, when the foot is resting on a surface, is directed towards the dorsal network through marginal veins (branches originating in the GSV and SSV) and runs, therefore, from the deep area towards the superficial. The second exception is the blood contained in the tributaries of the saphenous-femoral junction; it runs from the abdomen towards the groin.

An efficacious and rigorous interpretation of Doppler signals is necessary for a correct interpretation of the significance of the recorded trace in accordance with the manoeuvre used for obtaining it. Particularly nowadays no distinction is made by the majority of the operators between flow recorded in muscular systole and in muscular diastole; no distinction between the Doppler signals obtained under Valsalva and through compression-relaxation manoeuvre; no distinction between traces recorded in standing or in supine position, and/or by active and passive muscular elicitation. Only by decomposing and recognizing the phases of venous drainage of the lower limbs it will be possible to obtain correct information.

# 1. Venous Return in the Absence of Muscolar Activity

In the absence of muscular activity, basal venous return occurs due to the gradient that exists between residual venular pressure, that is, what remains of the initial push imparted by the heart to the circulating blood, and right atrial pressure.

We know from Chapter 1 that the area of the section of the vessels resulting from the confluence of several branchings is always smaller than the sum of the areas of the sections of the branchings. Therefore, according to Castelli's law, the flow velocity in the vessels of destination is always higher than that in the branchings.

If we apply Bernoulli's law and the Venturi effect, every vessel performs an aspiration action on its branchings. In fact, since flow velocity is higher, pressor energy is lower, and this creates an aspiration gradient.

# 2. Venous Return in Muscolar Systole

When a person begins to walk, the blood contained in the deep veins undergoes a significant acceleration in the antegrade direction and consequently reaches a high velocity due to the sequential action of the plantar pump and muscle contraction.

With an ultrasound probe positioned at the saphenous level, it is easy to verify with a sequential compression pump for the foot and calf that even the blood contained in the saphenous trunks undergoes an acceleration in the antegrade direction, but that the velocity attained is lower than that of the deep circle. Following the same principle and applying the concept of the Venturi effect (see Chapter 1) it is possible to observe a slower flow in the N3 compartment than that seen in the N2 compartment, leading to the physiologic hierarchy of venous drainage from N3 to N1.

This effect is due primarily to the lesser transfer to the superficial vessels of the energy from muscle contraction, and also to the reduced effect of the plantar pump (which involves only the 10% of blood departing from the foot), and to the greater flow resistance (Figure 3.1).

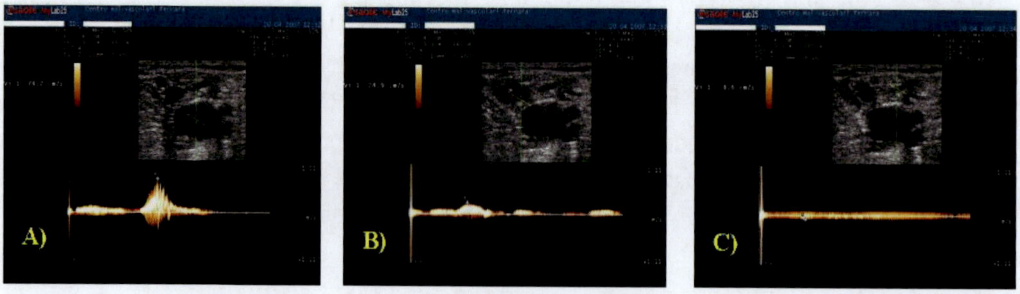


Figure 3.1. Decreasing velocities from N1 to N3, due primarily to the lesser transfer of energy from muscle contraction to the superficial vessels In A the Doppler sample is placed in the femoral vein (N1), in B in the saphenous vein (N2), and in C in the tributaries of the sapheno-femoral junction (N3).

At the level of the collaterals the effect of the pump is minimal, and it is completely absent at the level of the dermal plexuses, where there is only residual venular pressure. The average flow velocity is 0.05 cm/sec in the plexuses, 10-20 cm/sec in the saphenous trunks, and 20-40 cm/sec in the deep veins.

Figure 3.1 illustrates Doppler measurement of flow velocity as sampled in the N3 compartment (Figure 3.1 C), in the GSV (Figure 3.1 B) and the adjacent femoral vein (Figure 3.1 A) during muscular systole. Since the peak systolic velocity recorded in the femoral vein is at least twice as great in the GSV and more again as great in the N3 compartment a gradient is generated that causes the hierarchical emptying from N3 to N1.

## 3. The Hierarchy of Compartment Emptying

An unwritten but certainly not unimportant law is that which regulates the order of blood drainage and emptying in the various compartments of the venous system of the lower limbs. The emptying of the compartments, as explained in chapter 2 takes place by means of energy gradients that are activated during muscular systole.

Muscle contraction applies different amounts of energy to compartments AC1, AC2, and AC3, depending on their anatomical organization and their connections to muscular fasciae.

Muscle contraction brings about an energy application that is converted into levels of kinetic energy that differ in the respective compartments, as described in the preceding paragraph (Figure 3.2).

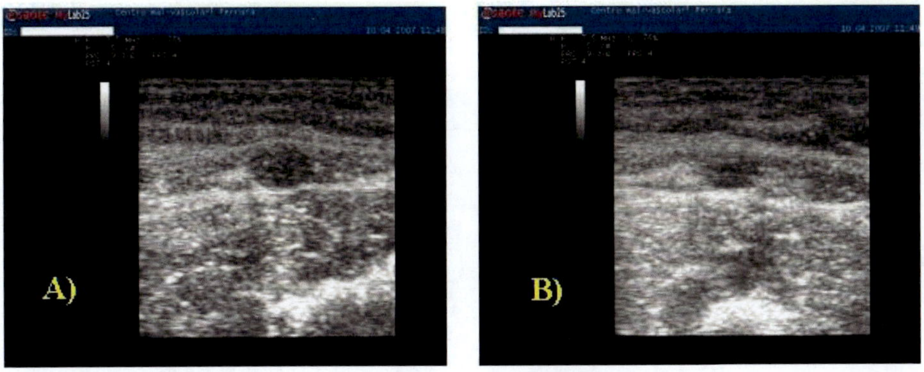


Figure 3.2. A) N2 compartment in absence of muscular activity and B) in muscular systole as an example of energy transfer through a "pliers-like" effect of the fasciae.

The different energy levels in the three compartments determine the hierarchy of emptying, so that compartment AC3 can empty into both compartments AC2 and AC1, while compartment AC2 can empty only into compartment AC1 (Figure 3.3, Figure 3.4a).

Whenever the hierarchical order of emptying is subverted, there exists a pathological situation due to a condition that annuls the physiological energy gradients. This concept is very important since it guides conservative and hemodynamic therapies that are aimed at restoring the emptying hierarchies (Figure 3.3b).

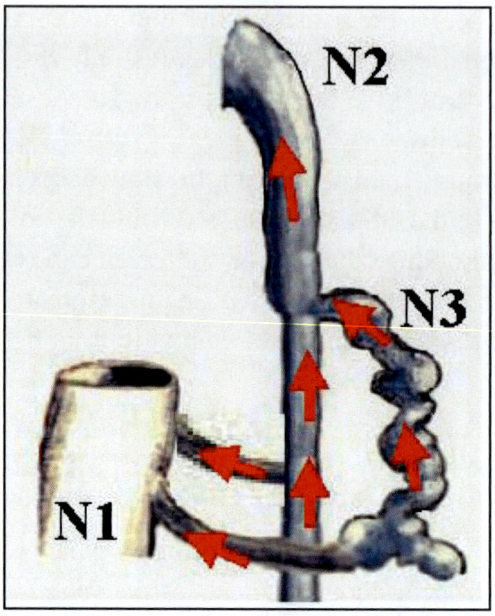


Figure 3.3. The hierarchy of compartment emptying, where N3 can empty into both N2 and N1, while N2 can empty only into compartment N1.

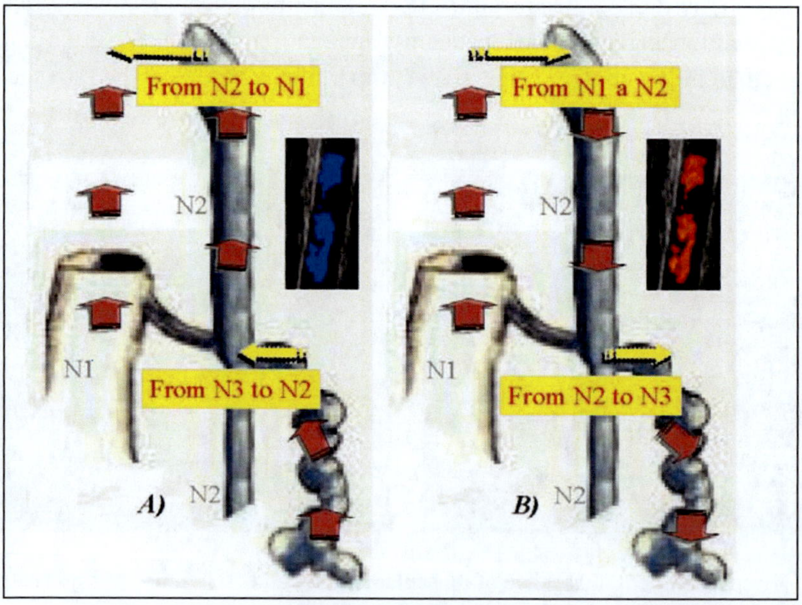


Figure 3.4. A) The hierarchy of compartment emptying. B) The hierarchical order of emptying subversion in a frequent condition of chronic venous disease.

It should be emphasized that, according to this novel concept, even a drainage inversion from compartment AC2 to compartment AC3 is considered pathological. In the traditional anatomical concept, the superficial system is considered as one unit, not being subdivided by the superficial fascia into the two compartments that we have identified.

Consequently, superficial refluxes are considered to be all the same, which leads to the loss of many diagnostic details that aid in identifying venous shunts, which we will learn about in the following chapters.

## 4. Venous Return in Muscolar Diastole

During muscular relaxation there occurs, at a deep level, a drop in pressure, the magnitude of which depends on whether the veins considered are intermuscular or intramuscular [26,59,78,135,183-184,193].

The latter, in fact, collapse completely upon muscle contraction, and so, upon muscle relaxation, they act as "sponges," exerting an aspiration effect upon the blood contained in the nearby veins, be they superficial or deep. As for intermuscular veins (tibial-popliteal-femoral axis), which do not collapse completely upon muscular contraction but rather decrease in caliber, the pressure drop upon relaxation is minor. Nevertheless, at the end of the contraction (telesystole), there occurs an antidromic gravitational gradient, relative to the above-standing hematic column, with a consequent closure of the valvular planes.

At the level of the superficial circle, the saphenous trunks act in the same way as the deep intermuscular veins.

Under physiological conditions, the distance between the valvular planes of the superficial distal network is decidedly greater than that of the deep vessels [14,17,27,28,234]. Thus, at the level of the leg during movement, hydrostatic columns are formed that are higher in the superficial network, with a consequent gradient directed toward the deep vessels (Figure 2.5). In accordance with the so-called principle of communicating vessels, there is blood flow from the superficial network towards the deep circle through the perforating veins.

The flow induced by this gradient in the superficial network, provided only to those segments having perforations, is not generally detectable by Doppler testing, probably because the velocities attained are less than 6 cm/sec.

About 25 seconds after the end of muscular contraction, in the absence of successive contractions, a pressor equilibrium is reached between the superficial and deep veins, in relation to the opening of the valves in all of the districts, perforating included, and the system returns to basal conditions again [135,193].

In order to reach this equilibrium, it is indispensable that the subject remain perfectly still, but such a situation, in orthostatism, is more theoretical than real. In fact, a few oscillations are sufficient to lower the filling pressure in the superficial network. This demonstrates that the flows entering the superficial venous system are physiologically much smaller than the flows exiting towards the deep venous network. In other words, the system presents a basic equilibrium that is actually unbalanced in aspiration, thereby creating its own functional reserve.

## 5. The Five Phases of Venous Return in Accordance to Muscular Pump

To summarize the subject of superficial venous network drainage, we can identify, from a hemodynamic point of view, five phases, three of which are hydrostatic, and two of which are hydrodynamic:

a) telediastolic (end-diastolic) phase, the instantaneous hydrostatic phase that immediately precedes muscular contraction;
b) systolic phase, the hydrodynamic phase during which occurs drainage of the superficial network towards the deep vessels and towards the center;
c) telesystolic phase, the instantaneous hydrostatic phase that immediately precedes muscular relaxation;
d) diastolic phase, the hydrodynamic phase during which occurs diastolic drainage from the superficial network towards the deep vessels, though not at a velocity detectable by Doppler; and
e) equilibrium phase, the hydrostatic phase during which the system is in basal conditions.

As regards the pressure that acts upon the venous walls, that is, lateral pressure, we recall that in the hydrostatic phases the systemic energy is all of the potential type, pressor and gravitational, and there exists no component of kinetic energy. In keeping with Bernoulli's theorem, the lateral pressure is, therefore, maximal. In the hydrodynamic phases, instead, the systemic energy is represented by both components. In accordance with Bernoulli's theorem, lateral pressure is, therefore, inversely proportional to flow velocity, and thus lower in the deep venous system.

## 6. The Establishment of Flow

As discussed above, the establishment of flow, regardless of its direction, depends upon the contemporary presence of two factors:

a) an energy gradient, generally of the pressor type; and
b) system compliance, so that the gradient applied can last for the time necessary to overcome inertia and start the flow.

Physiologically, the saphenous trunks present, according to the principle of communicating vessels, a retrograde segmental emptying in the diastolic phase. However, this retrograde flow is not detectable by Doppler, probably because the superficial hydrostatic columns, though larger than the deep ones, are not very high due to the continence of the valvular planes. Therefore, the flow velocities attained are modest.

*What happens in the case of valve incontinence?* The hydrostatic column can reach such a height that it induces a gradient able to cause, compatibly with the compliance of the system, a diastolic retrograde flow of high velocity, and thus Doppler-detectable [58,102,129,146,151,152,172].

The compliance of a hollow system, as previously stated, depends on the physical characteristics of the material of which it is made, on its geometric characteristics, and on its degree of filling.

As for the physical characteristics, the saphenic faces behave as if they were constructed of a relatively rigid material due to the reinforcing layer created by the splitting of the muscular fasciae.

As regards the geometric characteristics, since veins are tube-shaped, compliance is correlated primarily to the length of the valveless segment.

Finally, as for the degree of filling, the compliance of the venous system presents a double-phased pattern: at low volumes, when the system is empty, compliance is high; at high volumes, when the system is full, compliance is low.

This being a hydrodynamic system because blood circulates in the veins, the degree of filling is correlated to two categories of factors:

a) the initial volume, essentially in relation to the posture of the subject: in standing, the degree of filling is maximal; in supine it is modest; and with the legs raised, it is practically zero.
b) the relationship between entering flow and exiting flow, essentially correlated to the presence of an escape point in the system: if the system does not have escape points, the compliance is very low because it fills up immediately; if, instead, the system has an escape point, the compliance is very high because it can empty continually.

## 7. Reflux and Re-Entry

The escape point, that is, the connection between the venous segment that is the source of the diastolic retrograde flow and the vessel destined to receive it, constitutes the system's re-entry of retrograde flow [14,28,30,49,53-54,100-105,234,252,255-256,260,270,278,282].

The concept of re-entry does not include only the strictly anatomical aspect, that is, the connection between two vessels. The hemodynamic aspect must also be included, that is, the existence of a re-entry gradient that, for retrograde flows, is nothing other than an increment in the already illustrated, physiological antidromic gravitational gradient that causes diastolic drainage of the superficial network.

Obviously, the creation of a gradient between two vessels presumes that one of the two (that destined to receive the retrograde flow) presents lower pressor values as a consequence of fragmentation of the hydrostatic column on the part of functioning valvular apparatus.

In fact, if this were not the case, hydrostatic columns of different heights could not be created, and consequently there would be no gradients (Figure 3.6 A,B).

Once the presence of a reflux at the level of the superficial aces has been ascertained by echo-Doppler, the hemodynamic significance must be determined. *First of all, how do we define reflux?* A reflux is a flow that is inverted with respect to the physiological direction. Thus, it is a centrifugal flow directed away from the heart when we consider the axial vessels in compartments AC1, AC2, and AC3, and a flow directed toward the surface when we consider a perforating vein.

We must remember that venous drainage of the lower limbs occurs from the plexuses to the superficial collaterals of compartment AC3, from these towards the saphenous systems (AC2), and finally from the latter towards the deep venous circle (AC1), or even directly from the collaterals (AC3) to the deep venous circle (AC1).

The described course constitutes normal venous drainage of the lower limbs. If, in the normal hierarchical order of drainage through the various compartments, there is a vessel that runs longitudinally with incontinent valvular apparatus, it is possible to find a diastolic retrograde reflux at that level. This example represents a reflux with an escape point, if we define an escape point as the point in which there is a jump between compartments that subverts the hierarchical order of emptying. In this case, we can document the presence of a retrograde flow or reflux although the blood from AC1 or AC2 does not shunt into the AC3 compartment in which we have observed the phenomenon. Cases of this type are commonly described even in limbs that are nonpathological or in particular functional moments, e.g., following prolonged orthostatism, at the end of a hot summer day, etc. Some studies report its common occurrence even among surgeons and operating room personnel, but this does not render it synonymous with illness.

If, instead, even the flow coming from an anomalous rise in compartment contributes to the induction of diastolic reflux, that is, an inversed direction with respect to the normal hierarchical order of emptying (for example, AC1->AC2 or AC1->AC3 or AC2->AC3), the detected reflux is an expression of the presence of a reflux with an escape point and thus should be considered pathological (Figure 3.5).

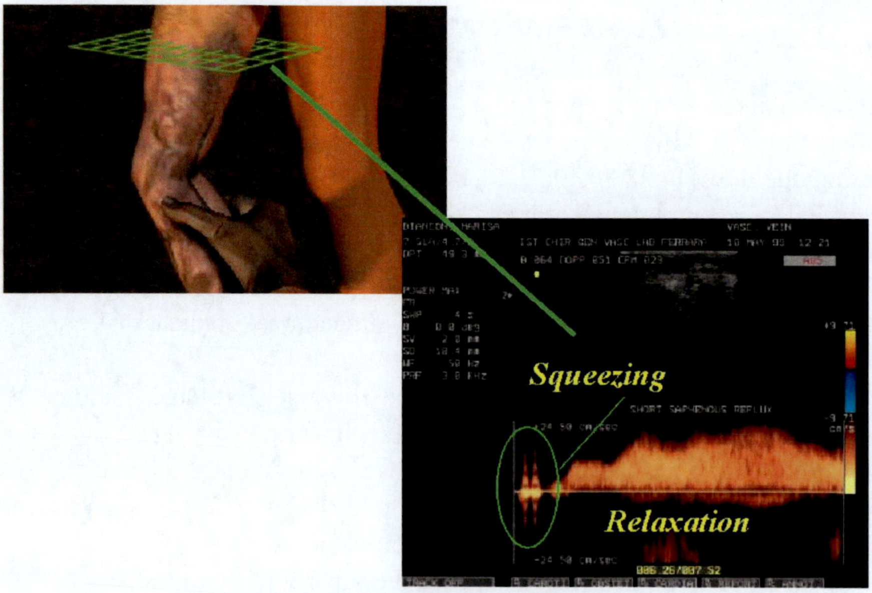


Figure 3.5. A reflux is a flow that is inverted with respect to the physiological direction and lasting more than 0.5 seconds. The phenomenon is related to the presence of a re-entry point.

As with the re-entry concept, the reflux concept includes not only the strictly anatomical aspect, that is, the existence of the "reflux point," which represents the obviously incontinent connection between two vessels, but also the hemodynamic aspect, that is, the existence of a reflux gradient, in this case diastolic. The rise in compartment (e.g., from the femoral to the saphena, AC1->AC2) can occur either because the deep pressure increases, as happens during the Valsalva maneuver, or because the superficial pressure decreases. In the latter case, the gradient occurs due to the combined action of two mechanisms. The first mechanism is represented by the already illustrated re-entry gradient that primes retrograde flow. The second is represented by the reduction in lateral pressure that follows an increase in retrograde flow velocity. In other words, once the retrograde flow is primed by the re-entry gradient, the consequent pressor drop sets the stage for the development of a gradient between the refluxing vessel and the vessel that feeds the retrograde flow.

Diastolic reflux occurs with analogous mechanisms, both at the level of the primary reflux point (that most proximal in the circle of the reflux system) and at the level of the secondary reflux points (those more distal).

It must be emphasized that a system having reflux is subject to hemodynamic overloading because it receives not only the quantity of blood coming from its tributary territory due to normal flow, but also the quantity of blood that comes from the hierarchically deeper compartment. The refilling pressures of such a system are high as a result, and this limits significantly the normal flow in the tributary territories.

Therefore, chronic venous insufficiency is to be considered hemodynamically as an "outflow pathology" because of the obstacles to outflow in the territories affected by reflux phenomena.

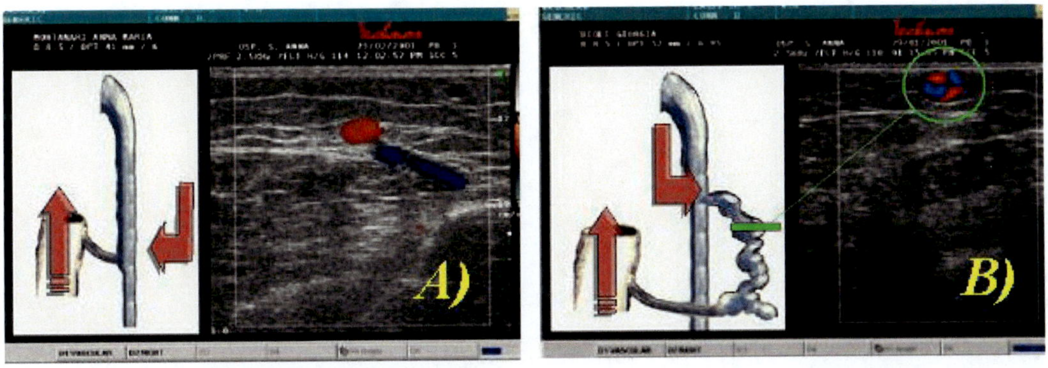


Figure 3.6. Re-entry flow into the deep venous system via perforating veins A) An example of re-entry focused on N2 and B) on N3. This finding determines different venous-venous type shunts and different CHIVA strategies (see chapter 9-10).

## 8. Private Circulation

The term "private circulation" identifies a vicious cycle of blood between superficial and deep networks, or even in only the superficial, that occurs in cases where a reflux and a re-entry are present contemporarily and the quantity of blood that refluxes during the muscular relaxation phase returns to the reflux point during the successive phase of muscular contraction [14,17,105,234,238].

Echo-Doppler studies of patients affected by varicose veins have shown, keeping in mind that in every case there is the presence of a re-entry, that the hemodynamic picture can be referable to one of the following situations:

a) refluxes associated with private circulations in the overwhelming majority of cases (more than 90%); or
b) absence of reflux, and therefore absence of private circulation, represented by the so-called outflow varices that are found in the segmentary incontinences of the saphenous collaterals that do not involve the origin of the collateral (if the latter were also incontinent, there would exist a compartment jump N2->N3 and therefore a reflux) and in those cases of post-stripping recurrence that do not present reflux points in the deep circle. Private circulations have been classified as Franceschi's shunt due to their course that is based on the compartments involved and will be described in the next chapter.

Chapter 4

# Chronic Venous Insufficiency: Definition and Patho-Physiological Mechanisms

*Claude Franceschi*
Saint Joseph and Pitié-Salpétrière Hospitals, Paris, France.

## 1. Definition of Venous Insufficiency

Venous function has three primary purposes: to drain tissues, to aid thermoregulation, and to refill the heart regardless of posture or muscular activity [4,14,34,93,105].

The venous system consists of all the organs necessary to the haemodynamic mechanisms of venous function. It adapts permanently the direction, flow, and pressure of blood return. It maintains a transmural pressure favourable to drainage, adapts superficial venous flow to the needs of thermoregulation, and modulates venous blood volume available for the heart. Thus, venous function depends essentially on the regulation of haemodynamic mechanisms.

The organs of the venous system are the pathways that transport venous blood from microcirculation to the right atrium, and the cardiac, thoraco-abdominal and valvulo-muscular pumps that move it.

Venous insufficiency is an acute or chronic incapacity of the venous system to ensure all or part of the functions previously defined. In haemodynamic terms, we can define venous insufficiency as the incapacity of the venous system to provide blood flow and pressure suitable for drainage, thermoregulation, and heart filling, whatever the subject's posture or muscular activity. It is the consequence of a permanent or transitory dysfunction of one or more of the components of the venous system. Insufficiency is generally identified by particular clinical symptoms according to the impaired function. For example, heaviness, pain, oedema, varicose veins, hypodermitis, and ulcers result from impaired venous drainage [2,3,87,184,193,194,222,231-233]. Intolerance to heat is related to disorders in venous flow adaptation to thermoregulation. Fainting in the standing position is caused by disorders of right heart filling. Light and/or beginning forms of insufficiency are often asymptomatic and can be detected only through instrumental testing.

Acute venous insufficiency is related to a major obstacle to blood flow, such as thrombosis. The most common form is represented by the phlegmatia cerulea, in which the absence of vicarious return stops arterial flow and induces an ischaemia.

Chronic venous insufficiency is generally related to the incapacity of the valvulo-muscular pumps to correct the negative effects of standing. Other causes (e.g., chronic venous occlusion, arterio-venous fistula, and congenital venous hypoplasia) are less frequent.

Haemodynamic physiopathology explains most mechanisms of venous insufficiency, clarifies the interpretation of instrumental investigations, and allows coherent therapeutic choices.

# 2. Haemodynamic Physiopathology of Venous Drainage

## 2.1. Tissue Drainage

Drainage of tissues is achieved by both venous and lymphatic systems. Venous drainage depends primarily on a major haemodynamic parameter called transmural pressure (TMP) [33,181,272]. TMP regulation is essential to tissue life. It eliminates catabolites that are toxic to cells and indirectly allows the surge of arterial blood. It plays a role in balancing the liquid compartments. Venous insufficiency owing to lack of drainage is due to an excess of TMP. It leads to cellular suffering from accumulation of toxic metabolites and ischemia from circulatory slowdown. It also increases the volume of the interstitial and cellular liquid compartment. Clinically, it results in such objective symptoms as oedema, hypodermitis, necrosis, and ulcer. There are multiple causes of excessive TMP, but they can be classified into two main groups: 1) too high venous pressure, and 2) too low external pressure.

## 2.2. Transmural Pressure (TMP)

Transmural pressure (Figures. 4.1) is the key to the haemodynamic drainage mechanism. It is the differential value between two opposite pressures [272]. One is the so-called external pressure (EP) that presses on the external side of the vessel wall. The other is the so-called internal pressure or lateral pressure (IP) that presses the internal side of the vessel wall. TMP, oncotic pressure, and permeability of the capillaries constitute the triad that determines the exchanges between the intra- and extra-vascular compartments. When IP of the capillary is low and/or extra-capillary pressure is high, TMP is low and favourable to drainage, and vice versa. The venous system cannot modify EP, but it can modify IP. Thus, the venous system must continually ensure an optimal TMP for drainage by maintaining a low venous pressure.

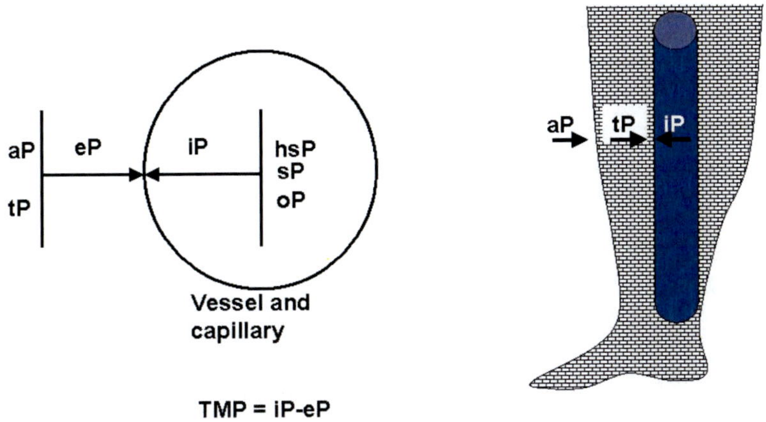


Figure 4.1. Trans mural pressure TMP. aP: atmospheric pressure. tP: tissue pressure. eP: external pressure. iP: internal pressure ( lateral pressure). hsP: hydrostatic pressure. sP: static pressure. oP: oncotic pressure (capillary vessel). TMP = iP-eP. TMP is the crucial parameter for tissue drainage and venous caliber and varies according to iP and eP modulators.

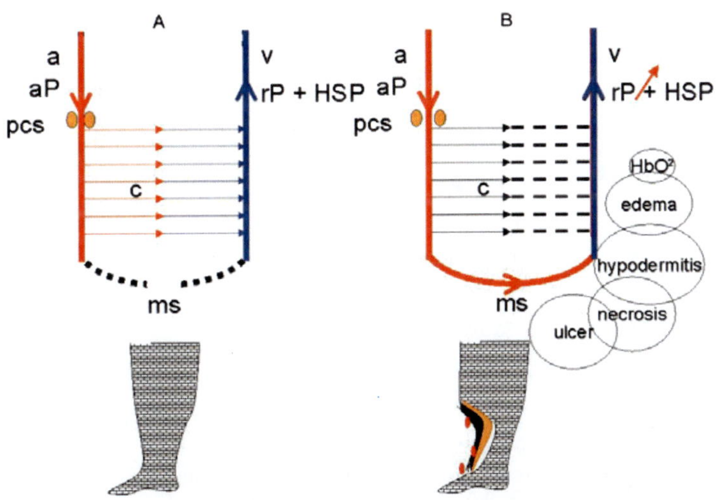


Figure 4.2. Microcirculation MC. a: arteriole v: veinule c: capillaries ms: micro-shunts aP: arterial pressure rP: residual pressure pcs: pre-capillary sphincter. rP=aP-MC Resistance. A: Normal status .B: Venous pressure rise increases TMP which opens pcs and ms with steal effect on the capillary flow and rP increase. That leads to tissue drainage impairment, flow capillary reduction until ischemia, tissue necrosis and hypodermitis. So the venous ulcer shows a paradoxal mix of necrotic tissue with red blood.

## 2.3. Oedema, Hypodermitis, and Ulcer from Venous Insufficiency (Figure 4.2)

When venous pressure increases, TMP increases so that liquids and metabolic wastes from the tissues cannot pass into circulation. Obstacles to the passage of liquids can cause oedemas. Intra-tissue accumulation of toxic metabolites, associated with capillary flow slowdown, are the key haemodynamic mechanisms possibly leading to trophic disorders [33,186]. The reactive vasodilation of arterioles and the opening of micro-shunts worsen tissue ischaemia in two ways: TMP increases because of residual pressure (RP) enhancement, and micro-shunts reduce capillary flow, thereby worsening cellular necrosis. The latter phenomenon explains the coexistence of oxygenated blood (red) with necroses in venous ulcers. Infection occurs because of the ideal culture medium that this type of ulcer represents. Recently, genetic and molecular mechanisms related to the inflammatory cascade explain individual differences in response to the above described mechanisms [264,279].

## 2.4. Correcting Excessive TMP

Because these drainage disorders due to venous insufficiency are related to excessive TMP, the logical solution is either to reduce IP or to increase EP.

## 2.5. Regulating Extra-Vascular Pressure to Correct Venous Insufficiency

Low EP is usually related to low atmospheric pressure (e.g., high altitude, air travel) and can be compensated by compression (bandage or stockings) [59,251]. Excessive IP can also be compensated by an increase in EP, but necessarily lower than the blood pressure in order not to cause ischemia. For this reason, external compression can be sufficient when IP is moderately high, but it cannot restore a completely satisfactory TMP when IP is very high. Thus, the beneficial effect of compression on drainage does not seem to result from the acceleration of venous return, which is negligible, but rather from the reduction in TMP.

## 2.6. Regulating Venous Pressure to Correct Venous Insufficiency

Venous pressure is made up of hydrostatic pressure (HSP), static pressure (SP), and dynamic pressure (DP). Reductions in HSP and SP decrease TMP. This effect can be obtained by acting on some or all of these components.

### *2.6.1. Components of Venous Pressure (Figure 4.3)*

Total venous pressure is the sum of HSP, SP, and DP. HSP is the pressure generated by the force of gravity. It is proportional to the acceleration of gravity (g), the density of blood (δ), and the height of the blood column (h). Expressed mathematically, HSP =δ gh. In other terms, the venous pressure at the level of the calf is proportional to the vertical distance from the calf to the top of the head. Therefore, HSP varies according to the posture. It is maximal in the standing position, close to zero in the lying position, and negative (lower than atmospheric pressure) when the feet are positioned above the level of the head. SP and DP are generated by the pumps of the venous system. DP is the dynamic energy $1/2\ \rho v^2$ (v = velocity of flow). The sum SP + DP is constant. So when SP increases, DP decreases, and vice versa. This is in accordance with the law of Bernoulli P = HSP+SP+DP = Constant. DP and SP change inversely according to flow resistance. The more flow resistance increases, the more circulatory speed decreases, and so SP increases and DP decreases. Thus, when a liquid is immobilized by high flow resistance, SP= SP+DP because DP is null (v=0). Conversely, when flow resistance decreases, DP increases with the flow velocity (v) and SP decreases (SP+DP=Constant). This drop in SP can be so significant (possibly to lower than atmospheric pressure) that it aspires the blood of the tributary veins (Venturi effect on drainage). However, HSP and SP play the major roles in tissue drainage [34,68,78,102-105,135,183].

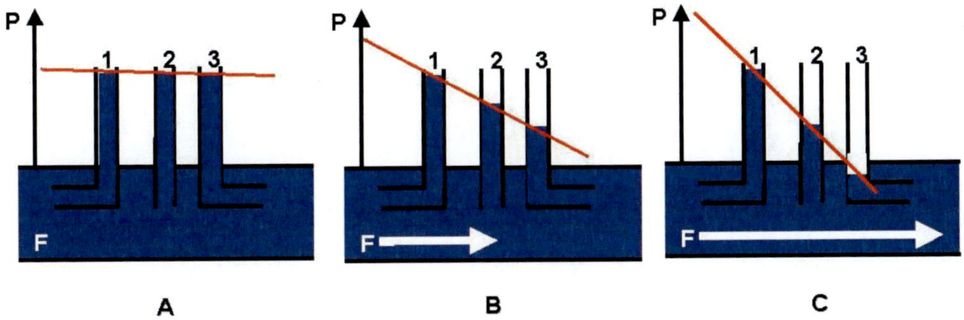


Figure 4.3, Pitot's tubes. Parameters of pressure. F: flow P: pressure. 1: P= Static pressure + dynamic pressure. 2: P= Static pressure.3: P= Static pressure - dynamic pressure ( Venturi effect). If 1,2 and 3, are catheters, one can see that for the same Total Pressure TP, the pressure values are different and depend on the orientation of their tip according to the flow F direction and velocity. The flow velocity in this case depends on the resistances to the flow. A: Flow velocity = 0, Resistance > or = TP, so all the TP is converted in Static pressure. B: Flow velocity = medium value, moderate Resistance <TP, so TP is converted. In tube 1 , were the tip is oriented in the opposite direction but parallel to the flow, the pressure value is related to the total pressure ie. dynamic pressure + lateral(static) pressure + hydrostatic (gravity) pressure where hydrostatic pressure is negligible because the tube is horizontal. In tube 2, where the tip is perpendicular to the flow, the pressure value is total pressure – dynamic pressure ie. represents the pressure applied against the wall of the tube. Venturi effect is shown in tube 3 were the tip is oriented in the same direction and parallel to the flow. This drawing up effect can be efficient for tributaries drainage but as far as the velocity is high enough. C: Flow velocity = high value, low Resistance <TP. TP converted in the same way as B, but lateral pressure is lower and Venturi effect more pronounced.

### *2.6.2. Regulating Lateral Pressure to Correct Venous Insufficiency*

IP is the sum of HSP+SP. It is the effective part of internal venous pressure that contributes to TMP. TMP = IP–EP. The modulation of IP can be achieved by modifications in HSP and/or SP.

### *2.6.3. Regulating Hydrostatic Pressure to Correct Venous Insufficiency (Figures 4.4a,b,c)*

HSP is usually the major variable in venous haemodynamics due to its strong influence on TMP. This explains the occurrence and aggravation of venous insufficiency in the standing position, that is, when HSP is maximal. Improvements in drainage through reductions in TMP can be achieved by either reducing or fractionating the height of the liquid column. Reductions in the height of the liquid column are obtained by changing the posture. HSP is maximum (around 90 mmHg) at the level of the ankle when the subject is in the standing position, close to null in the lying position, and negative (lower than atmospheric pressure), when the feet are higher than the head, as above reported.

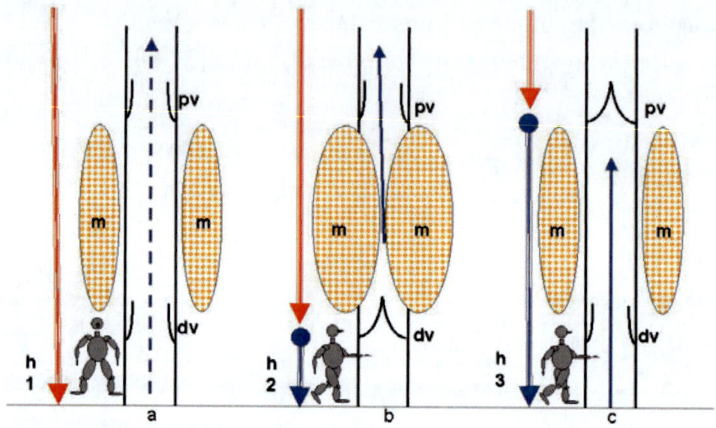


Figure 4.4. A)Physiological Dynamic Fractionation of Hydrostatic Pressure DFHP: alternate valve closure reduces hydrostatic pressure HSP by fractioning the height of the venous blood column. Effect of the valvulo-muscular pump VMP of the calf when walking HSP: Hydrostatic pressure. h: Height of venous blood column m: calf VMP muscles. Dv : distal calf VMP valve pv: proximal calf VMP valve. a: Standing immobile. No DFPH :VMP at rest. Open VMP valves. h1: maximum height. b :Walking. DFHP: distal VMP valve closed by VMP systole. h2 : reduced eight at the dv level c: :Walking. DFHP: proximal VMP valve closed by VMP diastole. h3 : reduced eight at the pv level.

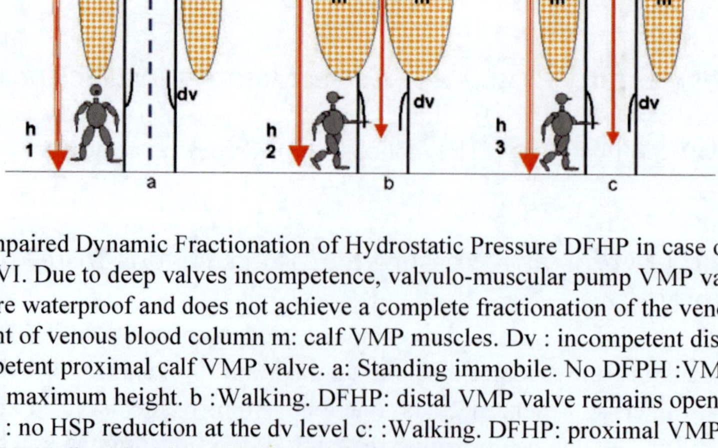


Figure 4.4. B) Impaired Dynamic Fractionation of Hydrostatic Pressure DFHP in case of deep venous incompetence DVI. Due to deep valves incompetence, valvulo-muscular pump VMP valve alternate closure is no more waterproof and does not achieve a complete fractionation of the venous blood column. h: Height of venous blood column m: calf VMP muscles. Dv : incompetent distal calf VMP valve pv: incompetent proximal calf VMP valve. a: Standing immobile. No DFPH :VMP at rest. Open VMP valves. h1: maximum height. b :Walking. DFHP: distal VMP valve remains open despite the VMP systole. h2 : no HSP reduction at the dv level c: :Walking. DFHP: proximal VMP valve remains open despite the VMP diastole. h3 : no HSP reduction at the pv level.

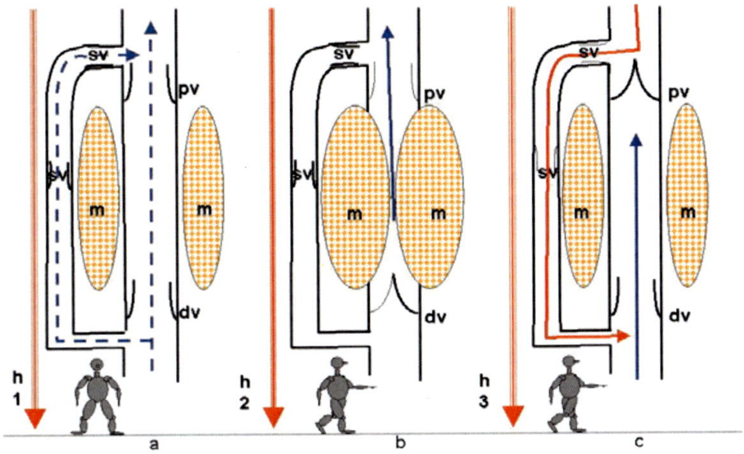


Figure 4.4. C) Impaired Dynamic Fractionation of Hydrostatic Pressure DFHP in case of superficial venous incompetence SVI. Despite deep valves waterproof closure, correct DFHP is not achieved in case of superficial valves incompetence, when the incompetent superficial vein shunts the deep fractionation. h: Height of venous blood column m: calf VMP muscles. Dv : competent distal calf VMP valve pv: competent proximal calf VMP valve. sv: incompetent superficial valves. a: Standing immobile. No DFPH :VMP at rest. Open VMP valves. h1: maximum height. b,c :Walking. DFHP: distal and proximal alternately closed by VMP systole and diastole but h2 and h3 are not fractionated because of the liquid continuity through the incompetent superficial venous shunt.

This constitutes a simple and effective method for controlling TMP, proved by its evident healing effect in everyday clinical practice. Fractionation of the liquid column takes place physiologically due to the so-called dynamic fractionation of hydrostatic pressure (DFHSP), as occurs when walking. When the subject is motionless in the standing position, the valves are open, and the column of venous blood remains in continuity, so that the HSP at the level of the ankle is maximal [102-105,193]. For this reason, standing motionless and sitting for prolonged periods compromise drainage and can lead to clinical consequences, as proved by clinical evidence, particularly in prolonged, motionless standing work conditions. Such conditions lead to a typical postural venous insufficiency. Fortunately, as soon as the subject moves or walks, the valvulo-muscular pump (VMP) of the lower limbs is activated. Alternating watertight closure of the distal valves (during the systole of the VMP) and proximal valves (during the diastole) dynamically fractionates the liquid column, and thus the HSP

Insufficient DFHSP represents the most frequent cause of chronic venous insufficiency (CVI) and is related to a defect in one or more of the VMP components, usually valvular incompetence [4,19,31,46,58,77,80,85,138,159,162,168,196,215,218,219,231,243,256]. In this case, CVI is proportional to the degree of valvular incompetence, which may affect deep and/or superficial veins, but in the large majority of cases affects superficial ones. Another defect of the VMP is deficit and/or lack of muscular contraction (muscular paralysis, joint ankylosis). Surgical correction of DFHSP impairment can be achieved either by valve repair [142,143,168,190,196], or by permitting permanent HSP fractionation [6,9,45,47,56,90-92,96,103,106,251,254,283].

### 2.6.4. Regulating Static Pressure to Correct Venous Insufficiency:

SP is part of IP, and thus of TMP. SP is maximal when flow is stopped by proximal resistance that obstructs it. On the contrary, SP is minimal when resistance is low. This is in accordance with the law of Bernoulli. At rest, SP depends on residual pressure (RP). RP is the arterial pressure transmitted to the venous bed through the micro-circulation. RP is equal to the arterial pressure (AP) value decreased by the loss of energy in micro-circulatory resistance (MCR). RP = AP-MCR = SP+DP. SP = RP-DP. DP = $1/2\ \rho v^2$ SP = AP-MCR-$1/2\ \rho v^2$. Therefore, TMP increases when MCR decreases and/or when proximal resistance to flow increases, and vice versa.

During muscular exercise, such as walking and running, venous pressure and venous flow increase through three mechanisms: increased cardiac output, decreased MCR, and VMP action. If the proximal resistance is low, TMP remains low and drainage remains good. For this reason, the athlete could develop varicose veins from excessive pressure and flow during training [237]. On the other hand, if the distal venous network does not manage to absorb correctly the energy of flow and pressures because of stenosis or occlusion, the subject may limp because of painful hypertension of the calf.

Correcting excessive SP can be achieved by two means: reducing venous flow resistance and reducing RP by increasing MCR. Flow resistance can be reduced by removing obstructions or bridging (by-pass) them. MCR can be increased by cooling the limb.

### 2.6.5. Draining Flow

Draining flow is central to venous function. It is indispensable to the economy of the drained organs. An acute or chronic obstacle in the venous path impairs drainage proportionally to the increase in SP. It appears clinically by restrictive syndrome. In *phlegmatia cerulea*, the venous obstacle is so resistant that it stops the incoming arterial flow as well. Proximal flow resistance increases venous pressure because the energy of RP is not consumed in blood motion (DP). It forces and dilates gradually the collateral veins that circumvent the obstacle [197]. This opening of collaterals decreases flow resistance and, therefore, the component SP of RP. Thus, RP explains not only the development of collateral varicose veins that circumvent the deep venous obstacles of post-thrombotic diseases, but also the development of superficial varicose veins after "therapeutic" occlusion or destruction of varicose or nonvaricose superficial veins [22,44,63,66,84,239,246,248].

### 2.6.6. Combined Correction of Drainage Defects

The various methods of TMP control can be combined to support drainage by optimizing the conditions. These methods include compression, posture, correction of the DFHSP, and removal of obstacles to the flow.

### 2.6.7. Flow Direction Significance

Flow direction is anterograde when it is physiological, that is, generally in the direction of valve action. Flow direction is retrograde when it is reversed as compared to the usual physiological direction. The term retrograde is not univocal in that does not necessarily mean backward flow, or from the deep veins towards the superficial system. It may mean flow of normal drainage derived between two competent valves towards a normal entry into the deep system. This aspect will be clarified in the next chapters. The normal content of flow, anterograde or retrograde, consists of the blood draining the tissues that depend on it. This physiological flow may be overloaded by flows coming from other tissues, or venous compartments. These additional contents come from the deep network in the event venous blood deviation, due to open shunt (OS) or closed shunt (CS), as described in the next paragraph. It may also come from other superficial territories by pathways of derivation.

## 2.7. Concept of Shunt

A venous shunt (VS) is a pathway for venous blood deviation. A VS carries two different flows, the draining flow and the deviated (derived) flow. The significance of the shunt depends on the flow that is deviated, the starting point and the end point of the deviation. The starting point is called the leak point and/or reflux point (RP) and the end point is called the re-entry point (usually a re-entry perforating vein) [14,26,27,102-105,234].

### *2.7.1. Vicarious Open Shunt (VOS)(Figure 4.5)*

When the flow is deviated to by-pass an obstacle [44,102-105,197], there exists what is called a vicarious open shunt (VOS). This type of shunt is desirable because it by-pass blocked veins and thereby reduce resistance to drainage. It is made of shunting veins that by-pass an obstacle without blood re-circulation. It flows permanently under the effects of distal draining residual pressure and proximal cardiac and thoraco-abdominal aspiration. Its flow increases during valvular-muscular pump systole. It may be antegrade or retrograde.

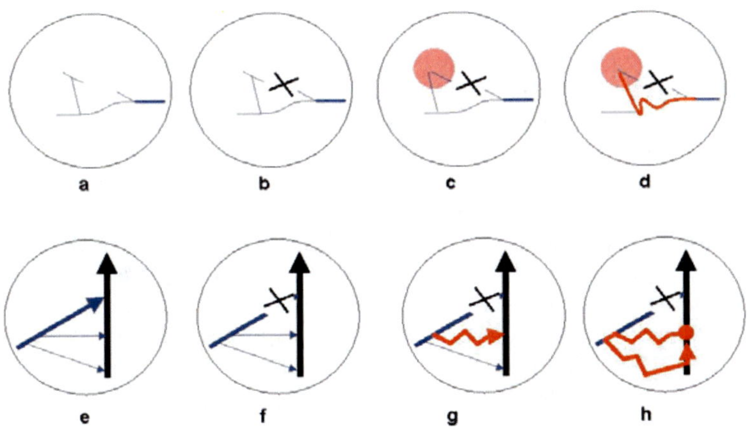


Figure 4.5. Superficial open vicarious shunts for superficial venous obstacles : Any venous draining flow suppression a ( phlebectomy, sclerosis, Laser…) raises the residual pressure in the previously drained territory, so that micro shunts are opened (matting) b , collaterals veins are forced and dilated c ( induced varicose recurrence). If the draining entry is suppressed f, the high residual pressure flow forces any collateral and reaches any perforating vein through which it drains g. In some cases, more than one perforating vein is reached and a closed shunt can be activated h. That is the key point of varicose recurrence after non haemodynamic therapy and explains why recurrent non haemodynamic therapies fail.

For example, a supra-pubic varicose vein that by-passes an occlusion in an iliac vein is an VOS [197]. The flow can be deviated because valve incompetence does not stop the flow inversion when the pressure gradient is physiologically inverted. This occurrence leads to two kinds of shunts according to the presence or absence of re-circulation.

### 2.7.2. Closed Shunt (CS)(Figures 4.6 a, 4.6 b)

When, in addition to the draining flow, the deviated flow re-circulates at each inversion of pressure gradient, as in a closed circuit, we call it closed shunt (CS) [26,30,49,53,105,234,238].

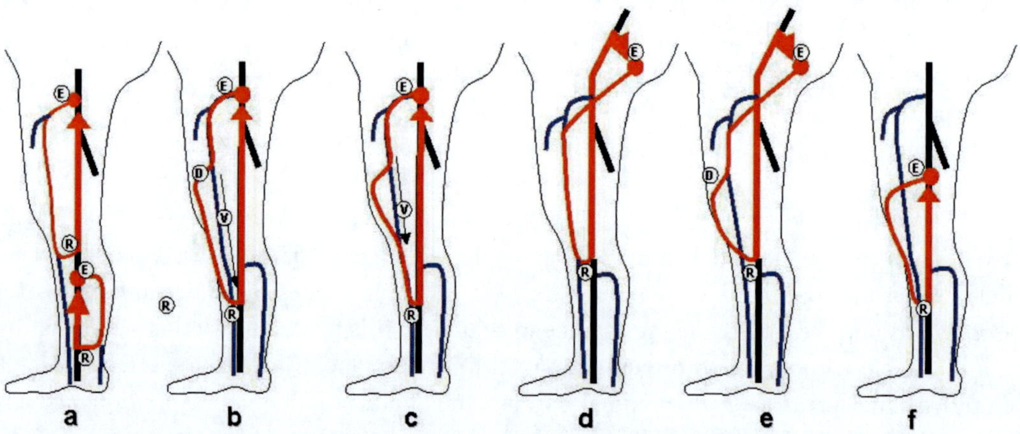


Figure 4.6 a. CS: Closed superficial-deep shunt by superficial incompetent collateral vein are activated by the valvulo-muscular pump diastole. E is the escape point where the retrograde flow refluxes from N1 into N2 or N3. R is the reentry point where the CS flow reenters into N1 where it comes from (Re-circulation). CHIVA procedure disconnects the CS at E and/or another place with or without devalvulation according to the type of CS. a: 2 CS type 1 (N1-N2-N1). Up: N2=GSV. Down:N2=SSV. In both, CHIVA disconnects the CS at E point. b: CS type 3a (N1-N2-N3-N1).E disconnection leaves a DOS. Simultaneous deconnexion at D would cure the DOS but permit not any draining of proximal great saphena and tributaries. So both disconnections can be done only if a devalvulation (arrow) in V is feasible to permit a draining flow to R. Otherwise, disconnection is done only at D (N3-N2 connection) which disconnects the DOS and impeaches the retrograde flow in the proximal GSV that drains its flow in an antegrade direction into the common femoral, despite its valve incompetence. In a second step, E shall be disconnected if a reentry point is developed and reflux reappears. That procedure is called CHIVA 2 ( 2nd step). c: CS type 3 (N1-N2-N3-N1).CHIVA procedure is equal to b. d: CS type 4 (N1-N3-N2-N1).E is one escape point out of the six pelvic escape points from the pelvic N1.( Perineal, Inguinal, Clitoris, Obturator, Superior and Inferior Gluteal points). CHIVA disconnects E. e: CS type 5 (N1-N3-N2-N3-N1).Similar to e, but the terminal superficial pathway is N3. So, E disconnection alone would leave in place a DOS. That is why it has to be completed by a disconnection at D. f: CS type C (N1-N3-N1). Escape and reentry points are connected with N3. CHIVA disconnects only at E.

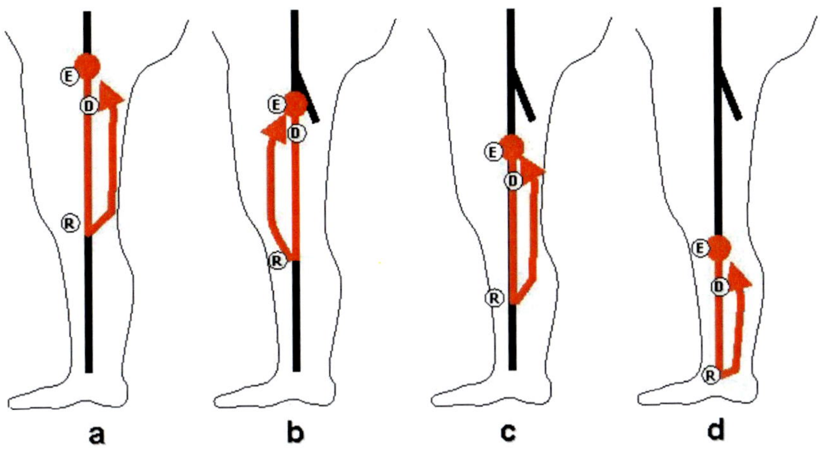


Figure 4.6 b. CS: Closed shunt by deep incompetent collateral vein. A deep CS is made of two collateral veins that drain the same territory and in which one of them is incompetent that lead to a retrograde refluxing flow in valvulo-muscular pump diastole. The escape point E is proximal and reentry point R distal. CHIVA consists in disconnection at D of the incompetent collateral so that DFHP is again efficient and the recirculation is suppressed.

Blood flow can be deviated because incompentent valves fail to stop the reverse flow. The flow inversion is elicited by reversed pressure gradient, usually during VMP diastole. This occurrence leads to two types of shunts, depending on the presence or absence of re-circulation. When, in addition to the draining flow, the deviated flow re-circulates at each inversion of pressure gradient, as in a closed circuit, a closed shunt (CS) is formed.

For example, an incompetent saphenous vein becomes a CS when it generates a closed circuit for deep venous blood. As a matter of fact, an incompetent GSV carries back the femoral blood from the sapheno-femoral junction to the deep veins of the calf through a perforating vein during the diastole, and continues to do so at each diastole. Thus, part of the deep venous blood remains "excluded" from the general circulation in a "private circulation." CS is activated by VMP diastole, as when walking. CS impairs drainage because it impairs the effect of the VMP on DFHSP.

The greater the efficiency of the VMP, the greater the diastolic flow. On the contrary, the lower the VMP efficiency, the less the diastolic flow. For this reason, in the case of totally inefficient VMP, as in rare case in which deep veins are totally incompetent, a dynamic test of VMP will not show any diastolic flow in the superficial veins, even if they are very large and varicose. Actually, during the diastole, total vein incompetence does not allow activation of the VMP and reduces venous pressure so that the gradient of the re-entry perforating vein is not favourable to inflow [19,58,252,258,260,262]. This phenomenon is illustrated by the Perthes test, which shows in the supposed case no reduction of varices when walking despite a tourniquet at the hip. It is also demonstrated by an unexpected lack of reflux duplex detection in superficial varicose veins during such dynamic tests as Paranà's manoeuvre [102].

### *2.7.3. Open Derived Shunt (ODS)(Figure 4.7)*

As previously noted, venous flow can be deviated into an incompetent vein because incompetence allows for flow inversion elicited by a reversed pressure gradient, usually during VMP diastole. This occurrence leads to two types of shunts, depending on the presence of re-circulation (CS) or its absence (ODS). When an incompetent vein carries draining blood from other territories in addition to its own territories during VMP diastole, without re-circulation or vicarious by-pass effect, an ODS is formed.

For example, an incompetent superficial vein generates an ODS when its retrograde flow toward the deep veins through a distal perforating vein consists of draining flow belonging not only to its own territory, but also to other territories. This is the case when an incompetent tributary of the GSV carries out the flow of the other competent tributaries, as seen in shunt type II [105,152].

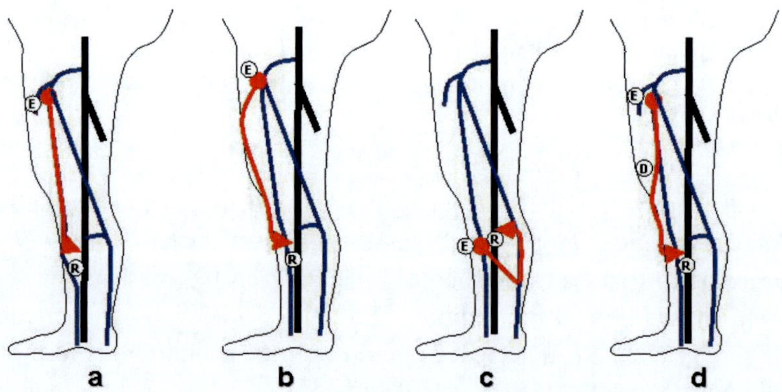


Figure 4.7. DOS: Derivated open shunt by superficial incompetent vein connecting with pumping out reentry. Retrograde flow in DOS is overloaded by the flow of the confluent superficial normal veins thanks to DOS incompetent valves that allow the diastolic pumping up of the valvulo-muscular pump connected with the reentry point R. No re-circulation because E and R points are connected with different networks. In CHIVA treatment, disconnection is done on DOS at E point excepted in shunt 2D (d) where it can be done at N2-N3 junction (D) . Examples: a- Shunt 0: N3-N2-N1. b- Shunt 2 a: N2-N3-N1 Shunt c- N2-N4-N2-N1 d- Shunt 2d: N2-N3-N1.

*2.7.4. Mixed Shunts (MS) (Figure 4.8)* which are VOS and CS that share the same escape point and part of their shunting veins. However, their re-entry points are in different locations, the CS re-entry being distal to the reflux point, and the VOS re-entry being proximal. An example is when an iliac venous occlusion is associated with homolateral great saphenous incompetence. The escape point at the sapheno-femoral junction acts as a VOS in systole, draining femoral flow towards the opposite femoral vein (re-entry point) through right and left arch tributaries (spontaneous Palma). The same escape point acts as a CS in diastole, spilling femoral flow into distal deep veins through retrograde saphenous flow and perforator re-entry. This is also the case in haemodynamic block of a superficial femoral vein. Popliteal flow may escape into the SSV, and then into Giacomini's vein, and re-enter the deep network through the sapheno-femoral junction in systole; it escapes also in diastole when great saphena incompetence distal to the Giacomini-great saphena junction allows retrograde flow until a distal re-entry [80,91,111].

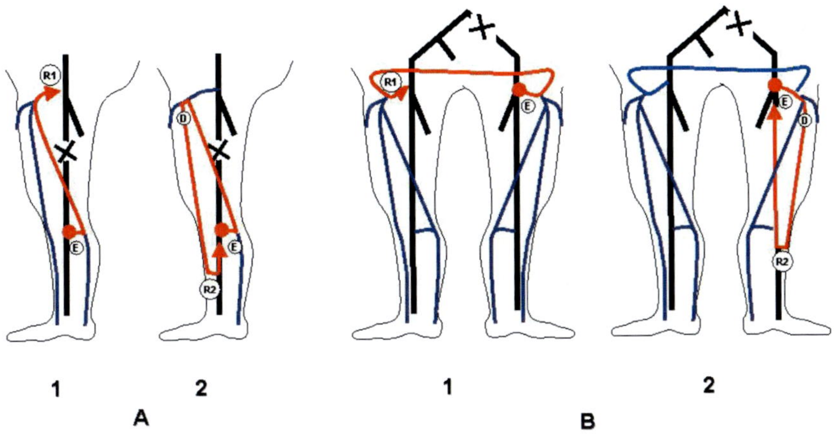


Figure 4.8. Mixed shunts (MS) and haemodynamic management. MS by association of vicarious open shunt VOS with closed shunt CS where initial venous pathways and the escape point E are common and terminal venous pathways and reentry point R are different (R1 for VOS and R2 for CS). VOS activation is enhanced by the valvulo-muscular pump systole VMP and CS is activated only by VMP diastole. The CHIVA treatment aims to spear the VOS and disconnect the CS. So the disconnection D has not to be done at E point, but beyond, where CS and VOS pathways diverge, at the beginning terminal CS pathway. A: MS due to association of incompetent great saphenous trunk and superficial femoral vein obstacle. 1: VOS systolic activation . 2: Closed shunt diastolic activation. They share sapheno-popliteal reflux, small saphenous arch retrograde flow and Giacomini vein antegrade (physiologic direction but pathologic flow). Beyond they flow in different directions. VOS flows proximally according to physiologic antegrade direction but abnormal content through the great saphenous arch then sapheno-femoral junction (R1). CS flows distally through the great saphenous trunk then antegrade through the perforating vein of the leg R2.CHIVA consists in disconnection not at E because of a mandatory spear of VOS but at D, i.e. on the CS pathway beyond its diversion from VOS. B: MS due to association of incompetent great saphenous arch and trunk and iliac vein obstacle. 1: VOS systolic activation . 2: Closed shunt diastolic activation. They share sapheno-femoral reflux and great saphenous arch retrograde flow. Beyond, VOS flow is retrograde through the great saphenous trunk then antegrade through a perforating vein of the leg R2.CHIVA consists in disconnection not at E because of a mandatory spear of VOS but at D, i.e. on the CS pathway beyond its diversion from VOS.

### 2.8. Non-Haemodynamic Causes of Venous Drainage Impairment

Permanent or transitory abnormalities of capillary permeability and/or oncotic pressure may be responsible for symptoms of venous insufficiency that are generally limited to oedema. They may be added to haemodynamic causes, particularly during pregnancy.

## 3. Pathophysiologic Significance of Shunts

Some types of venous shunts can involve drainage impairment and/or varicose veins, while others can improve both.

Analysing the varicose phenomenon, all types of shunts involve venous dilatation because they are veins overloaded by a pathologic flow in addition to physiologic. This dilatation is roughly proportional to the charge of the added flow, especially if significant turbulence occurs.

***VOS and ODS*** are overloaded proportionally to the drained territory. Theoretically, total flow cannot exceed the amount delivered by the territory.

***CS***. drains excessive flow that is not proportional to the flow of the drained territory, but rather to the activity of the VMP to which it is connected. The more the patient walks and runs, the more the flow and the greater the varicose dilatation.

Analysing the drainage of tissues we know that it depends on trans-mural pressure (TMP), and thus on resistance to flow and hydrostatic pressure.

***VOS*** is opened by residual pressure (RP), and so it is directly related to tissue drainage. It is necessary for drainage because it by-passes an obstacle, thereby reducing resistance to flow. The larger the VOS veins, the better the drainage. Thus, VOS represents a natural correction of drainage impairments and must be preserved.

***ODS*** does not interfere directly with drainage, but does so indirectly by disrupting DFHSP. The longer the incompetent vein, the worse the DFHSP.

***CS*** disrupts TMP regulation through DFHSP impairment and excess volume/pressure due to VMP re-circulation charge.

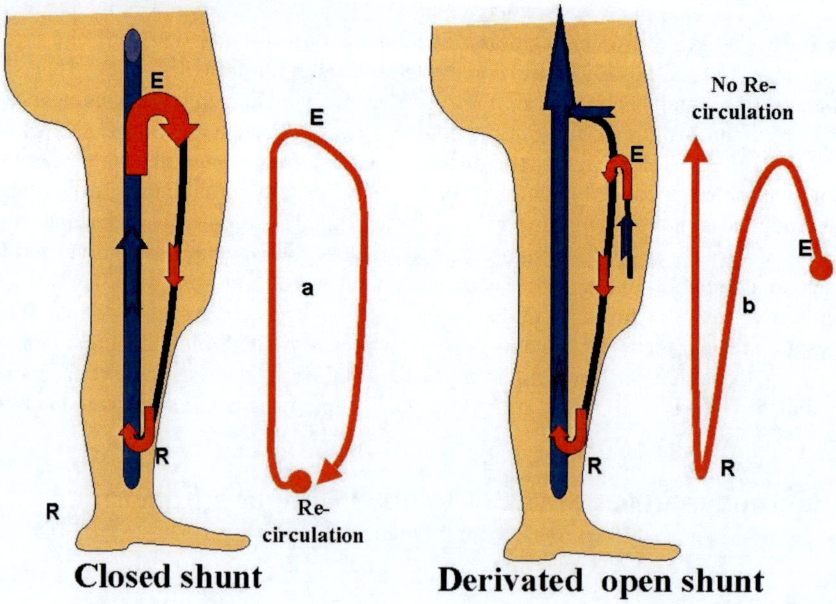


Figure 4.9. Venous Shunts: Closed Shunt (CS) and Derivated open shunt DOS activated in diastole. E:Escape point. R:reentry point. a: re-circullating circuit, part of blood returns to its source through E.. b: no re-circulating circuit, no blood returns to its source.

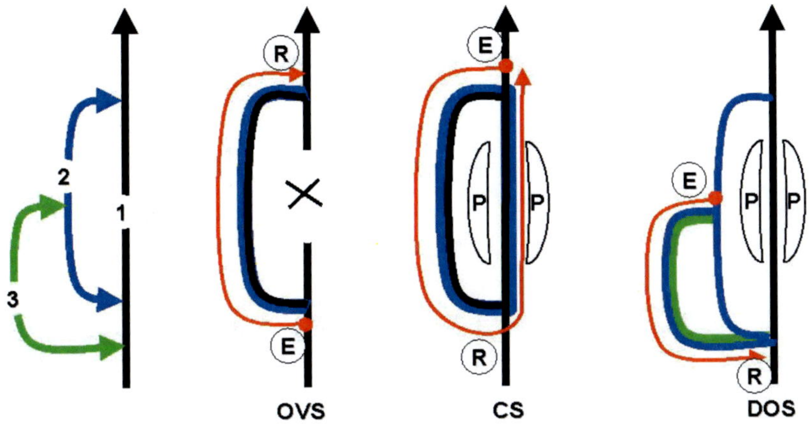


Figure 4.10. VENOUS SHUNTS PRINCIPLES: 1,2,3: Competent interconnected veins draining their own territory without shunts. E: escape point. R: reentry point. P: valvulo-muscular pump at diastolic phase. A venous shunt is made of a vein overloaded by any flow depending on other territories. OVS: Open vicarious shunt: vein 2 by-passes an obstacle in a collateral vein 1 and so carries out two flows: its physiologic draining flow and an overloading flow from the vein 1 territory distal to the obstacle. The escape point E is distal to reentry R. VOS flow is permanent but enhanced by P systole. No re-circulation. CS: Closed shunt: during P diastolic aspiration, incompetent vein 2 allows a retrograde flow so that vein 2 drains properly its own physiologic flow despite its retrograde direction plus vein 1 flow refluxing through E that is proximal to R. So, vein 1 flow re-circulates at each P diastole. DOS: Derivated open shunt: during P diastolic aspiration, incompetent vein 3 allows a retrograde flow so that vein 3 drains properly its own physiologic flow despite its retrograde direction plus vein 2 flow refluxing through E. There is no recirculation because the distal reentry R is not connected with vein 2 but vein 1.

## 4. Haemodynamic Physiopathology of Deep Veins

Total occlusion of the deep veins of the lower limbs by thrombosis is exceptional (phlegmatia cerulea). Most of the time, occlusion is partial. Clinical manifestations depend on the severity of the restrictive syndrome. Usually, the restrictive syndrome decreases thanks to the recanalisation of thromboses and development of collateral veins (e.g., VOS) brought about by residual pressure [78,135,168,197]. Unfortunately, the recanalisation of thromboses often destroys the valves. Coexistence of competent and incompetent parallel deep veins may constitute a deep closed shunt (CS). This occurrence is more frequent in cases of double superficial femoral veins. Valvular incompetence leads to a lack of DFHSP and its consequences on TMP, and therefore on drainage. An obstacle may be dynamic without thrombosis. This occurs, for example, when the calibre of a superficial femoral vein is too narrow to absorb the flow ejected by the calf when the subject is walking. In this case, the superficial femoral vein is "naturally" by-passed from the popliteal vein to the common femoral vein thanks to a collateral pathway. This pathway is made up of a succession of short saphenous vein, Giacomini veins, and proximal great saphenous vein that absorbs the excess flow during the systole of the calf's VMP (figure 4.11). These vicarious veins are often tortuous and dilated and are called varicose veins. Klippel-Trenaunay Syndrome is another example of when a large varicose vein compensates for an aplasic deep vein, such as aplasic popliteal and superficial femoral veins.

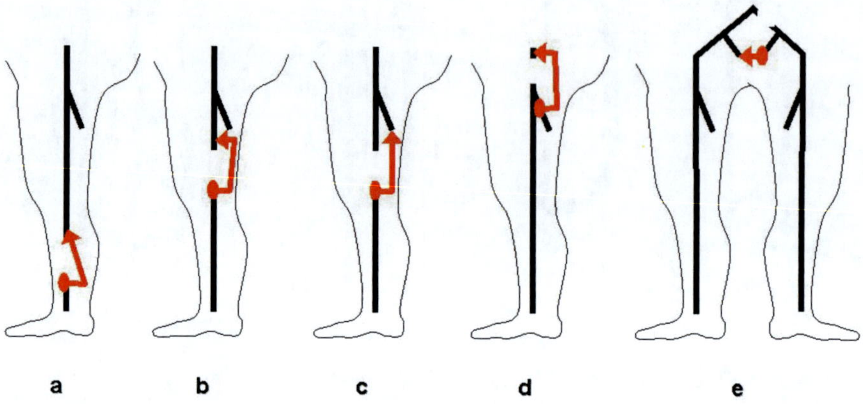


Figure 4.11 A) Deep open vicarious shunts for deep venous obstacles :Flow enhanced in systole: examples: spontaneous deep by-pass for vein obstruction or agenesis: a: peroneal vein by-passing tibial veins. b: superficial femoral collateral vein by-passing superficial femoral vein c: deep femoral vein by-passing superficial femoral vein.d: hypogastic and deep femoral veins connection by-passing external iliac vein. e: hypogastric veins connection by-passing common iliac vein. Those spontaneous by-pass improve the bad haemodynamic condition due to venous obstacles. So they have to be recognized to be speared especially in venous malformations where inappropriate embolization or avulsion can worsen the venous condition.

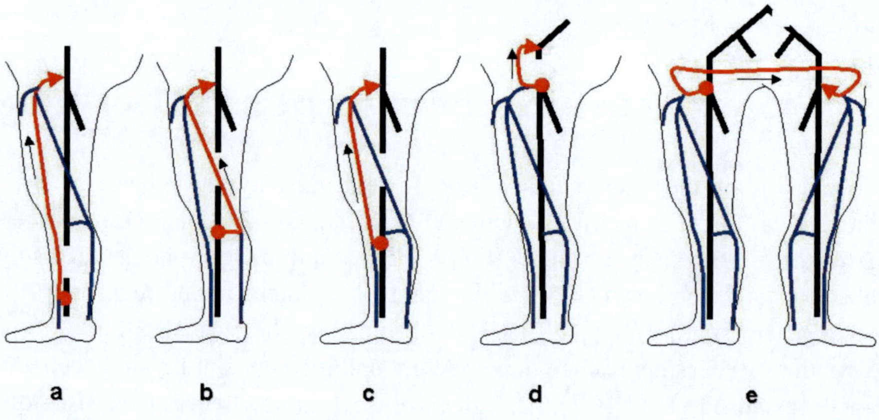


Figure 4.11 B) Superficial open vicarious shunts for deep venous obstacles : Flow enhanced in systole: examples: spontaneous superficial by-pass for vein obstruction or agenesis: a: great saphena vein by-passing tibial veins. b: Giacomini vein by-passing superficial femoral vein c: proximal great saphena vein by-passing superficial femoral vein. d: great sahenous arch and superficial epigastric vein by-passing iliac vein. e: external pudendal veins connection by-passing by-passing common iliac vein (spontaneous Palma operation). Those spontaneous by-pass improve the bad haemodynamic condition due to venous obstacles. So they have to be recognized to be speared especially in venous malformations where inappropriate embolization, sclerosis, laser or avulsion can worsen the venous condition.

# 5. Haemodynamic Physiopathology of Superficial Veins

## 5.1. Calibre of Superficial Veins and Varices

The calibre of the superficial veins depends on TMP and compliance [1,10,12,74,75,275-277]. The external pressure (EP) that limits dilation varies according to the topography of the superficial veins. The trunk of short and great saphenous and Giacomini veins (network N2) are located in a fascia duplication that limits dilation. The superficial veins (epifascial) located between the skin and the fascia (networks N3 and N4) dilate more easily, having a lower EP due to the smooth surrounding tissue [8,57].

Superficial veins (N2, N3, N4) drain all the superficial tissues of the lower limbs. At rest this drainage is provided by cardiac and thoraco-abdominal pumps. In addition the superficial network also drain the majority of the foot tissues, especially when the plantar pump (PP) of Lejars is activated [18]. When the subject is walking, most of the flow is aspirated by deep VMP diastole; much less is aspirated during deep VMP systole by the Venturi effect. These pumps also drain deep venous blood by the dynamic vicarious effect when the major venous network is saturated (VOS). This saturation may be due to a significant but physiological flow (varices of the athlete) or to a pathological flow (arteriovenous fistulas).

When superficial veins by-bass deep vein occlusion, vicarious open shunts are formed.

These shunts may dilate proportionally to the vicarious flow until they become varicose. They may also be the pathway of a closed shunt (CS) when they allow re-circulation of deep venous blood by the closed circuit effect. A CS dilates superficial veins until they become varicose due to DFHSP impairment and/or shunt flow excess. When the subject is walking, HSP remains too high and the flow energy delivered into the CS by the VMP action of the calf is partially converted into turbulence that stresses the wall and increases lateral pressure. Turbulence occurs when the shunt flow is too high for the calibre of the vein. According to Reynolds' law related to viscous liquids, when velocity reaches a critical value, laminar flow becomes turbulent. When the varicose calibre reaches a value such that velocity is lower than the critical Reynolds' value, turbulence disappears and flow becomes laminar again; the varicose calibre does not increase further but remains stable. This means that, contrary to common belief, walking increases varicose veins, especially when due to CS, and also explains why varicosity progresses for a while and then remains stable for a long period. Superficial veins are necessary for the drainage of superficial tissues related to their physiological territory, even if they carry a supplementary flow, as in VOS, CS and ODS. An accurate therapy for varices has to consider draining flow and focus on the causes of excessive flow and pressure, based on the above described haemodynamic mechanisms. Systematic vein destruction may lead to recurrences because of drainage necessity (RP) of surrounding tissues, either by vein re-opening in the case of closure (ligation, sclerosis, laser, closure, etc) or by varicose by-pass (iatrogenic VOS).

The most frequent varices of lower limbs are related to CS.

# 6. Haemodynamic Physiopathology of Perforating Veins

Perforating veins (PV) and crosses drain the superficial tissues by connecting the superficial networks (N2, N3, N4 and N5) to the deep network (N1) by piercing the muscular fascia. The physiological direction of the superficial venous flow is from superficial networks to the deep network. This direction is determined by the orientation of the valves and the gradient of pressure. When deep pressure is lower than superficial pressure, the valves remain open and the superficial blood is drained into the deep network. When this gradient is inverted because deep pressure is higher than superficial pressure, the valves shut and prevent flow inversion [79,89,107,113,125,137,138,150,177,178,195,212,256,278]. In other words, PV valves do not interfere directly with physiological drainage. This gradient is oriented in the physiological direction during the diastole of the various venous pumps, cardiac pump (CP), thoraco-abdominal pump (TAP), and VMP. It may also be oriented in this direction during the systole of the VMP when deep blood reaches a sufficient speed to aspire blood from PV by the Venturi effect. However, during the systole, the pressure gradient is generally inverted, and flow in tributaries is stopped if the valves are competent. If the valves are incompetent, flow direction is inverted. This backward flow can be the reflux point (RP) of either an open or closed shunt. The diameter of junction and PV depends on the same haemodynamic conditions as previously described for superficial veins. Most of the time, a large-calibre junction or PV is not due to systolic outflow from deep veins, as generally thought, but rather to the combination of DFHSP impairment and excessive CS flow. For example, in a CS such as a saphena that is incompetent from the sapheno-femoral junction to a distal PV of the leg, the large calibre of the RP (junction) and re-entry point (distal PV) depends on the energy of the diastolic flow of the VMP of the calf; an ulcer or hypodermitis may be centred by a large PV at the re-entry point. A dynamic test of VMP shows an inflow during the diastole. This means that the large PV is not responsible for trophic disease, as is commonly believed, even if a dynamic test sometimes shows an outflow during the systole, because usually the outflow is much less than the inflow (compensated outflow). Evidence of this is the complete healing of ulcer and hypodermitis after cross-ligation without ligation of the PV. A PV is pathogenic when its diastolic flow is retrograde during a dynamic test. This demonstrates that PV calibre depends on flow, independent of its direction or pathogenic responsibility. The haemodynamic significance of a PV depends on its function according to the type of shunt. In fact, regardless of its calibre, a PV may be the leak point or the re-entry point of a CS or VOS. Haemodynamic analysis is indispensable to any therapeutic strategy. For example, ligation would be erroneous at the PV (leak point and re-entry point) of an open shunt, at the re-entry point of a VOS, or at the re-entry point of a CS or ODS. In addition, PV are necessary to drainage of the superficial tissues related to their physiological territories, even if they carry a supplementary flow, as in VOS, CS and ODS.

# 7. Haemodynamic Physiopathology of the Cardiac Pump

The heart is the principal pump of the venous system [34]. The venous system supplies the cardiac pump in volume and pressure according to physiological needs due to the heart's active and passive capacities. The cardiac pump increases volume, flow and pressure in the venous system through the action of the left ventricle during the systole, and decreases them through the action of the right ventricle during the diastole. This suffices for the various functions of the venous system in the lying down position because HSP is almost null. On the other hand, it is not sufficient in the motionless standing position, *i.e.*, when HSP is maximal and the VMP is not active. Moreover, the progressive sequestration of blood in the venous system may cause an "intravenous haemorrhage" draining of the cardiac pump (falls of the sentinel). One can deduce that prolonged standing in a motionless position is not physiologically correct. One can also say that the great majority of venous pathologies affect the subject in the standing position and disappear when he or she lies down.

On the other hand, when the right cardiac pump is defective, right ventricle diastolic pressure increases. Thus, TMP in the lower limbs increases with cardiac resistance to the venous flow, causing venous oedemas of cardiac origin.

# 8. Haemodynamic Physiopathology of the Thoraco-Abdominal Pump

The thoraco-abdominal pump (TAP) modulates intrathoracic and intra-abdominal pressure during breathing [34]. This pressure is communicated to the right auricle and the retro-peritoneal veins and transmitted to the veins of the lower limbs. Usually, during inspiration, diaphragm contraction is simultaneous with relaxation of the abdominal muscles, and vice versa during expiration.

The Valsalva manoeuvre (VM) is different from respiratory movements [46,48,241]. It is equivalent to defecation or to holding a heavy weight while standing. It consists of blocking the TAP in the proto-systolic position by simultaneous contraction of diaphragm and muscles of the abdomen. VM reverses the pressure gradient, thereby causing reverse flow in incompetent veins. Valsalva manoeuvre is positive when it reverses the flow in any vein, and negative when it does not. It may involve a reverse flow in a venous segment of a lower limb even if the venous flow proximal to the abdomen is normal thanks to competent valves. The reason is that a pressure wave is transmitted even in the absence of flow motion. For example, a VM may be positive in the safeno-femoral or safeno-popliteal junction even if iliac or femoral valves are competent. Normally, VM stops all flow during contraction, and flow reappears during relaxation. This is important to note, particularly when investigating tributaries of the saphena magna junction. The normal flow of junctional tributaries is anterograde, descending to the junction, but it has to stop during VM contraction and reappear at the following relaxation. It is VM negative. When the tributary is fed by a leak point related to a CS, VM also evolves an anterograde flow, descending to the cross, but it is pathological because it occurs during contraction. It is VM positive. This Valsalva effect explains how constipation and heavy weight handling may interfere with CVI.

Intra-abdominal hyperpression may be chronic, particularly in obese patients, and responsible for venous insufficiency of the lower limbs.

# 9. Haemodynamic Physiopathology of the Valvulo-Muscular Pump

## 9.1. The Valvulo-Muscular Pump (VMP)

The VMP acts by volume and pressure variations of the venous blood. These variations are due to skeletal contraction (systole) and relaxation (diastole) of the muscles that surround the deep veins (N1) of the lower limbs. Venous valves complete the VMP. They determine flow direction. Proximal valves open in systole and close in diastole, which permits systolic blood expulsion and prevents diastolic reflux. Distal valves close in systole and open in diastole, which permits distal blood diastolic aspiration and prevents systolic reflux. Therefore, flow direction of the VMP depends on the valvular competence.

Epifascial and intrafascial veins of the superficial network (N2, N3, N4) are not surrounded by muscle, and therefore do not participate in VMP systo-diastolic action. However, their drainage depends for largely on VMP. The VMP receives systolic flow from the foot when the plantar pump is activated. Most of its flow is aspirated by deep VMP diastole. Much less is aspirated during deep VMP systole by the Venturi effect. The VMP not only helps the venous system to evacuate excessive blood flow brought in by the arteriolo-capillary vasodilation that accompanies muscular effort, but it also dynamically fractionates the hydrostatic column of pressure (DFHSP), thanks to the alternating closing of distal and proximal valves. This fractionation makes possible standing for a long time with a normal TMP in the lower limbs, provided that the muscles are activated.

It is included that DFHSP work will be the more effective as muscular activity will be important, because DFHSP increases as muscular activity increases.

It is also understandable that any degradation of the various elements of the VMP, such as valvular incompetence and/or muscular inactivity (paralysis, ankylosis), may be responsible for a lack of DFHSP and the clinical consequences thereof.

## 9.2. Concept of Shunt and VMP

A shunt is a venous pathway that deviates and carries all or part of a venous flow that is not intended to drain. These shunts are known as vicarious and open (VOS) when they compensate for an obstacle. Since VOS are activated by cardiac and thoraco-abdominal pumps, they are permanently activated. VOS are overloaded by extra flow when the systole of the VMP is activated. In contrast, closed shunts (CS) are not permanently activated. They cause venous blood recirculation in closed loop only when the VMP diastole back-aspirates blood from the leak point to the re-entry point. In short, VOS is a spontaneous and permanent healing by-pass of the venous network, and CS is a temporary spontaneous pathogenic by-pass activated only when the subject is walking.

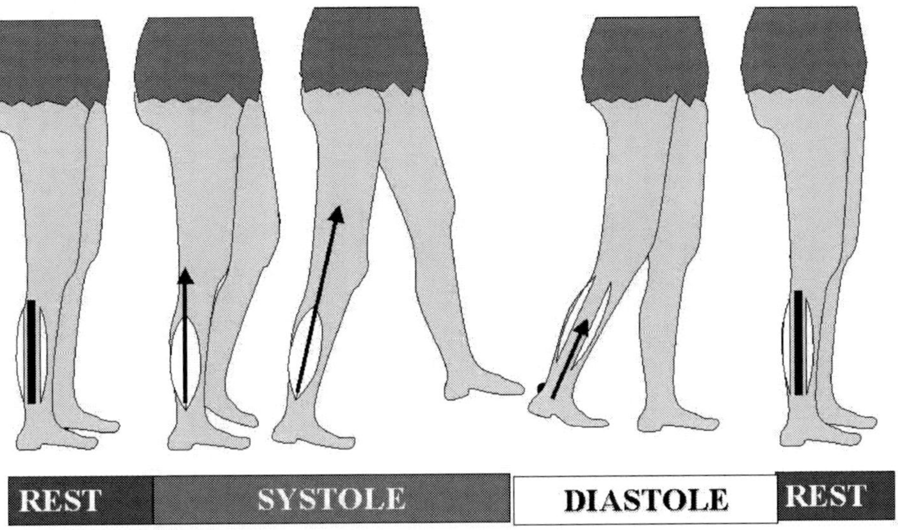


Figure 4.12 A) Schematic normal valvulo-muscular (VMP) behaviour when walking. Rest: relaxed VMP pump, veins dilated, slow cardiopete flow due to heart pump, thoraco-abdominal pump and residual pressure. Systole: cardipete VMP ejection. Diastole: cardipete VMP admission.

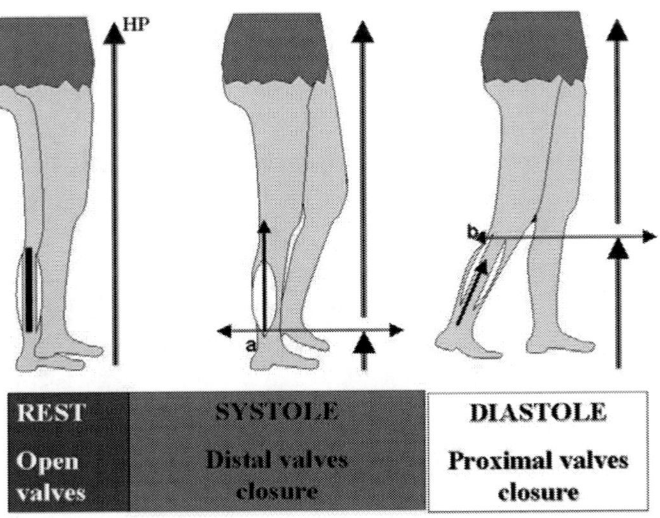


Figure 4.12 B) Schematic normal Dynamic Fractionation of the Hydrostatic Pressure by the valvulo-muscular pump (VMP) when walking. Rest :Maximal Hydrostatic pressure (HP) ,relaxed VMP pump , veins dilated, opened valves, slow cardiopete flow due to heart pump, thoraco-abdominal pump and residual l pressure. Systole: Fractionation of HP at the distal valves level (a) ,cardipete VMP ejection. distal valves closure and proximal valves opening Diastole: Fractionation of HP at the proximal valves level (b), cardipete VMP admission.

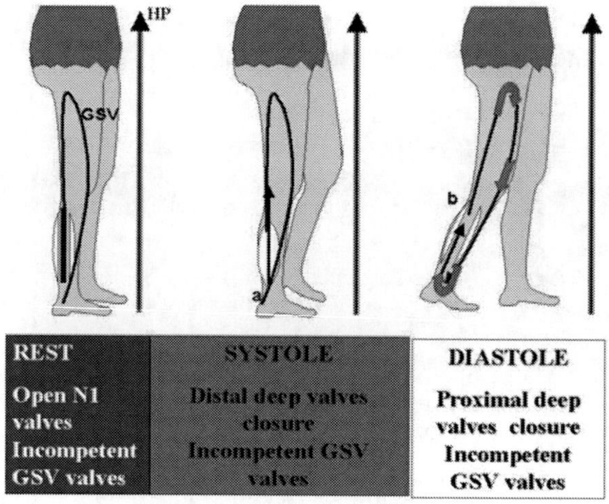


Figure 4.12 C) Schematic impaired Dynamic Fractionation of the Hydrostatic Pressure by the valvulo-muscular pump (VMP) when walking in case of closed shunt (CS) by incompetent great saphenous vein (GSV) and competent deep veins (N1). Rest :Maximal Hydrostatic pressure (HP) like normal ,relaxed VMP pump , veins dilated, opened valves, slow cardiopete flow due to heart pump, thoraco-abdominal pump and residual l pressure. Systole and diastole : despite a correct closure of distal valves (a) and proximal valves (b) ,cardipete VMP ejection and admission at N1, the HP fractionation fails because the deep column is shunted by an incompetent GSV.

## 9.3. DFHSP and the VMP (Figure 4.12)

The VMP is essential to the DFHSP that ensures a low TMP in the standing position. This effect is proportional to VMP action [19,23,78,135,183]. When the body is in the standing position and "totally motionless," VMP is at rest and HSP is not fractionated. This condition is only theoretical (except in artificial situations, as the body hanged by the neck or in the Tilt test manoeuvre) because in practice, even in a stiff standing position, muscles move to maintain the equilibrium and a low, but not null, DFHSP. The DFHSP effect increases with increasing movement, as walking and than running. Conversely, DFHSP is impaired proportionally to muscular inactivity (paralysis, ankylosis) and/or valvular incompetence that alters VMP efficiency.

## 9.4. CVI, Varices, Posture, and the VMP

HSP at the ankle is lower in the sitting position than in the standing position because the height of the liquid column is less. Thus, the incidence of HSP should be less when sitting. In reality, sitting for a long period is as bad for drainage as standing immobile for the following reasons: standing in an immobile position is usually not as prolonged as sitting, and DFHSP is active, though weak, during standing, while it is null while sitting. On the other hand, the sitting position does not increase varices in the case of CS, thanks to VMP inactivity.

### 9.5. Varices and the VMP

When active, the VMP adds flow and pressure to the venous network, so it overloads not only normal veins, but also venous pathways of shunts (VOS, ODS, and CS) that become varicose with time.

The relationship between varicose veins and the VMP in the presence of CS is spectacularly demonstrated in patients in whom varicosity disappears in a limb when affected by paralysis. Venous incompetence without CS may cause severe drainage disorders in the absence of varices. In other conditions, such as dilated saphenous vein, in which the valves are necessarily incompetent, no diastolic back flow will be detected upon Doppler testing if the VMP is totally impaired because VMP efficacy is necessary to activate CS. The more efficient the VMP is, the more reverse diastolic flow will occur.

### 9.6. Claudication (Limping), Restrictive Syndrome, Capacitive Syndrome, and the VMP

In the case of a severe occlusion of the proximal veins of the lower limbs, patients may complain about limping because of calf pain. This is due to an excess of pressure, the energy of which cannot be consumed because of flow resistance. This pressure has two components: residual pressure (RP), which is increased by microvascular dilation due to muscular stress reflex, and pressure delivered by the VMP. In cases of severe incompetence without any significant occlusion, patients may not bear compression (bandage or stockings) well because calf tissues are squeezed between the excessive venous pressure (which is not corrected in the absence of DFHSP) and the external compression.

## 10. Haemodynamic Physiopathology of the Plantar Pump

The plantar pump consists of the venous volume of the sole modulated when walking by compression against the ground (systole) then relaxation (diastole). It drains superficial tissues and partially the deep tissues because perforating veins of the foot are constitutionally incompetent and allow the passage of deep blood into the superficial network. It represents the most important part of the flow carried by saphenas throughout walking periods. Its physiological importance seems to be limited to the drainage of the foot [18].

## 11. Haemodynamic Physiopathology of Venous Calibre and Varices (Figure 4.13, Figure 4.14)

Varices are defined as tortuous and dilated veins. They are not the cause of CVI, as is still believed by most phlebologists, but rather the consequence of flow and pressure perturbations in the venous system [69,94,95,268]. In short, they are a symptom, not the cause, of venous insufficiency. They involve four haemodynamic causes. The first is tortuous dilation due to vicariousness of one or more occluded veins, such as the occlusion of deep and/or superficial veins in so-called vicarious open shunts (VOS). The second cause is varicose veins related to a diverted open shunt (DOS). The third is hyperflow induced by arterio-venous fistula. The fourth and most frequent cause are varices of superficial veins induced by closed-shunt hyperflow.

Dilation depends on flow and pressure. The more compliant the vein, the greater the dilation will be. Venous dilation regresses totally or partially when the responsible flow and pressure are reduced.

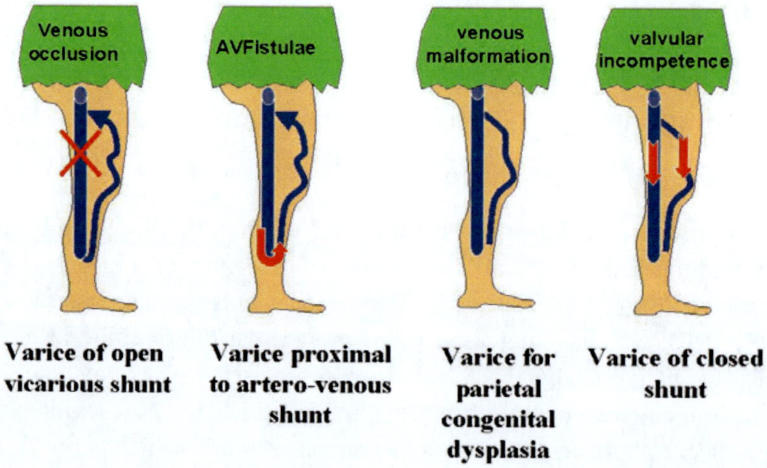


Figure 4.13. Varicosities: tortuous, visible and dilate vein. It is not the disease but the symptom of various causes. Here, four similar varices for 4 different etiologies i.e four different diagnosis and therapy.

### 11.1. Process of Venous Dilation

There are two processes of vascular dilation. The first depends on TMP and compliance. The second is related to the change from laminar to turbulent flow.

### 11.2. Dilation, Varices, TMP and Compliance (Figure 4.15)

The calibre of veins depends on the TMP value and on the active or passive resistance of the walls to the parietal tension (T). T = TMP . r, where r is the radius of the vessel (Laplace law). The parietal factors that determine the distensibility or compliance are made of different components, either passive such as elastin and collagen, or regulated such as smooth muscular cells. The muscular fibres of the media are subjected to neuro-humoral control, ensuring changes in tone, vasoconstriction or vasodilation according to the body's requirements for thermoregulation and cardiac haemodynamics.

Compliance is not constant, but varies with the degree of extension. Compliance (C) is the ratio of volume and pressure [1,10,12,34,73-75,187,261,276,277]. This function is described in deep in the chapter 3.

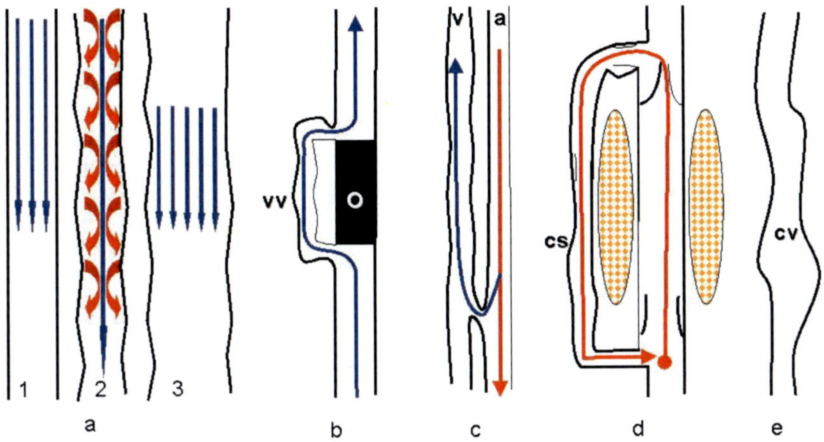


Figure 4.14. Haemodynamic physiopathology of the varices. a: high velocity changes laminar flow into turbulent flow according to Reynolds law .The resulting turbulences hit the wall of the vessel and so enlarges it. 1: laminar flow 2: when the flow velocity increases turbulences appear. Turbulences hit the walls and increase the diameter of the vessel. 3: Vessel enlargement does not reduce the flow volume but decreases the flow velocity until low values so that the flow comes back to laminar and the enlargement stops. b: in case of obstacle o, high velocity in vicarious vein vv causes varices. c: high velocity and high pressure in arterio-venous av fistulae causes varices. d: high velocity in closed shunts cs when walking causes varices. e: congenital varicose veins cv ( venous malformation) is not due to haemodynamic but structural cause.

## 11.3. Dilation, Varicose Veins, and Turbulence (Figure 1.5)

Independent of TMP, i.e. of the pressure, circulatory turbulence itself, typical of venous reflux, may cause tortuous dilation. According to Reynolds' law, the circulatory mode of viscous liquids, such as blood, changes from laminar to turbulent when the flow exceeds a critical velocity. As long as the flow is adapted to the calibre of the vein, velocity is less than critical. If the flow increases for any reason and surpasses the critical velocity, it becomes turbulent. Turbulence disperses part of the blood's kinetic energy against the vessel wall. With time, the stressed wall loses its viscoelastic resistance, widens, lengthens and becomes tortuous (varicose veins). The degree of dilation is proportional to increased velocity and turbulence. When the varice reaches such a calibre that flow velocity drops below critical despite the unchanged high flow, the circulatory mode becomes laminar again and the calibre is stabilized as long as high flow remains the same. This theoretical process is illustrated by clinical findings and explains why varicosity can remain stable for many years after a period of progression.

### 11.4. Dilation, Varicose Veins, Tissue Pressure, and Fascias

Dilation of the deep and superficial veins depends on TMP, circulatory mode and compliance, but it can be limited by the surrounding tissues that contribute to extra-vascular pressure. Dilation of the deep veins (N1 network) is limited by the muscular masses contained in a closed aponeurotic bag. The saphenous trunk and Giacomini's vein are protected from excessive dilations because they are located in a fascial compartment, composed by the deep and the superficial fascia. The veins located above the muscular fascia (N3 and N4 networks) dilate more easily because they are contained by low extra-vascular pressure (subcutaneous tissues, skin and the atmospheric pressure).

## 12. Venous Physiopathology and Cardiac Haemodynamics

The venous system is able to respond to the variable flow volume needed for cardiac preload while venous pressure remains steady thanks to its blood volume (four times greater than arterial), great compliance, and a remarkable viscoelasticity. A prolonged motionless standing position may cause accumulation of excessive blood volume in the venous sector (intravenous haemorrhage), such that cardiac preload is impaired and fainting with vagal reaction may be induced. This is favoured by excessive volume in the venous sector (varices) and potentiated by neuro-vegetative dystonia. Fainting occurs frequently during phlebologic examinations in which the patient remains standing and motionless for a long time. Prevention consists of blood volume reduction, either by the pumping action of the VMP or by leg compression.

## 13. Haemodynamic Physiopathology and Thermoregulation

The venous system interferes with the thermoregulatory function by controlling the exchange of calories between the superficial venous blood and the environment. In order to reduce the core temperature, superficial veins dilate and superficial venous flow increases due to the reduction of micro-circulatory resistance. A reverse process is activated to increase core temperature. This regulation may induce negative side effects.

Actually, when microcirculatory resistance (MCR) decreases, TMP in the superficial venous system increases with the flow and the residual pressure. For this reason, thermoregulation can worsen an already diagnosed venous insufficiency. Some typical clinical examples can be seen in the haemodynamic venous conditions of professional cooks exposed to high temperatures in prolonged motionless standing posture and aggravation of CVI symptoms in summer.

Chapter 5

# SHUNT'S CLASSIFICATION

*Claude Franceschi*
Saint Joseph and Pitié-Salpétrière Hospitals, Paris, France.

## 1. SUMING UP THE CONCEPTS EXPRESSED SO FAR

We have seen, as stated in chapter 3 and 4, that there is a hierarchical order of emptying in the venous networks, based on physical laws and levels of kinetic energy; in addiction, in the previous chapters, we illustrated the mechanisms leading to the DFHSP, which is at the end the most important factor in determining the lower limb venous drainage.

Venous shunts and primary CVD generally speaking involve abnormal flows that, with their different pathway, are just the consequences of an impairment of the DFHSP and of venous compartments order of emptying.

Furthermore, we have classified the venous networks into five categories, N1 to N5, according to their anatomo-functional significance. Network N1 represents deep veins located in the AC1 compartment. Network N2 represents sub- and intra-fascial superficial veins located in the AC2 compartment, i.e., saphenous trunks and Giacomini's vein. Network N3 represents supra-fascial superficial veins located in the AC3 compartment, i.e., saphenous and extra-saphenous tributaries. Network N4 represents superficial veins located in the AC3 compartment that link different regions of the saphenous network. N4 Longitudinal (N4L) vertically links two regions of the same saphenous network, such as GSV or SSV. N4 transversal (N4T) transversally links the GSV network to SSV. N5 represents the microcirculatory venous network.

Normally, superficial venous blood flows from superficial into deeper veins. Thus, superficial venous blood leaves the micro-circulation N5, flows into the superficial network N3, then into N2 and finally N1, according to the direction of the valves as well as to the levels of the energy gradient produced by muscular contraction; sometimes, directly from N3 into N1.The majority of shunts inverts this normal direction, that is, blood flows from deeper to more superficial veins.

We have highlighted in chapter 4 as venous shunts are those veins that deviate venous blood from its normal pathway, more often during muscular relaxation. VS have in common the fact that they carry two different flows: physiologic draining flow and abnormal flow, or shunt flow (SF). They differ not only in blood origin abnormal venous pathway, and destination of the deviated flow, but also in their systolic or diastolic activation by the valvulo-muscular pump (VMP).

Shunting veins may be any deep and/or superficial vein. A shunt may be made of a venous segment and/or a succession of different segments of different veins. The shunting flow direction may be partially or totally normal (antegrade) or reverse (retrograde). The content of shunting flow may be re-circulating blood or not.

Moreover we have identified four main types of shunt: VOS, CS, ODS and MS.

ODS and CS can be classified according to the venous segments that usually constitute the venous shunting pathways, in order to standardize the anatomical-functional venous cartographies, mappings and consequent therapeutic strategies.

It is possible to consider a first operative classification and a more recent one, coming from an evolution of the same previous one.

For educational purposes we suggest to approach the first following classification, leaving the new shunt description to the reader interested in approaching the deepest aspects of this.

### 1.1. First Classification

The vast majority (90%) of 'private circulations' or veno-venous shunts that involve the saphenous trunks [39,77-80] are included in one of the following types [105]:

a) Type 1 Shunts (constituting about 30% of varicosity networks): N1 > N2 reflux; the superficial segment of the 'private circulation', from reflux point to reentry, is represented exclusively by the incompetent saphenous trunk. The reentry perforator, detectable on Doppler, is located on this saphenous trunk. Therefore, the 'private circulation' follows a N1 > N2 > N1 route.

The principal variants of type 1 shunts (SH 1) may be represented as SH 1 + 1 and SH 1 + N3 shunts. In Figure 5.1, first diagram, we find a superimposed SH 1; in the second a N3 collateral is draining part of the refluxing blood while the saphenous perforator is emptying only a part. The characteristic feature is the reduction in saphenous diameter (detectable on sonogram) below the origin of N3. If this did not occur, then we would have a simple SH 1 with emergence of a collateral at the level of the reentry.

b) Type 3 Shunts (constituting about 60% of varicosity networks): N1 > N2 reflux; the superficial segment of the 'private circulation', from reflux point to reentry, is not represented exclusively by the incompetent saphenous trunk. Instead, part of the 'private circulation' is constituted by a N2 (N3 or N4T or N4L) collateral located distally from the origin where the saphenous vein has at least one competent segment. The intervening saphenous segment between the reflux point and the origin of the collateral should not have any reentry perforator that is detectable on Doppler. Different hemodynamic models of type 3 'private circulation' are possible.

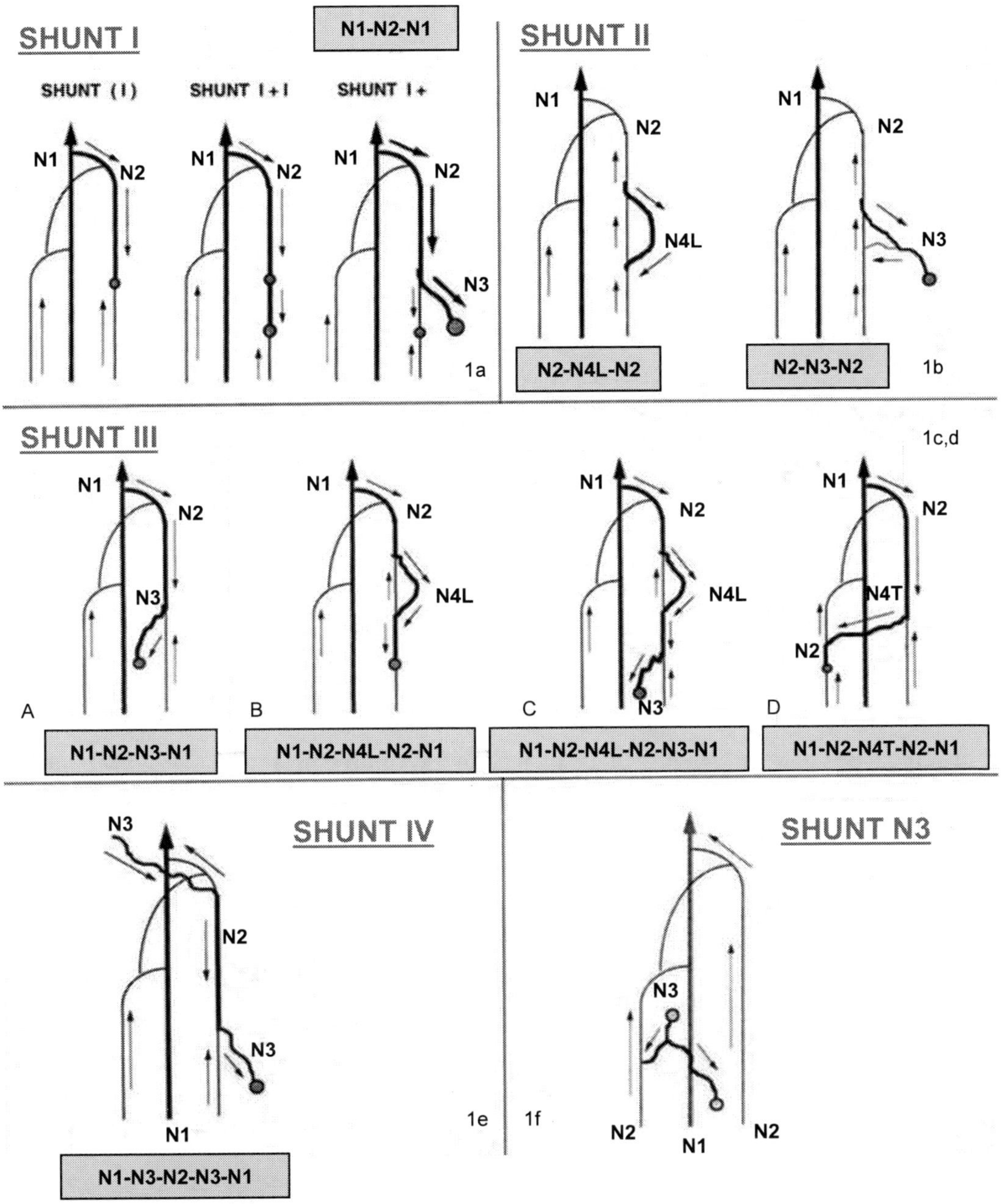


Figure 5.1. a-b-c-d-e-f. Types of 'private circulation' or veno-venous shunts; 1a: type 1 shunt with reentry on the saphenous trunk, and variations; 1b: type 2 shunt without reflux from the deep circulation, with compartmental regurgitation N2>N4>N2 or N2>N3>N2; 1c-d: type 3 shunt with reentry located on an extrasaphenous perforator, and variations; 1e: type 4 shunt with reflux from the pelvic circulation; 1 f: N3 shunt with reflux from an incompetent perforator and reentry on an extrasaphenous perforator. Reflux from an incompetent perforator does not necessarily give rise to a 'private circulation'.

As Figure 5.1c, Example A shows, refluxing blood starts from the N3 collateral and reenters through a perforator located on the collateral (N1 > N2 > N3 > N1).

In Example B, blood emerges from a N4L collateral, flows back again into the saphenous vein and reenters through a perforator located on the saphenous (N1 > N2 > N4L > N2 > N1).

In Example C the reflux abandons the saphenous for a N4L route before reentering and discharging the reflux along a N3 branch (N1 > N2 > N4L > N2 > N3 > N1).

In Example D the refluxing blood follows a route from a N4T collateral to another saphenous trunk before reentering through a perforator from this trunk (N1 > N2 > N4T > a different N2 > N1).

In the remaining cases (10%) the 'private circulations' that involve the saphenous trunks are represented by:

c) Type 2 Shunt: reflux N2 > N4L or N2 > N3, with the 'private circulation' entirely accounted for by the superficial network. In these cases, reflux from the deep circulation is absent. There is however a 'private circulation': N2 > N4L > N2 or N2 > N3 > N2 (Figure 5.1b).

d) Type 4 Shunt: reflux N1 > N3, or a reflux from the deep circulation along a pelvic shunt to empty into the saphenous vein. A basic prerequisite is that at least the terminal valve of the saphenofemoral junction be competent.

Lastly, there are 'private circulations' that involve solely the saphenous collaterals:

e) "N3" Shunt: reflux N1 > N3, or directly from an incompetent perforator, with reentry through a perforator located on the collateral (P/N3). The saphenous trunks are not affected by the 'private circulation'.

In some types of veno-venous shunt, such as overlapping type 1 shunts or type 3 shunts, in addition to the primary 'private circulation' supplied by the primary reflux point, there are also secondary 'private circulations' supplied by secondary reflux points, which are of significant hemodynamic importance. In type 3 shunts the secondary 'private circulation' is initiated by the N2 > N4L reflux, i.e., the reflux at the origin of the collateral. Of course, if the reflux is a N2 > N3 type, there is no secondary 'private circulation' since reentry into the saphenous is absent. In superimposed type 1 shunts it is the incompetent perforators that start the secondary 'private circulation'.

### 1.2. Revised Classification

The European CHIVA study group proposed in 2002 a more detailed and revised classification [179]. This offers the possibility to recognize the wide majority of pattern that can be easily recognized under duplex investigation. However, most of the CHIVA group in Europe still continue to adopt the above described classification for superficial venous insufficiency.

## 2. Deep Shunts

Deep shunts are CS or VOS but never ODS.

# 3. Superficial Shunts

Superficial shunts are superficial shunting veins that deviate only superficial venous flows when ODS is activated. They can deviate deep or superficial flows if VOS or CS.

## 3.1. Shunt 0:

Shunt 0 is an ODS or a VOS where, contrary to shunt 2 (N2-N3-N1), the drainage direction is normal (N3-N2-N1), even if flow in the N2 segment is retrograde. For example, when only the sapheno-femoral junction valve is competent and distal valves are incompetent, tributaries of the arch are drained during the diastole in a distal perforator of the saphenous trunk through a retrograde flow, by ODS effect. The same drainage direction is carried out not only in diastole, but permanently through the distal perforator by VOS effect after the sapheno-femoral junction is disconnected in shunt 1.

The retrograde flow in N2 is fed by antegrade N3 draining tributaries with distal reentry R into N1 activated by the valvulo-muscular pump diastole without re-circulation. The haemodynamic condition are very good even if not properly normal and so doesn't any therapy. In the figure above, N2 is the great saphenous upper trunk and arch is incompetent except in the terminal sapheno-femoral junction valve that is competent. The same type 0 can be described when any superficial draining flow is oriented from N2 to N1 or N3 to N1 or N3-N2-N1 without any flow oriented N1-N2.

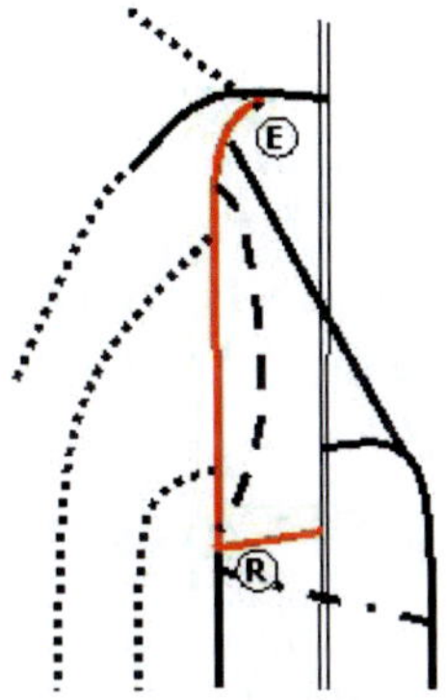


**Shunt 0**

DOS: N3-N2-N1

Legend- CS: Closed shunts. E: Escape points. R: reentry points. D: Disconnection point. V: Devalvulation point.

Resuming, shunt 0 is a reflux in the GSV trunk with re-entry and no re-circulation because there is no EP from N1. It is a VOS or an ODS N3-N2-N1.The more frequent cases of observation are:

1. Reflux in GSV with competent terminal valve, and thus without change of compartment. The reverse flow detectable in the GSV is due to a gravitational gradient of the column ending in a RPV located distally in the saphenous trunk.
2. Reflux in the GSV after SFJ disconnection. Again, the reverse flow is a draining and asymptomatic flow without change of compartment. This is the normal outcome following CHIVA 1 procedure.

Shunt 0 can be often detected at duplex examination, in normal and/or asymptomatic subjects. This pattern may usually be detected at the end of a busy day in standing or sitting position in individuals like surgeons, hairdresser, waiter, etc…during summer.

Pathophysiologic explanation should include increased volume in the GSV with opening of distal perforators located on the trunk in order to favour inward flow to the deep veins. This creates a segmental retrograde flow for a recruitment effect.

Thus, Shunt 0 can be considered a physiologic pattern due to functional reasons of drainage.

It is noteworthy that Shunt 0 is the desirable outcome of the so-called CHIVA 1 surgical procedure.

## 3.2. Shunt 1:

Shunt 1 is a saphenous CS made of N1-N2-N1 succession.

The retrograde flow in N2 is fed by reflux from N1 through E and antegrade N3 draining tributaries with distal reentry into N1 activated by the valvulo-muscular pump diastole with re-circulation. CHIVA disconnects E, which results as Shunt 0. E is the sapheno-femoral junction in **shunt 1a**, sapheno-popliteal junction in **shunt 1b**, any perorating vein connected with N2 in **shunt 1c**.

Therefore shunt 1 is a reflux in an incompetent segment of the GSV trunk with a distal re-entry perforator connected to the trunk, similar to shunt 0 but with re-circulation caused by a proximal EP connected with N1, either at the SFJ or at any incompetent perforator connected with the trunk.

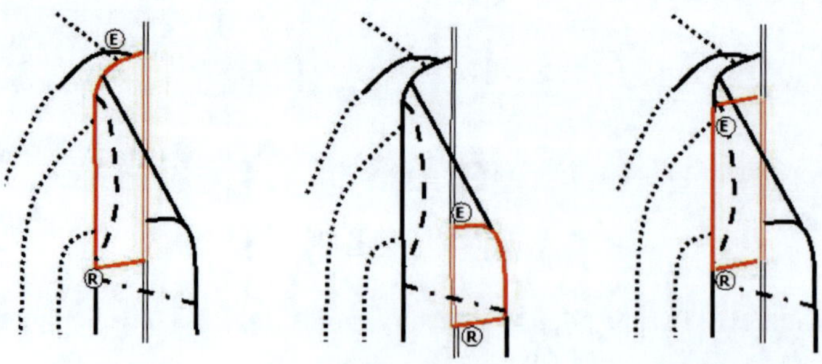


**Shunt 1a** CS: N1-N2-N1 **Shunt 1b** CS: N1-N2-N1 **Shunt 1c** CS: N1-N2-N1

## 3.3. Shunt 2:

Shunt 2 is a shunt made of N2-N3-N1 or N2-N4T-N2-N1 or N2-N4L-N2-N1 succession. The saphenous trunk proximal to the EP can be incompetent except at the SFJ.

Shunt 2 are derivated open shunts DOS except shunt 2C that is a CS. **Shunt 2a** is any N3 incompetent tributary fed by N2 flow (E is the N3-N2 confluence) activated by VMP diastole through R connected with N1. **Shunt 2b** is an incompetent N4T tributary that connects the GSV trunk with the SSV trunk. **Shunt 2C** is an incompetent N4L tributary. **Shunt 2d** is an incompetent N2 segment that extend to N3 and then to extra troncular R. CHIVA procedure consists in disconnection at E except in shunt 2d where disconnection is done at N2-N3 junction (D).

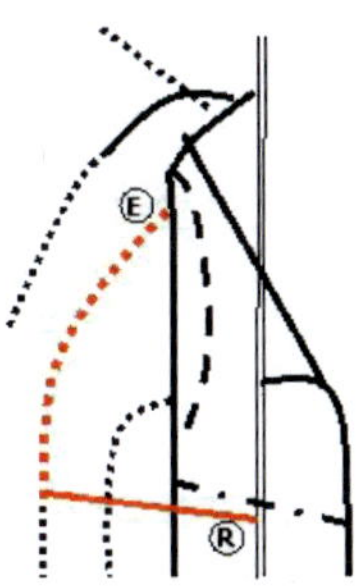


**Shunt 2a**
DOS: N2-N3-N1

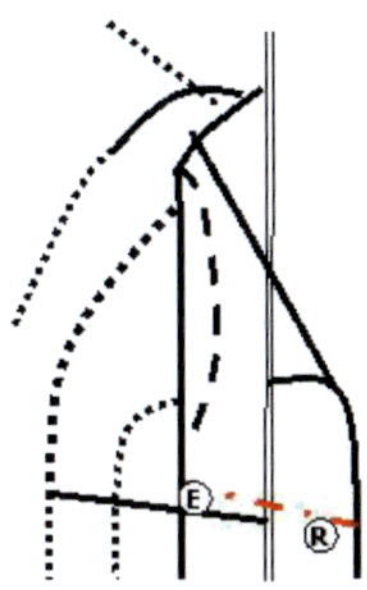


**Shunt 2b**
DOS: N2-N4T-N1

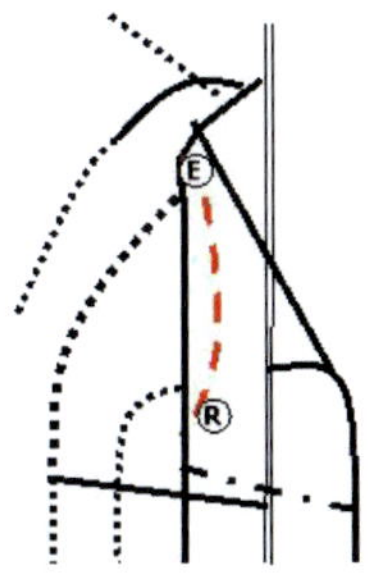


**Shunt 2c**
CS: N2-N4L-N2

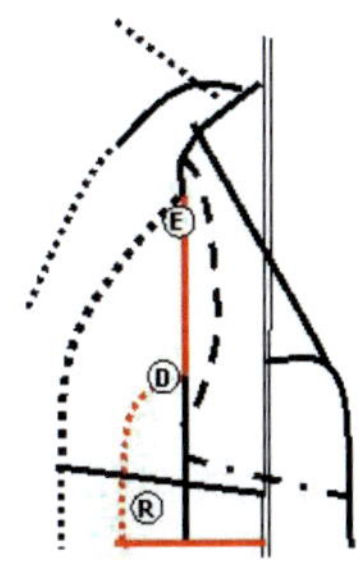


**Shunt 2d**
DOS: incomp N2-N3-N1

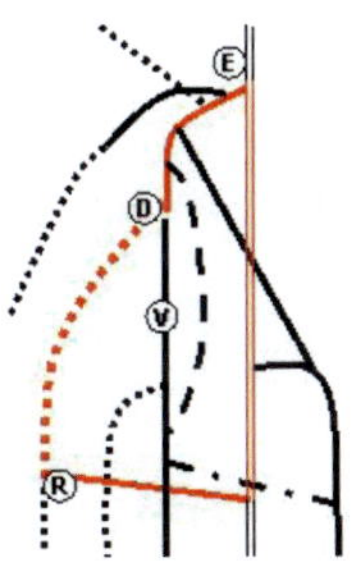


**Shunt 3a**
CS: N1-N2-N3-N1

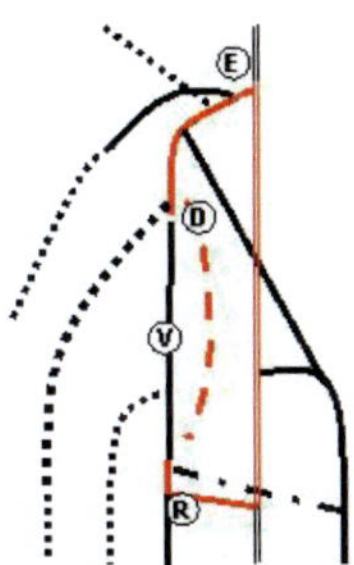


**Shunt 3b**
CS: N1-N2-N4L-N2-N1

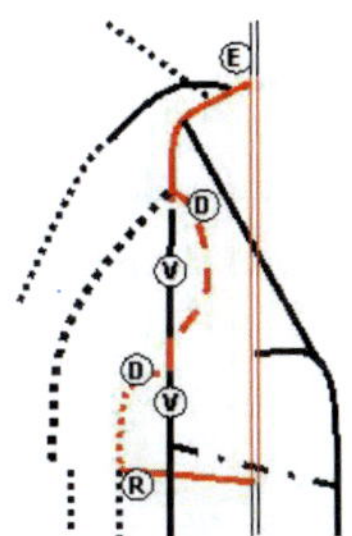


**Shunt 3c**
CS: N1-N2-N4L-N2-N3-N1

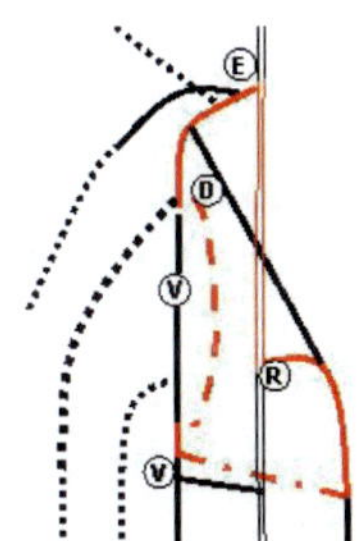


**Shunt 3d**
CS: N1-N2-N4L-N4T-N2-N1

## 3.4. Shunt 3:

Shunt 3 is a saphenous CS made of N1-N2-N3-N1 or N1-N2-N4L-N1 or N1-N2-N4L-N2-N3-N1succession.

Like shunt 1, it is CS except that its shunting veins are made not only of a GS trunk segment, but also of tributaries N3 and/or N4, and a re-entry perforator can be connected with N3.

The retrograde flow in N2 is fed by reflux from N1 through E and antegrade N3 draining tributaries then connected with incompetent distal reentry into N1 activated by the valvulo-muscular pump VMP diastole with re-circulation.

## 3.5. Shunt 4:

Shunt 4 is a CS made of N1-N3-N2-N1 succession, where N3 is fed by an EP connected with N1, usually pelvic, and feeds N1 through N2.

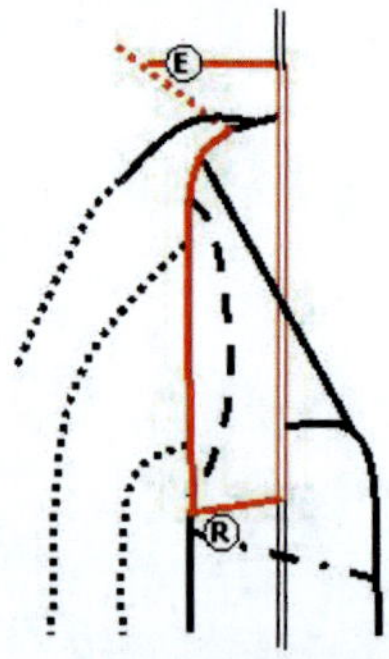


**Shunt 4**

CS:N1,N3,N2,N1

## 3.6. Shunt 5:

Shunt 5 is a CS made of N1-N3-N2-N3-N1 succession, thus similar to a CS except that N2 is prolonged by another N3 before re-entering N1.

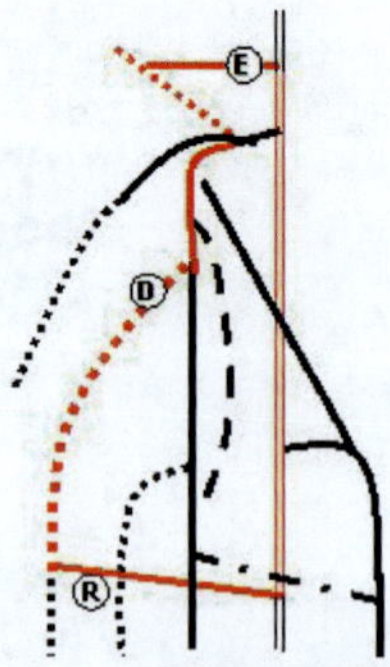


**Shunt 5**

CS: N1-N3-N2-N3-N1

## 3.7. Shunt 6:

Shunt 6 is a CS made of N1-N3 -N1 succession. Shunt 6 EPs may come out at any perforator location. They occur mostly in venous malformations and in varicose recurrences, particularly after stripping.

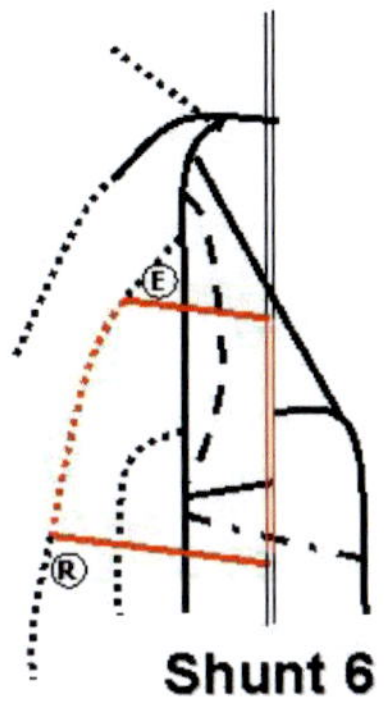


**Shunt 6**

CS: N1-N3-N1

## 3.8. Composite Shunts:

Composite shunts are made of different connected shunts; for example, Shunt 1 + 2 and so on.

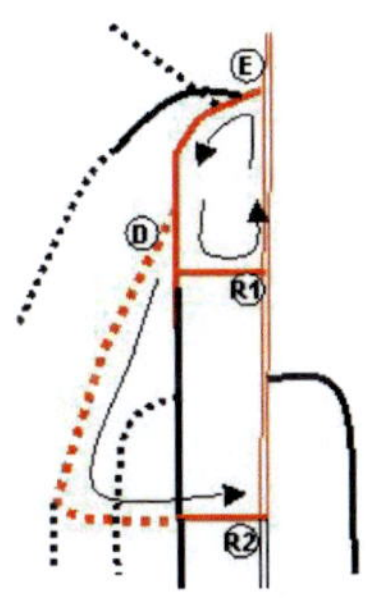


**Shunt 1+2**

Common E
2 different R

## 3.9. Mixed Shunts:

Mixed shunts (MS) are VOS and CS that share the same escape point (EP) and part of their shunting veins. Their re-entry points are located differently, that of CS being distal to the EP, and that of VOS being proximal. An example is when an iliac venous occlusion is associated with a homolateral great saphenous incompetence. An EP at the saphenous-femoral junction (SFJ) acts as a VOS in systole, draining femoral flow towards the opposite femoral vein (re-entry point) through right and left arch tributaries (spontaneous Palma). The same EP acts as a CS in diastole, spilling femoral flow into distal deep veins through retrograde saphenous flow and perforator re-entry. This is also the case in hemodynamic block at a superficial femoral vein. Popliteal flow may escape into the small saphena arch, then into Giacomini's vein, and re-enter in the deep network through the SFJ in systole. Popliteal flow also escapes in diastole when great saphena incompetence distal to the Giacomini-great saphena junction allows retrograde flow until a distal re-entry.

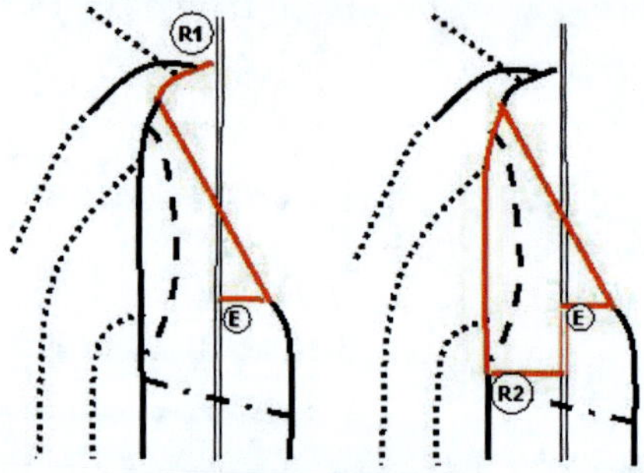


**Mixed Shunt**

VOS+CS

*Chapter 6*

# PELVIC SHUNTS

***Claude Franceschi***
Saint Joseph and Pitié-Salpétrière Hospitals, Paris, France.

## 1. PELVIC ESCAPE POINTS

Pelvic escape points (PEP) represent an important source of varicose veins [161]. They are defined according to their location and the tributaries of the hypogastric veins that feed them. Superior and inferior gluteal veins feed the superior and inferior gluteal points (SGP and IGP) at the buttocks; the obturator vein feeds the obturatory point (OP) at the groin; the round ligament vein feeds the I point (IP) at the superficial inguinal orifice; and the internal pudendal vein feeds the P point (PP) at the perforator of perineal location. Pelvic veins on one side of the body communicate, vertically and horizontally, with the corresponding veins on the opposite side through numerous plexuses. That is why a closure of one or more pelvic veins cannot completely correct the refluxes at PEPs. In the same way, PEPs are connected to any vein at the same side and at the opposite side. Consequently, any varice of the lower limbs can be due to any escape point, at the same or the opposite side.

### 1.1. I Point (IP) and P Point (PP)

They come out much more specifically in women during and after pregnancy. The reasons are the excesses of venous pressure due to fistulae effect of the placenta, pelvic vein compression by the voluminous uterus, and the hormonal status that modifies venous compliance. Usually, they are associated with intra-pelvic varicose veins, such as varicocele of broad ligaments. This association is not necessarily one of cause and effect. On the one hand, pelvic varicose veins after pregnancy are virtually constant, but varices of the lower limbs are not. On the other hand, retrograde phlebography in pelvic varicese does not show IP or PP constantly, and the embolization of pelvic varices does not stop the escapes through

IP and PP [161]. These points are not precisely identified by phlebography but rather by duplex-scan [106].

## 1.2. I Point (IP)

IP escape in women consists of the re-opening of the embryological duct of Nuck during pregnancy. This duct re-opening links the incompetent vein of the round ligament of the uterus (equivalent to sinus pampiniformis in males) with the tributaries of the saphenous arch and leads to closed shunts 4 and 5. As several anastomoses connect in particular the external pudendal vein not only with ipsilateral tributaries of the great saphenous arch, but also with controlateral tributaries, varices of the right limb can be due to left I point and vice versa. IP can also feed vulvar varices through connections with labial veins, which are tributaries of the perineal vein (Figure 6.2a,b). IP is located about 2cm above the arch of the great saphenous vein, medially to the the epigastric vein (Figure 6.1). The diagnosis is not constantly reliable with phlebography. Color Doppler in the standing position shows a characteristic backflow during VM. In males, reflux through the IP corresponds to varicocele outflow.

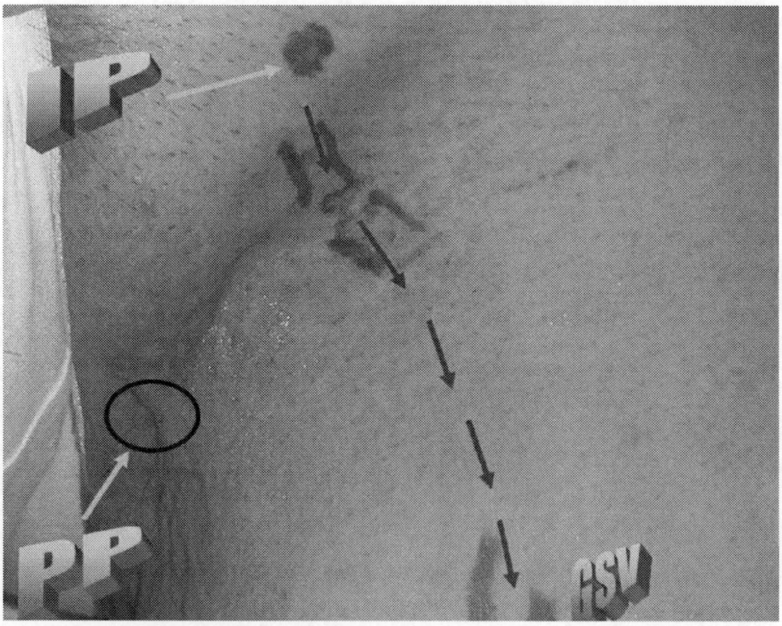


Figure 6.1. IP and PP pre-operative mapping.

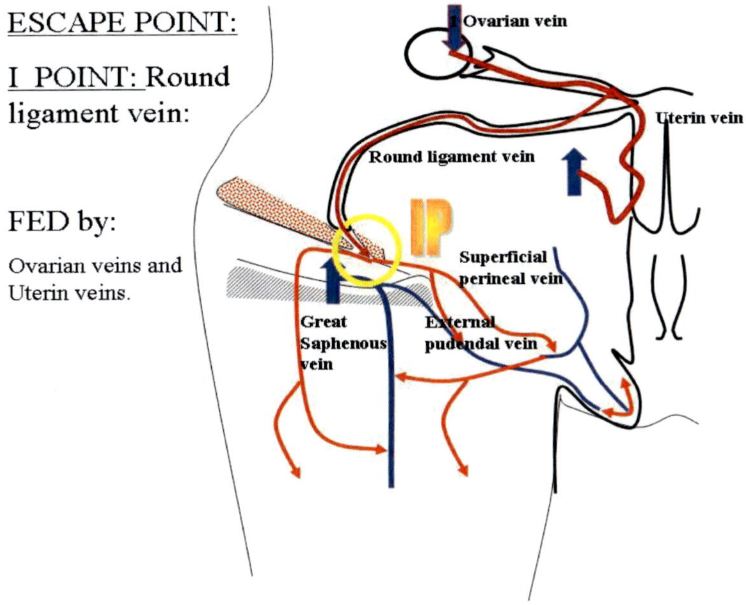


Figure 6.2a. Veins Anastomosis leading to IP.

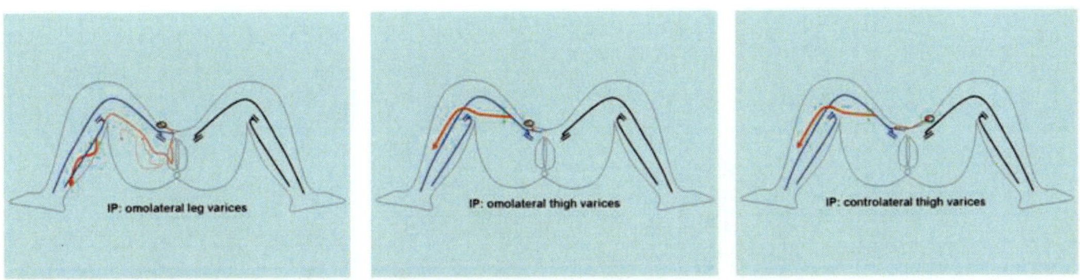


Figure 6.2b. Varices of the limb fed by pelvic shunts linked to IP.

## 1.3. P Point (PP)

PP escape in the perineal vein of women receives labial veins than perforates the superficial perineal fascia at a P point that is located at the posterior edge of the transversal muscle of the perineum. PP skin projection is at the junction of the posterior fourth and the anterior fourth of the external edge of the labia major. PP can feed vulval varices, perineal varices, and closed shunts 4 and 5. Due to transversal anastomosis, it can also feed the same varices on the opposite side (Figure 6.3 a,b). As for IP, PP is not always evident in retrograde pelvic phlebography, but can be diagnosed reliably by duplex-scan, which shows reflux at PP during VM [106]. The standing position is not easy for duplex-scan of PP. The best position is gynecologic. The investigation must be superficial and not intra-vaginal. A superficial probe, preferably equipped with a high resolution probe (10 Mhz or more), or with a water interface filing a surgical glove is simply put on the skin of the perineum.

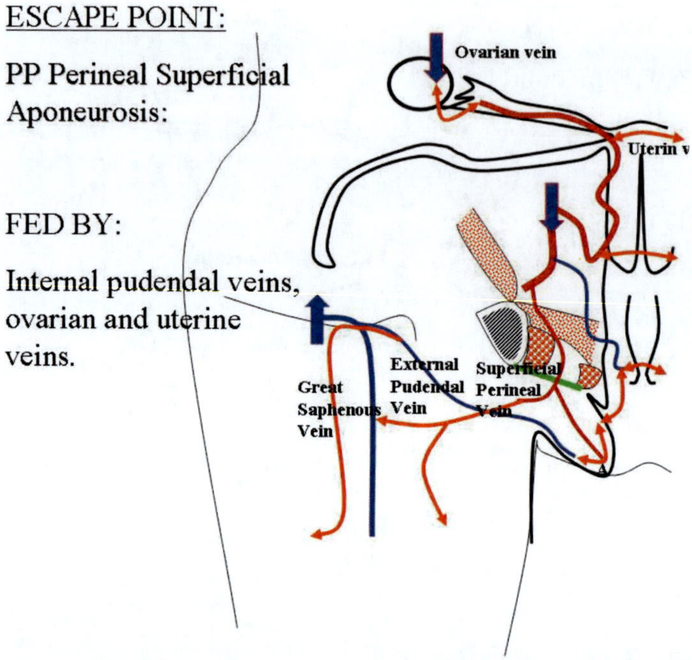


Figure 6.3a. Veins Anastomosis leading to PP.

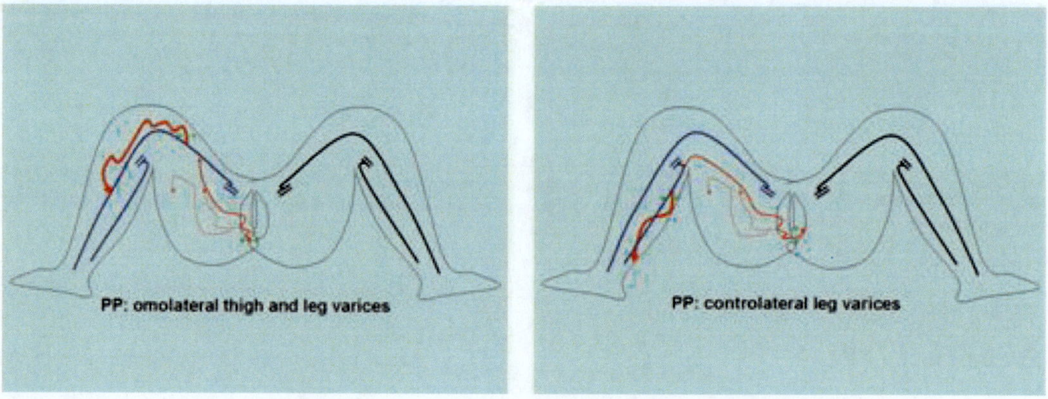


Figure 6.3b. Varices of the limb fed by pelvic shunts linked to PP.

## 1.4. Obturator Escape Point

The oburator vein (OV) emerges in the thigh through the obturator orifice and usually connects with the common femoral vein. Thus, in the majority of cases, a possible reflux is absorbed by a competent deep network, with neither varices nor clinical symptoms in the limb. Sometimes, however, the OV connects with the arch of the great saphena, in which case reflux in OV can involve closed shunts 4 or 5.

## 1.5. Superior Gluteal Escape Point (SGEP)

SGEP usually comes out at the middle of the buttock and connects congenital varices of the persistent external vein and/or the arch of the small saphena. It sometimes causes a closed shunt 3 or 5 that involves the small saphena.

## 1.6. Inferior Gluteal Escape Point (IGEP)

IGEP also occurs, particularly in congenital venous malformations. It usually emerges either at the inferior edge of the buttock or at the popliteal fossa when it feeds varices of the sciatic nerve.

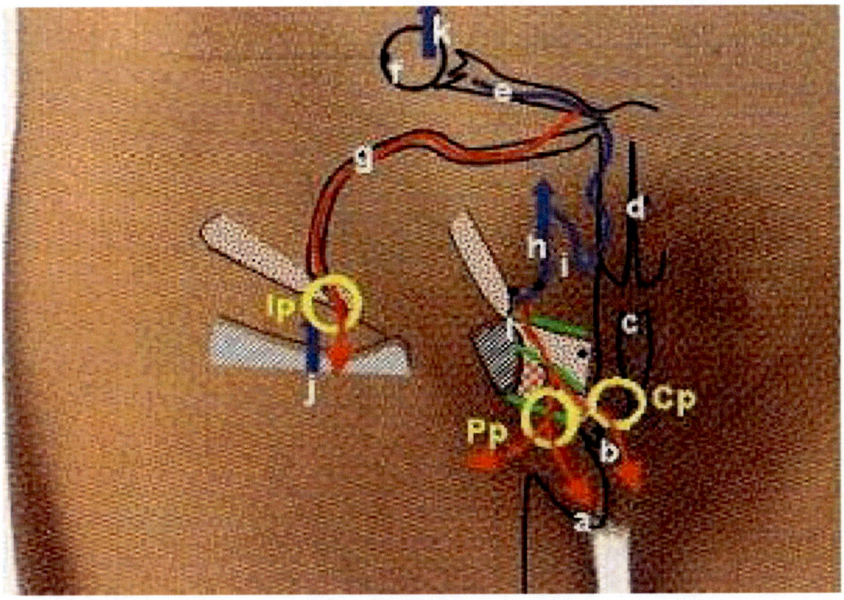


Figure 6.4 A) Visceral pelvic escape points and feeding veins. a: labium major. b:labium minor + clitoris. c: rectum. d: uterus. e: fallopian tube + tubo-ovarian vein. f: ovary. ground ligament of uterus and its vein. h: hypogastric vein. i: uterine vein. j: great saphena h: hypogastric vein. k: ovarian vein. l: internal pudendal vein. Ip: Inguinal point: reflux location at the superficial inguinal ring is due to round ligament vein (g) incompetence fed by one more out of the visceral tributaries (I ,e) of the hypogastric vein( h) and/or ovarian vein ( k). This reflux can feed superficial varices anywhere in the ipsi-lateral limb but in the opposite too either in the labium major (a) through superficial connections with superficial tributaries of the internal pudendal vein (l). Pp: Perineal point: reflux location at the superficial perineal fascia perforation at the posterior edge transversum muscle, in correspondence with the fourth posterior part of the external edge of the labium major, due to the perineal vein incompetence fed by the internal pudendal vein (I) of the hypogastric vein( h) and/or ovarian vein ( k). This reflux can feed superficial varices anywhere in the ipsi-lateral limb but in the opposite too either in the labium major (a) through its labial posterior tributary. Cp: Clitoris point: reflux location at the superficial perineal fascia perforatio next to the proximal clitoris, due to the incompetence of the superficial vein of the clitoris fed by the internal pudendal vein (I) of the hypogastric vein( h) through the incompetent bulbo-clitoridis vein. This reflux can feed superficial varices anywhere in the ipsi-lateral limb but in the opposite too either in the labium major (a) through its labial anterior tributary.

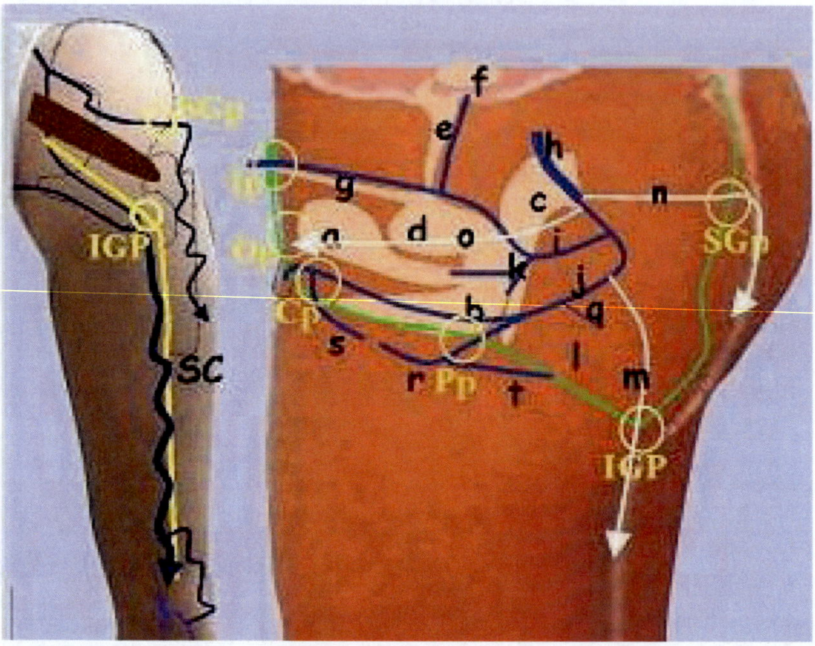


Figure 6.4 B) Three parietal pelvic venous escape points and feeding hypogastric tributaries. a: bladder. b:vagina. c: rectum: uterus. e: fallopian tube + tubo-ovarian vein. f: ovary. g:round ligament of uterus and its vein. h: hypogastric vein. i: uterine vein. j: internal pudendal vein k: vesico-vaginal veins.l: fascia superficialis m: inferior gluteal vein. n:superior gluteal vein. o:obturator vein. P: bulbo-clitoridis vein. q: inferior haemorroidal vein r: labialis posterior vein. s: labialis anterior vein.t: superfificial perineal vein.SC: sciatic nerve and its varicose vein. SGP: Superior gluteal point: reflux location fed by the incompetent superior gluteal vein (n) into a superficial gluteal vein through a fascial perforation. This reflux can feed superficial varices anywhere in the ipsi-lateral limb and connect with any perineal tributary. IGP : Inferior gluteal point: reflux location at the middle of the buttock inferior fold fed by the incompetent inferior gluteal vein (m). This reflux can feed superficial varices anywhere in the ipsi-lateral limb and connect with any perineal tributary but frequently deep varices around the sciatic nerve and then surface in the popliteal region. Op: Obturator point: reflux location at the groin where the obturator vein connects distally with the great saphenous arch or the common femoral vein , fed by the incompetent obturator vein (o) connected proximally whith the hypogastric vein (h) or with the internal pudendal vein. This reflux can feed superficial varices anywhere in the ipsi-lateral limb, but particularly through its coonection with the great saphenous arch. Otherwise, if the distally connection is unique with the common femoral vein, superficial veins cannot be overloaded.

## 1.7. Venous Shunts in Congenital Venous Malformations (CVM)

Usually, CVM of lower limbs make different presentations under different hemodynamic conditions. Shunts are either VOS, in cases of more or less extended deep venous aplasia, or CS, particularly when embryologic veins persist after birth. In some cases, both VOS and CS can be associated in mixed shunts. These mixed shunts can be overloaded not only by the shunting flow, but also by cutaneous malformations, such as superficial angiomas.

*Chapter 7*

# The CHIVA Strategy and Other Conservative and Hemodynamic Treatments


***Claude Franceschi***

Saint Joseph and Pitié-Salpêtrière Hospitals, Paris, France.


## 1. CHIVA Definition

CHIVA is a French acronym for a type of treatment: Conservatrice et Hemodynamique de l'Insuffisance Veineuse en Ambulatoire, which means conservative and hemodynamic treatment of venous insufficiency in ambulatory care [100-106]. The original goal of CHIVA was the preservation of the superficial venous capital for further possible arterial by-pass necessity, thus any aggressive treatment of the superficial venous network was avoided. However, the fact that varices and most other venous disorders are treated by lying down and, above all, by raising the legs suggests that any treatment that can control hydrostatic pressure, including positioning, deserves great medical interest. Most varices and venous insufficiencies are postural because they are triggered by positions in which hydrostatic pressure is too high and not physiologically corrected because of an impairment in dynamic fractionation of hydrostatic pressure (DFHSP). Such impairment is usually caused by superficial and deep closed shunts (CS) or superficial derived open shunts (DOS) due to venous incompetence that disrupts DFHSP control by the valvulo-muscular pump (VMP). Since valve repair or prosthesis is neither easy nor feasible to date, interruption at or immediately under escape points should repair the VMP and suppress pathologic shunt flow. At the same time, these interruptions fractionate permanently and dynamically the column of pressure. Furthermore, and in order to fragment better the hydrostatic column in long incompetent superficial veins, other interruptions immediately under possible competent perforators connected with those veins are performed. This means that CHIVA restores venous physiology in walking patients by maintaining a low distal venous pressure due to renewed VMP efficiency and its effect on DFHSP and blood drainage. Ultimately, venous disorders and varices are supposed to heal. Venous disorders caused by excessive transmural pressure (TMP) should heal due to restoration of DFHSP and venous drainage repair. Varicose calibres should decrease to normal thanks to aggressive shunt flow suppression and efficient VMP blood aspiration. These theoretical hypotheses have been confirmed by numerous publications since their initial presentation at Precy-sous-thil France in October 1988, at which time a text was published entitled Theorie et pratique de la Cure Conservatrice et Hemodynamique de l'Insuffisance Veineuse en Ambulatoire [105].

# 2. Fundamentals of the CHIVA Strategy

## 2.1. Strategy, Tactics, and Definitions

Strategy is the intellectual concept of the actions that have to be taken in order to reach a goal according to a theoretical model. Tactics are the material means selected to perform the actions according to the strategy. In this field, successful strategy relies on understanding venous pathophysiology, and the efficiency of the tactics depends on the quality of the material means. For example, an arterial by-pass can fail because of a mistaken strategy (wrong indication according to the arterial pathophysiology knowledge) or because of a bad tactic (faulty prosthetic material or surgical error). Many CHIVA failures are either due to disrespect or misunderstanding of the strategy or inadequate material means. For this reason, both a clear understanding of the theory and adequate training are necessary to perform CHIVA.

## 2.2. Fundamental Rules of Strategy

CHIVA strategy is conservative not only to preserve the venous capital for further arterial by-pass, but also because vein destruction involves hemodynamic disorders. Actually, venous destruction precludes the drainage that causes tissue suffering and varicose recurrence by vicarious effect. CHIVA strategy is hemodynamic because it restores proper distal venous pressure. As a matter of fact, CHIVA reduces lateral pressure and consequently transmural pressure (TMP) by restoring DFHSP through disconnection of closed shunts, suppressing pathogenic shunt flows, and preserving beneficial vicarious shunts. CHIVA strategy is focused on the re-entry quality, that is, on its ability to drain the venous network properly in order to avoid the effects of drainage preclusion. For this reason, limited venous interruptions are preferable to extensive ones, even if the immediate aesthetic outcomes are less satisfactory. Actually, aesthetic outcomes improve with time, long-term results are much better, and recurrences are much fewer with limited interventions. Clearly, however, any removal or occlusion of nondraining or redundant veins is not contrary to CHIVA strategy, which consists of the following principles:

A. Preservation of deep and superficial draining flows even in varicose veins.

B. Disconnection of deep and superficial CS and superficial DOS in a way that blocks the shunting flow WITHOUT precluding the draining flow.
C. Fractionation of the hydrostatic pressure column WITHOUT precluding the draining flow.
D. Adaptation of the re-entry efficiency to the needs of draining flow.
E. Minimization of venous interruptions. The less the veins are interrupted, even in extended varicose, the better the long-term results. The more the veins are destroyed, even if varicose, the better the short-term results but the worse the long-term [100-106].

### *2.2.1. Preservation of Deep and Superficial Draining Flows Even in Varicose Veins*

Any venous flow, even in varicose veins, is composed totally or partially of physiologic draining blood from tissues. Any blockage of that draining flow involves upstream tissue suffering including capillaro-venular overload (telangiectasias and micro-varicosities). Collateral veins, overloaded and dilated by the force of draining flow, act as natural venous by-passes that circumvent a blockage and allow for physiologic drainage of the upstream tissues. In this way, a vicarious open shunt (VOS) is formed. VOS can be elicited by a functional block, thrombosis, sclerosis, ligation or removal, the latter two being the reason for recurrent varices after disrespect of draining flows. There is no indication for VOS destruction, even if VOS is an unsightly varice. However, it is obvious that removal or occlusion of non-draining or redundant veins is compatible with CHIVA strategy.

### *2.2.2. Disconnection of Deep and Superficial Closed Shunts (CS) and Superficial Derived open Shunts (DOS) in a way that Blocks Shunting flow WITHOUT Compromising Draining Flow*

**2.2.2.1.** ***Disconnection of deep closed shunts (CS).*** The principle of CHIVA in deep veins is disconnection of the shunting deep incompetent vein at its junction with the deep competent but shunted vein. Thus, during VMP systole, the distal flow is totally injected into the competent vein and does not flow back again during the diastole. Also, correct dynamic fractionation of hydrostatic pressure (DFHSP) is once again possible. The competent shunted vein can be close to or distant from the incompetent shunting. It is sufficient that the blood drained by the incompetent vein can be transported by the competent one. If it cannot be, disconnection of the incompetent deep vein is obviously contraindicated because it would be hazardous to physiologic drainage. For example, the incompetent collateral of a double superficial femoral vein can be successfully blocked if the other one is competent. An incompetent superficial femoral vein can be blocked only if the deep femoral vein is competent and participates to the drainage of the calf. The same reasoning applies to deep shunts of the calf. An incompetent posterior tibial vein, for example, can be interrupted if the competent fibular vein can drain the tibial territory and vice versa.

**2.2.2.2.** ***Disconnection of superficial closed shunts (CS).*** Superficial veins can shunt other superficial or deep veins in closed circuit either open circuits.

*2.2.2.2.1. Superficial veins shunting other superficial veins in closed circuit.* This type of shunt is usually not much overloaded because it is not connected directly with the deep network, so it is not much activated by the VMP. However, its disconnection at the escape junction can reduce its calibre. Furthermore, this shunting vein can be destroyed when redundant. It corresponds to shunt type 2.

*2.2.2.2.2. Superficial veins shunting deep veins in closed circuit.* These represent a major cause of chronic venous insufficiency and varicose veins. They are classified in shunts type 1, 3, 4, 5, and 6 according to the patterns of the superficial veins that shunt the deep veins. CHIVA strategy attempts to disconnect the closed shunts at the escape point without affecting the physiological blood drained by the shunting vein. Therefore, particularities of disconnections depend on the hemodynamic configuration of each CS. Disconnection at the escape point (i.e., at the N1-N2 junction) has to take into account the shunt's ability to provide for efficient re-entry for the proximal tributaries. If it can, N2 can be disconnected immediately beneath the junction. If not, N2 will be disconnected at the junction.

2.2.2.2.2.1. Shunt 1 CHIVA strategy: Shunt 1 is N1-N2-N1. It can involve the great or small saphenous veins. One has to make sure that these shunts are not just the diastolic phase of a mixed shunt because the strategy would be different.

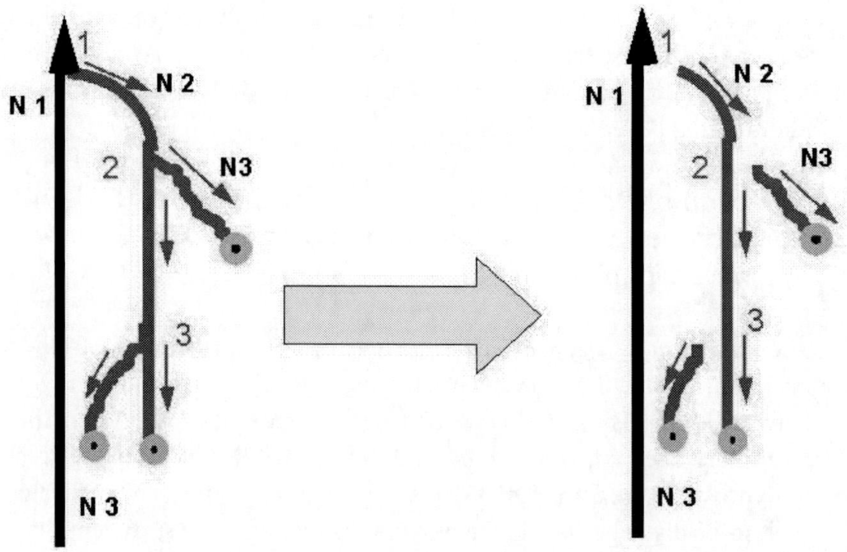


Figure 7.1. Shunt type 1+N3 and associated CHIVA 1 procedure.

2.2.2.2.2.1.a. Shunt 1 in great saphenous vein (GSV): When the sapheno-femoral junction (SFJ) is the escape point (EP), GSV is precisely disconnected at the GSV. This disconnection could be made immediately beneath the arch in order to drain the arch and its tributaries through the SFJ. This is not because of the risk of recurrence by the arch tributaries. As a matter of fact, at this point aspiration is weak (no VMP), and terminal valve incompetence does not prevent excessive pressure in the deep network (from coughing, defecating, lifting heavy loads, etc.). For these reasons, the arch and its tributaries are better drained by distal re-entry.

When the escape point is an incompetent perforator connected to the saphenous trunk, it remains preferable to disconnect the perforator itself when the corresponding VMP is not efficient. This is the case in the thigh. On the contrary, in the lower region of the leg, disconnection can be performed at the saphenous trunk immediately beneath the incompetent perforator thanks to the efficiency of calf VMP. This efficiency can be assessed by Doppler, which shows whether or not there is an inflow during VMP diastole while N2 is compressed by a tourniquet or a finger.

2.2.2.2.2.1.b. Shunt 1 in small saphenous vein (SSV): Usually the RP is at the saphena-popliteal junction (SPJ).Theoretically, the shunting SSV has to be disconnected at SPJ. In fact, Giacomini vein (GV) hemodynamics allow disconnecting of the SSV immediately beneath its junction with GV because GV can function as a vicarious pathway in case of flow-pressure excess in the popliteal vein, thereby preventing recurrences through forced perforators of popliteal fossa.

2.2.2.2.2.2. Shunt 3 CHIVA strategy: Shunt 3 is N1-N2-N3-N1. It can involve the great or small saphenous veins. One has to make sure that these shunts are not just the diastolic phase of a mixed shunt because the strategy would be different. Shunt 3 differs from shunt 1 by N3 segment interposition between N2 and the re-entry point (REP). The strategies are also different. Actually, disconnection at the junction as in shunt 1 is problematic because it would disconnect a closed shunt at N1-N2 but leave a derived open shunt (DOS) N2-N3 called shunt 2. N3 would be less overloaded because CS shunting flow would have been interrupted and the pressure column would have been fractionated at the arch, but overload would still be excessive because of the remaining shunt 2. Disconnection at both N1-N2 and N2-N3 junctions would disconnect both shunts 1 and 2, but N2 draining flow would be precluded because there would be no available re-entry points (REP) on its track. Even if this approach is conservative, disconnects the shunts, and fractionates the hydrostatic pressure, double disconnection in shunt 3 is not CHIVA because it does not allow draining flow. In order to carry out a correct CHIVA in shunt 3, two different procedures are possible. The first is limited to one disconnection at N2-N3 that stops the shunt 1 and 2 shunt flows. In that case, N2 and N3 drain no more shunt flows. N3 is retrograde but drains only its territory, and hydrostatic pressure is fractionated at the N2-N3 junction. N2 is antegrade due to no efficient *re-entry* on its track, but it is still subjected to the previous nonfractioned column of hydrostatic pressure because of no N1-N2 fractioning. N2 segment submitted to excessive hydrostatic pressure explains two phenomena: 1) calibre is partially reduced due to shunt flow suppression but does not return completely to normal, and 2) in some cases a previously small and inefficient perforator located on this N2 segment can enlarge, so that N2 flow is reversed and the previous shunt 3 is converted to shunt 1. In the latter case, the induced shunt has to be corrected, like any shunt 1, by a disconnection at the N1-N2 junction. This procedure is called CHIVA 2 because it may need of two different procedures planned when the duplex investigation confirms the transformation of type 3 shunt into type 1. The latter consists of disconnections at both the N1-N2 and N2-N3 junctions associated with distal N2 devalvulation until an efficient re-entry is represented by one or more perforators.

2.2.2.2.2.3. Shunt 4 CHIVA strategy: Shunt 4 is a CS N1-N3-N2-N1. EP at the N1-N3 junction is usually a pelvic escape point, gluteal, obturatory, inguinal (I point) or perineal (P point). Disconnection must be performed only at the EP.

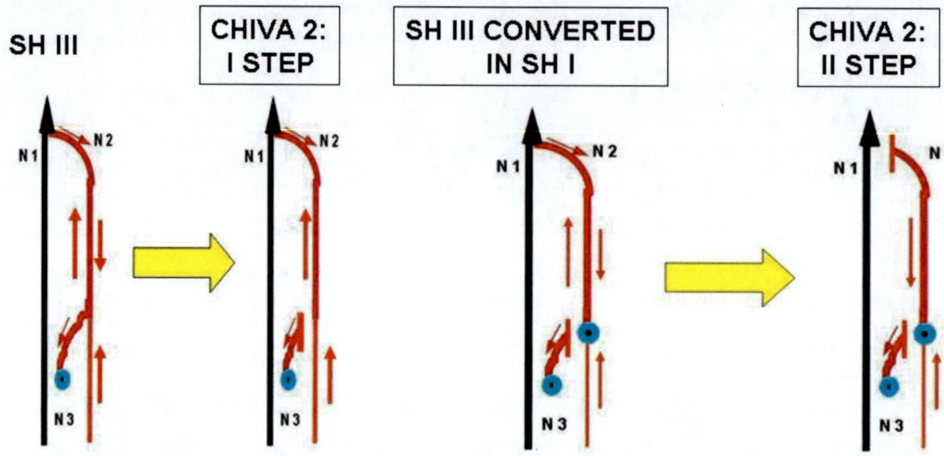


Figure 7.2. CHIVA II first and second step for Shunt type III.

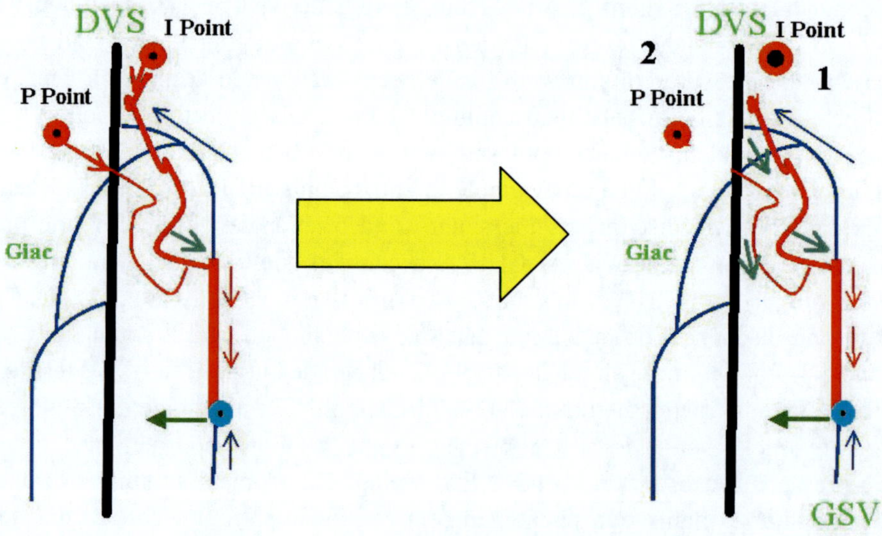


Figure 7.3. Shunt type IV and associated CHIVA procedure.

2.2.2.2.2.4. Shunt 5 CHIVA strategy: Shunt 5 is a CS N1-N3-N2-N3-N1. As in shunt 4, EP at the N1-N3 junction is usually a pelvic escape point, gluteal, obturatory, inguinal (I point) or perineal (P point). Disconnection must be performed not only at the N1-N3 EP, but also at the N2-N3 in order not to leave a shunt 2.

2.2.2.2.2.5. Shunt 6 CHIVA strategy: Shunt 6 is a CS N1-N3-N1. EP can be a pelvic escape point or any other EP. This shunt can appear in congenital malformations but is more usually seen in recurrences following removal of varices and saphenas.

**2.2.2.3.** ***Disconnection of a mixed shunt (MS):*** A mixed shunt is composed of two shunts: a vicarious open shunt (VOS) and a closed shunt (CS) that share the same EP and distal segments of the shunting veins. Their REP and proximal segments are different. REP of VOS is proximal to LP, and REP of CS is distal to LP. As VOS has to be preserved and CS disconnected, the disconnection cannot be at LP but only at the distal venous segment of CS where it diverges from the distal venous segment of VOS.

**2.2.2.4.** ***Disconnection of superficial derived open shunts (DOS):*** DOS are shunts 2, N2-N3-N1. Disconnection of DOS is done simply on N3 at the N2-N3 junction.

**2.2.2.5.** ***Disconnection of composite shunts:*** Practically speaking, most shunts are composite in that a shunt 1 can be connected to a shunt 2 and so on. Sometimes the REP of one shunt is not efficient enough, and drainage is also provided by the REP of an associated shunt. Therefore, any shunt can be disconnected as long as its disconnection does not preclude any draining flow in the associated shunt. For this reason, the proper REP of every associated shunt has to be assessed by dynamic tests. For example, when a composite shunt is shunt 1+2 (N1-N2-N1-N2-N3-N1), disconnection can be carried out at N1-N2 and N3-N1 as long as REP in N2 is efficient. If REP in shunt 1 is not obviously efficient, this composite shunt can be assimilated to a shunt 3 and treated by CHIVA 2 or CHIVA devalvulation. In another case, two EPs can be superimposed and be drained by the same distal REP (N1-N2-N1-N2-N1). Fractionation can be done immediately at the upper EP. It may be also done beyond the lower EP even if refluxing during diastole, but only if testing shows it to be efficient enough as REP. Thus, under appropriate conditions, a previous EP can be transformed into REP.

### *2.2.3. Static Fractionation of Hydrostatic Pressure Column WITHOUT Compromising Drainage*

Disconnection of CS and DOS shunts also allows for static fragmentation of the column of hydrostatic pressure. Sometimes the incompetent segment disconnected from the shunt is too long and high, so it needs a complementary fractionation. As this fractionation must not preclude drainage, every remaining subsegment of vein must have a REP.

### *2.2.4. Adaptation of the Re-Entry Efficiency to the needs of Draining Flow*

Re-entry is the place where shunt flow rejoins its physiologic pathway. After CS or DOS disconnection, flow is limited to the draining flow but can be too great for the capacity of the REP, either because its calibre is too small or because downstream aspiration is too weak. REP is efficient when it allows a correct drainage of the network that converges on it, that is, when its calibre is sufficient and downstream aspiration is correct.

When more than one REP drain a CS or DOS, hemodynamic assessment of each perforator is performed by diastolic flow velocity registration in the shunting vein while other veins that carry the same flow to other re-entries are blocked. An inefficient re-entry leads to tissue suffering, telangiecstases, and vicarious varices.

### *2.2.5. Superficial CS and Deep Venous Incompetence*

In cases of superficial CS or DOS, the greater the efficiency of the VMP, the more the diastolic flow. On the contrary, the lower the VMP efficiency, the less the diastolic flow. That is why, in cases of totally inefficient VMP, as when the deep veins are totally incompetent, dynamic tests of VMP will not show any diastolic flow in the superficial veins, even if they are very large and varicose. Actually, during the diastole, total incompetence does not allow the VMP to reduce venous pressure, so the gradient of the re-entry perforating vein is not favorable to inflow. This is illustrated by the Perth test, which shows no reduction of varices when walking despite a tourniquet at the hip. It is also demonstrated by an unexpected lack of reflux in superficial varicose veins during dynamic tests, such as Paranà maneuver. The CHIVA strategy is to correct before deep incompetence occurs, through disconnection in case of deep closed shunt or valve repair if there is total incompetence without any CS, followed by disconnection of superficial shunts.

Superficial disconnection without deep incompetence correction makes no haemodynamic sense because no HDSFP cannot be achieved

## 2.3. Post Chiva Controls

After CHIVA, clinical and instrumental tests have to be interpreted according to CHIVA patterns.

*2.3.1. Regression of Clinical Symptoms:* is favored by walking. All functional symptoms and oedemas related to venous insufficiency, such as postural pains and heaviness, should disappear or diminish during the first postoperative days. Ulcers should close within few weeks. Hypodermitis should disappear in the course of several weeks. Pigmentation should regress after several months, up to two years. The caliber of varicose veins should return to normal within a few days or weeks, depending upon their pre-operative size.Thus, clinical outcome cannot be definitely assessed until some weeks or months after the procedure.

*2.3.2. Post-CHIVA Echo-Doppler Assessments:* Valsalva maneuver has to be negative at the operated shunts. Retrograde flow during dynamic tests does not necessarily signify a failure. Poor systolic but significant diastolic retrograde flow attests to shunt 0, thus a correct drainage [6,45,47,56,255].

*2.3.3. Air PLethysmography Assessments:* The pressure-volume relationship in the leg has to normalize according to the efficiency of the procedure [251].

## 2.4. Post-Chiva Iterative Procedures

Except for CHIVA 2, no further procedures usually have to be performed. Actually, in complex cases such as multi-shunts in venous congenital malformations, it is better to spread the cure over two or more operations every six months in order to avoid excessive interruptions and to clarify the situation progressively.

## 2.5. Short and Long Term Results

The less the veins are interrupted, even in extended varicose, the better the long-term results [56]. The more the veins are destroyed, even if they are varicose, the better the short-term results but the worse the long-term. It is preferable to spread CHIVA over two distant procedures, thereby delaying to the second operation those complementary interruptions that are not obviously safe for drainage. This is the case, for example, when in a shunt 1+2, the REP in shunt 1 is not obviously efficient. This composite shunt can be assimilated to a shunt 3 and treated by CHIVA 2. These iterative operations, when necessary, are not difficult because they are ambulatory, brief, and performed using local anaesthesia.

Obviously, complete removal or closure of all varicose veins results in immediate aesthetic success. Telangiectases, micro-varicosities and vicarious varices that appear over time are not due to a “natural” evolution of the varicose disease, but rather to long-term complications of nonhemodynamic procedures. On the contrary, hemodynamic procedures like CHIVA preserve the veins, even if varicose, in order not only to spare the venous capital for further arterial by-pass, but also to restore correct venous function. The so-obtained correct venous function progressively cures varicose veins and trophic disorders and prevents further recurrence. The time necessary for healing ranges from several days to several weeks, and the varicose veins remain visible during that period. Patients accept this delay for a better final outcome.

### *2.5.1. Chiva and Recurrence*

Varicose recurrence is usually imputed either to an incomplete destruction of superficial veins (especially incomplete resection of the arch of great saphena or small saphena and its tributaries) or to the natural evolution of varicose disease. Actually, thanks to pre- and post-operative echo-Doppler findings, the problem can be identified as one of four conditions.

***Same varices reappear:*** Varicose reappearance over time (of the same varices as before the therapy) constitutes true recurrence. An example is when an occluded or caliber- reduced varicose vein becomes permeable and dilated again. In this case, recurrence could be due to the forcing of veins by draining flow because of inefficient re-entry or an inefficient interruption. If the recurrence is due to an inefficient REP, it is better not to repeat any interruption at the same point, but rather check another one beyond a better REP. If the recurrence is due to a tactical (material) interruption failure, a more reliable technique is necessary.

***Remaining varices:*** Some or all of the varices may be left untreated by the therapist e.g., when some or all of varices remain immediately after therapy. In this case, a complementary CHIVA can be performed.

***Varices in different territories:*** Varices different from those previous to therapy can be due to an independent varicose evolution, e.g., when new varices of previously normal small saphena occur after therapy of great saphena. Here, too, complementary CHIVA can be carried out.

***Iatrogenic varicose veins:*** Varices may be induced by previous therapy, so that one can call them long-term iatrogenic complications. For example, it is not rare to notice new varices without any leak point but made only of vicarious veins. This occurs because previous draining normal or varicose veins were destroyed. In the case of superficial VOS due to drainage preclusion, static fractionation is possible only if intermediate perforators (REP) are found on their track. In the case of CS created by anarchical VOS that open incompetent perforators, CHIVA has to disconnect them. Unfortunately, most cases of recurrence after venous removal are VOS without much intermediate REP, which reduces the therapeutic possibilities.

# 3. Particular CHIVA Strategies

When venous pressure increases, transmural pressure (TMP) increases so that liquids and metabolic wastes from the tissues cannot pass into circulation. An obstacle to the passage of liquids involves the appearance of oedemas. Intra-tissue accumulation of toxic metabolites associated with capillary flow slowdown is responsible for trophic disorders. The reactive vasodilation of arterioles and the opening of micro-shunts worsen tissue ischemia in two ways: 1) TMP increases because of residual pressure (RP) enhancement; and 2) the opening of micro-shunts steals capillary flow, thereby worsening cellular necrosis. This explains the coexistence of oxygenated (red) blood with necroses in venous ulcers. Infection occurs because of the ideal culture medium that this type of ulcer represents. CHIVA has to reduce TMP through lateral pressure reduction. Disconnection of shunts and fractionation of pressure have to be done with the utmost attention to drainage of the damaged tissue. However, those sites that theoretically have to be interrupted but that involve inflamed tissues must not be touched at the first operation. The first procedure is performed only at sites having healthy tissues. A second procedure is performed at the remaining sites when their trophicity is improved by the first procedure. Actually, correct and long-term durable interruptions cannot be obtained in inflamed tissues.

## 3.1. Congenital Venous Malformations

Examination is necessary to identify which varicose and/or incompetent deep and/or superficial veins are CS, DOS, VOS, mixed shunts, or NON draining malformative vein. In these multiple and complex situations where, in addition to shunting flows, superficial "physiologic" flows are increased by superficial angiomas, interruptions must divided into multiple operations in order to correct hemodynamic disorders in the most efficient, accurate, and safe manner.

# 4. CHIVA MAPPING

Mapping is a schematic design that depicts the venous anatomo-functional configuration of each patient. Flow direction according to the *systole-diastolic* phase of dynamic tests and Valsalva maneuver is indicated by an arrow for each depicted vein. Data are obtained through echo-Doppler. In this way EP, shunting veins, REP, and occluded or removed veins can be identified and analyzed in order to plan an appropriate CHIVA strategy. Only echo-Doppler allows such mapping and thus a correct CHIVA strategy.

Clinical examination is not sufficient to assess accurately different types of shunts. Use of an ultrasound duplex scanner is mandatory because it is the only noninvasive instrument able to show in real time the anatomy of the venous network and, contemporaneously, venous flow direction and velocity in any position and during any dynamic maneuver.

## 4.1. Valsalva Manoeuver (VM)

Positive VM, that is an antegrade or retrograde flow elicited by thoraco-abdominal and diaphragm contraction, evidences a deep incompetence when in deep veins and a closed shunt CS when in superficial veins. Escape point is checked upstream. Valsalva maneuver is negative in VOS and DOS [46,48,241].

## 4.2. Manual or Pneumatic Squeezing of the Calf

It can evidence reflux upon relaxation but can be false negative when squeezing is performed incorrectly or when the aspiring VMP sector is not involved by compression. Moreover, squeezing compresses superficial veins, which does not occur during physiologic VMP motion [102,148,150].

## 4.3. Dynamic VMP Activation

Paranà maneuver allows a "physiologic contraction" and, at the same time, facilitates ultrasound scanning in the standing immobile position due to an isometric reflex contraction of the muscles of the lower limbs to a slight push-pull at the patient's waist. Flow is activated by VMP systole and /or diastole [102].

*4.3.1. In the superficial network,* diastolic flows are elicited by the VMP in CS and DOS. Systolic flows are elicited in CS, VOS and DOS. Diastolic velocity is proportional to the shunting flow. Diastolic and systolic flow directions are usually opposite in CS and

DOS but can be the same *as* CS that involve Giacomini vein. In the case of multiple REPs in CS or DOS, the efficiency of the REPs proximal to the terminal can be assessed by diastolic flow velocity while compressing the terminal re-entry. This assessment is useful to the hemodynamic therapeutic strategy. Reflux time, Psatakis index, or dynamic reflux index (DRI) measurement can evidence reflux only when systolic and diastolic flow directions are opposite. Flow directions remain pathologic even when pressure and velocity return to normal but remain inverted after shunt disconnection. In this case, flow direction is abnormal but no longer pathogenic. In some cases, the flow in great incompetent varicose saphena cannot be activated by diastole when the VMP is disabled because of total deep venous valve incompetence. That is why valve incompetence allows retrograde flow only if the pressure gradient is inverted, that is, when the VMP is efficient. In other cases, diastolic reflux occurs while deep venous veins are refluxing, too. This means that there remains an efficient valvulo-muscular portion connected to the shunt. In other words, the greater the superficial diastolic reflux, the better the VMP efficiency.

*4.3.2. In the deep network,* systolic and diastolic flows are elicited by the VMP. Diastolic flow evidences a proximal valve incompetence without deep CS when diastolic flow volume is less than or equal to systolic, or when DRI $\geq$1. Deep CS is demonstrated when diastolic flow volume is greater than systolic, or DRI >1, because, as explained previously, CS carries deviated flow in addition to normal during diastole. Detection of deep CS is the central goal of deep venous incompetence investigation because it is determinant for hemodynanamic therapeutic strategy.

## 5. Other Conservative and Hemodynamic Treatments

CHIVA can be associated with other hemodynamic and conservative techniques but is incompatible with nonhemodynamic techniques [43,98,99,126-128,153,154]. In order to reduce transmural pressure (TMP), those methods affect lateral or external pressure. Surgical and medical treatments can be classified into two categories, according to whether they are in accordance with hemodynamic principles or not. TMP is the central parameter of the regulation of venous function. Consequently, treatments must restore a TMP that is favorable to drainage and an optimal venous capacity. The therapeutic action must consist of either increasing extra-venous pressure or decreasing intra-venous pressure.

### 5.1. Increase in Extra Venous Pressure

An increase in external pressure reduces TMP and thus supports drainage and the reduction of venous caliber. This can be obtained by an increase in atmospheric pressure, which is maximal at sea level. Generally, however, increases in EP are obtained through passive external compression with rigid or elastic bandages, but also by immersion in a water bath or even in a mercury bath. Sometimes active pneumatic compression is used. In all cases, the goal is reached when the TMP is corrected. Such applied external pressure cannot exceed the arterial blood pressure because of the risk of ischemia. Also, when intravenous pressure is very high, strong external compression can be painful due to the crushing of tissues between excessive intravenous and external pressures. Therefore, external compression is appropriate only when the intravenous pressure is not too high. The hemodynamic effects of rigid and elastic bandages differ in two ways. Rigid application increases VMP efficiency during systole because it confines the content of the pump in a rigid container, but it is less efficient at rest. Elastic application cushions the hemodynamic effects of the systole and is more efficient at rest. For these reasons, rigid application is preferred for subjects who walk. In any case, compression represents a logical and effective hemodynamic treatment for venous insufficiency. It is free of side effects except when overdone, and it can be applied alone or associated with other treatments. Because of its direct effect on TMP, compression also constitutes also a major preventive treatment under temporary physiological conditions, such as presence at high altitude, long-term standing or sitting, and pregnancy.

## 5.2. Reduction of Venous Pressure

Reduction of venous lateral pressure (LP) decreases TMP, thereby improving drainage, venous size, and venous caliber. LP depends on HSP and the lateral component of residual pressure (RP).

### *5.2.1. Postural Therapy:*

At the ankle, HSP is maximal in the motionless standing position, low in the lying position, and negative (lower than the atmospheric pressure) when the foot is raised above head level. Therefore, posture can control TMP by action on the HSP. So, lying and, moreover, raising lower limbs support drainage and decrease venous caliber.

### *5.2.2. Thermo-Therapy:*

Heat increases RP by reducing microcirculatory resistance and increases LP as well. Thus, cooling the legs reduces LP.

### *5.2.3. Valve Repair or Valve Prosthesis:*

In cases of deep venous valvular incompetence without any shunt, the theoretical treatment consists of valvular repair or valvular prosthesis [142,168,265-267]. Unfortunately, these techniques have need of improvement. In most cases, only postural and compressive therapy can be applied.

## 5.3. External and Lateral Pressure-Associated Correction

Treatments for venous insufficiency by TMP correction often combine external pressure increase with LP reduction. This occurs when one walks into the sea because the external effects of compression by water are combined with maximal atmospheric pressure, with LP reduction caused by reduced superficial flow from thermoregulation, and with DFHSP induced by walking. It is also the case when an imperfect correction of closed shunts is supplemented by compression.

# 6. Tactic Material Means in CHIVA

Which are the best procedures to achieve the strategic decisions? In other words, which are the most accurate, efficient and lasting material means to perform flow interruptions at the right places according to strategic needs? How not to confuse tactic failure with strategic error? Is a forced or by-passed interruption due to an inappropriate tactic or a mistaken strategy?

## 6.1. Surgery

First of all, a previous precise marking under duplex ultrasound by an operator aware of the surgical necessities is indispensable. Venous short resection (1 to 4 cm) associated with nonresorbable ligation and nonresorbable closure of the perforated fascia seems to be the most precise, efficient, and long-lasting material means to date. Simple nonresorbable ligations are seldom forced and reopened. Multiple ligations with nonresorbable thick thread seem to resist better. Resorbable venous ligation after section could favor a recanalisation due to inflammatory angiogenetic effects.

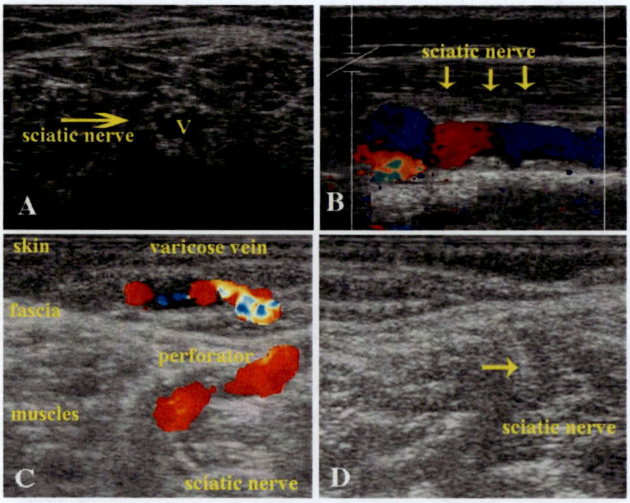


Figure 7.4. Sciatic nerve varices and its therapy by echo-guided sclerotherapy. The sciatic veins are deep veins and lay within the sciatic nerve The nerve was easily visible on ultrasound imaging because of thickening of the neural sheath and dissection of the nerve fibres by the dilated vessels (Figure A transversal access, B longitudinal access. C varicose veins ot the lateral aspect of the leg fed by reflux coming from sciatic veins through a perforator Please note in D) the echo coming from the foam reaching its target in an area not so easily reachable by surgery.

## 6.2. Endovenous Procedures

Endovenous procedures, such as sclerotherapy, laser, and radiofrequency, are not yet appropriated for precise, limited, and lasting interruptions. Nevertheless, they are useful when surgery is not feasible, as for example in sciatic nerve varices where surgery is not suitable for the great risk of iatrogenic nerve damage [199].

*Chapter 8*

# HAEMODYNAMICS OF VENOUS INSUFFICIENCY: ASSESMENT TECHNIQUES

***Claude Franceschi*[1] *and Paolo Zamboni*[2]**
[1]Saint Joseph and Pitié-Salpétrière Hospitals, Paris, France;
[2]University of Ferrara, Italy.

Functional investigations measure the various haemodynamic parameters of the venous system.

## 1. VENOUS PRESSURE MEASUREMENT

### 1.1. Invasive Pressure Measurement

Invasive pressure measurement of distal venous pressure is independent of the orientation of the endovenous sensor when the subject is motionless. This is because circulatory velocities are too low to create sufficient dynamic energy, and total pressure is roughly equal to lateral pressure (LP). On the contrary, when the subject is moving, circulatory velocity is no longer negligible, and measurement has to take into account the angle of the sensor to the flow (tubes of Pitot). However, despite some overlaps, ambulatory venous pressure is widely considered the gold standard assessment of venous function [19,23,26,58,135,183].

### 1.2. Non-Invasive Pressure Measurement

#### *1.2.1. Doppler and Sphygmomanometer:*

Measurement of venous pressure is performed at the ankle with a sphygmomanometer. Although this type of assessment is incapable of providing an accurate pressure value, it provides an indicative value for assessing the presence of venous disorders. The sphygmomanometer is inflated to 120 mmHg and deflated immediately. Venous pressure is the pressure value when the posterior tibial venous flow is heard at the Doppler. The sphygmomanometer has to be deflated immediately in order to avoid any overevaluation of venous pressure. This pressure is normally lower than 30 mmHg in the supine position. It rises in the case of a proximal haemodynamic obstacle to the venous flow. A comparative measurement at both ankles prevents misleading due to artefacts. The Authors think that such a procedure may produce an additional parameter, i.e., the time of appearance of venous flow after sphygmomanometer deflation, which is probably related to refilling time. However, the significance of this parameter in clinical practice has not yet been assessed [13].

### *1.2.2. Ultrasonographic Derived Venous Pressure (Zamboni Pressure):*

The relationship between vein volume and pressure (venous compliance) is known to be linear after completion of the filling phase, in which the vein is distended by the increase in blood volume. However, during the filling phase, the volume/pressure relationship is not linear. Rather, there is a significant increase in volume with little change in pressure. The volume/pressure relationship becomes linear starting at pressure values around 20 mmHg, that is, near the completion of the filling phase.

Because of the particular anatomical and structural configuration of veins related to their function, vein diameter reflects vein volume. This assumption is confirmed by our demonstration of linearity in the filled saphenous vein, starting at a pressure value of 20 mm Hg, and also by the pressure/diameter relationship of the GSV in patients affected by primary venous insufficiency. This observation has allowed us to describe a new, ultrasonographic method of determination. We have experimented with a non-invasive method for extrapolation of saphenous AVP values from a diameter/pressure curve. This can be obtained by drawing a straight line from the point of initial venous distension (20 mmHg) that best approximates the two pressure/diameter values determined noninvasively and measured effectively under different hydrostatic conditions (sitting and standing).

In clinical practice, if the venous system is able to empty with exercise, we can document reductions in both vein diameter (assessed by ultrasound) and vein volume (expressed by RVF), as in the clinical Perthes test. By contrast, if the system is unable to empty satisfactorily due to impaired muscle pump function or another cause, we cannot document a significant reduction in vein diameter and/or volume (and, of course, in AVP since these three parameters are linearly related after the filling phase).

The ultrasonographic technique is simple, non-invasive and thus easily repeatable, and performed with equipment widely used for vascular investigations.

Minor errors in diameter assessment could occur due to the fact that the probe is held manually, thus the accuracy of the ultrasonic measurement is strictly operator-dependent. However, this is a general limitation of ultrasound techniques [258,259,260,262,284].

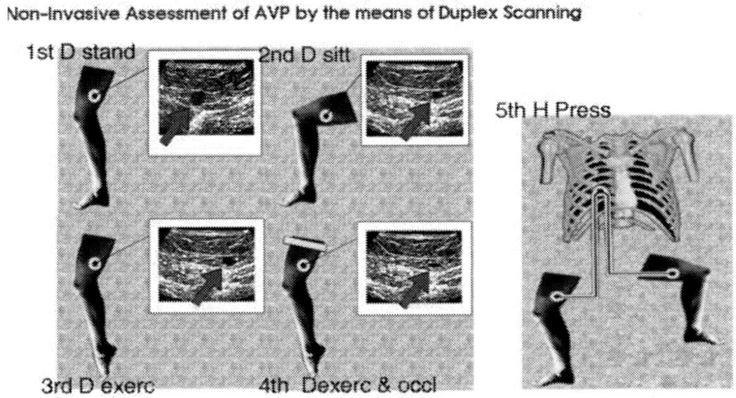


Figure 8.1A. ULTRASONIC MEASUREMENT OF DIAMETER OF THE SAPHENOUS VEIN IN DIFFERENT CONDITIONS. ASSESSMENT OF THE HYDROSTATIC PRESSURE. Diameter and pressure were first measured in two different hydrostatic positions: sitting and standing. The two values of diameter (D1, D2) were measured by duplex scanning in a saphenous segment of the thigh. P1-2 is the pressure of the hydrostatic column, i.e. the distance between the heart level and the point of saphenous diameter measurement in quiet standing (P1) and in sitting position (P2) according to the formula P = p x g x h. At 37 °C and with an ambient pressure of 1 atm, p x g can be considered a constant. Consequently, P1-2 (mm Hg) is equal to 0,7723 x h, where h is the distance (in cm) between the heart level and the point of measurement

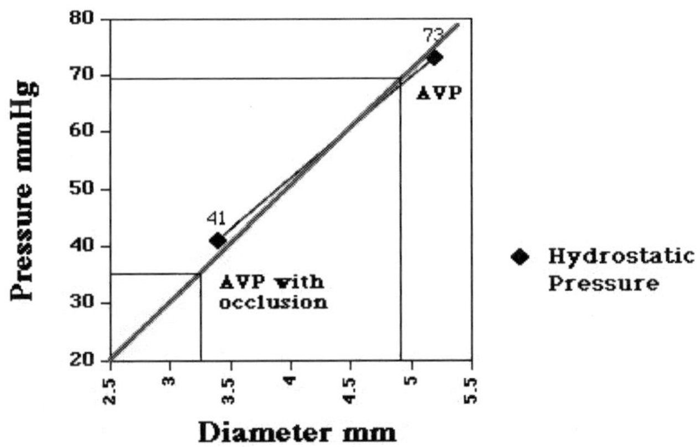


Figure 8.1B. EXTRAPOLATION OF AVP FROM A LINEAR DIAMETER-PRESSURE CURVE (ZAMBONI'S METHOD): Extrapolation of ultrasonic AVP values from a diameter/pressure curve of the saphenous vein. Zero point of the curve is arbitrarily considered a pressure value of 20 mmHg (P0). This is the lowest level of pressure from which the saphenous diameter/pressure relationship at the thigh can be approximated to a straight line. Hence, the axes intersection was set to 20 mm Hg in order to shift the reference system to the minimum level from which the diameter/pressure relationship was demonstrated to be linear. By drawing a straight line from this zero to the middle point of the segment joining the two diameter/pressure values measured in sitting and in standing position (Fig 8.1A), a linear diameter/pressure curve can be drawn for each patient. This is the line that starts from the point of initial venous distension (20 mm Hg) and best approximates the two pressure/diameter values non invasively determined in different hydrostatic conditions. Subsequently it is necessary to assess the GSV diameter after 10 consecutive tip-toe movements, both with and without external tourniquet occlusion of the proximal saphenous vein. (Fig. 8.1A). The two values of GSV diameter after exercise are plotted on the diameter/pressure curve previously created, allowing the extrapolation of two AVP values, respectively with and without sapheno-femoral reflux elimination, as shown in Figure 8.1B.

### *1.2.3. Postural Venous Cardiac Controlled Impairment Assessment, or Tilt Test:*

The subject lies on a table inclined close to vertical in order to test his vagal reaction to lower limb extreme venous stasis, given the totally motionless standing position, that is, without VMP support. The operator has to be careful not to elicit a malign vasovagal syndrome [5].

### *1.2.4. Leg Oedema Volume Measurement (LEVM):*

It assesses variations in edema of the lower limbs. Many means of measurement have been proposed: mercury volumetry, infrared volumetry, echo volumetry and water volumetry, magnetic resonance imaging (MRI), impedancemetry, and Leg-O-Meter. Volume varies with the causes of the edema [186,232].

### *1.2.5. Plethysmography*

***1.2.5.1. Mercury gauge plethysmography:*** measures variations of volume in the limb, based on derived limb circumference without prejudging it to its value of the pressures [89].

***1.2.5.2. Air plethysmography:*** measures variations in pressure and volume of the calf during stress tests, and thus variations in transmural pressure (TMP). It divides the venous function according to change in posture and activation of the VMP, permitting the derivation of four useful parameters [19,59]:

- total volume (TV), the amount of blood to be found in the venous reservoir; air plethysmography measures the change in volume (in ml air) produced by passage from the supine position with the leg raised at 45° to the standing position;
- venous filling index (VFI), the volume variation produced in a limb in a defined time by passage from the supine to the standing position; VFI is related to the severity of the reflux and is expressed in ml air/sec;
- ejected fraction (EF), the rate of reduction in TV after a single tiptoe movement; It reflects the calf muscular systole; and
- residual volume fraction (RVF), the rate of reduction in TV obtainable after ten tiptoe movements; this index is related to ambulatory venous pressure measurement.

We measured the changes in all of these parameters after CHIVA procedures (see chapter 12).

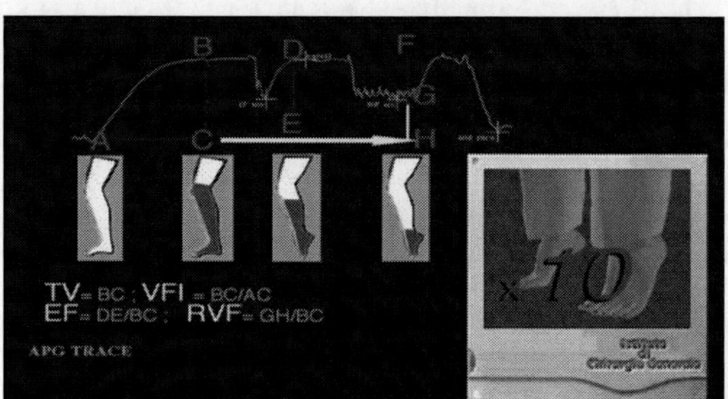


Figure 8.2. APG TRACE: The red color in the limb indicates the filling rate according to the different condition of volume measurement. The parameters are indicated in yellow and described in the text.

# 2. Flow Measurement

## 2.1. *Angiography,* or Dynamic Phlebography

It can assess the competence or incompetence of valves. However, the filling of veins depends on the point of introduction of the contrast, and contrast dispersion may be incomplete, especially where a "washing" effect occurs [143].

## 2.2. Doppler

It is an anatomical and haemodynamic non-invasive technique of major interest in venous investigation. It has allowed decisive progress in the comprehension of venous haemodynamic physiopathology and remains indispensable to an accurate diagnosis. Its accuracy_depends on the operator's expertise [61,72,151,159].

### *2.2.1. Antegrade Flows:*

*(AF)* are those in the direction of the valve's opening, as recorded by Doppler. However, normal direction is insufficient to indicate normal flow, since flow content, origin, and velocity must also be normal. AF can be recorded in open shunts and closed shunts, depending on the patterns of the particular shunt and the stress test or manoeuvre involved.

### *2.2.2. Retrograde Flows:*

*(RF)* are those in the opposite direction of the valve's opening, as recorded by Doppler. Such reversed flow direction is insufficient to indicate pathologic flow, and the content, origin, and velocity of the flow must be considered as well. Just as for AF, RF can be recorded in open shunts and closed shunts, depending on the patterns of the particular shunt and the stress test or manoeuvre involved.

### *2.2.3. Reflux Time:*

*(RT)* has to be > 0.05 m/*s* to be pathologic because a short proto-diastolic backflow is physiologic. RT lasts as long as the reflux but is not necessarily proportional to the importance of the reflux because the smaller the leaking valvular hole, the longer the RT, yet the importance of the reflux time is less. In addiction, RT is not proportional to the clinical class of severity of the disease. Finally, can be different in accordance with the manoeuvre used for eliciting reflux. For example, in the GSV is longer by using Wunstorf rather than squeezing manoeuvre [150,151,162,172,184,188].

*2.2.4. Psatakis Index (PI):* it is an index of reflux assessed in deep veins during compression-relaxation of the calf. PI = diastolic reflux velocity surface / systolic velocity flow surface.

It takes into account the reflux volume but not the flow and is considered pathological when it is >0.40. The limitations of PI are roughly equal to those of RT, for the same reasons explained above. Therefore, PI varies according to reflux volume but not to reflux flow rate [102].

*2.2.5. Dynamic reflux index (DRI):* it takes into account volume and flow rate of reflux, in order to avoid the limitations of RT and PI. DRI = [(diastolic reflux mean velocity)$^2$. diastolic reflux time] / [(systolic reflux mean velocity)$^2$. diastolic flow time]. Because DRI varies according to the reflux flow rate, it expresses more completely than RT or PI the degree or severity of reflux haemodynamics. Thus, for the same diastolic reflux volume, the higher the diastolic reflux flow rate, more the reflux volume between two steps while walking, and vice versa. When, for the same volume, the diastolic reflux flow rate is low, and consequently the reflux time is long, the systole of the successive step interrupts the reflux so that it is of minor importance during walking [58,184,224].

## 2.3. Infrared Plethysmography (IRP)

It measures the refilling time (RFT) of the deep network by the superficial one through the perforating veins after calf stress (VMP motion). This time is proportional to the volume of available superficial blood and to the gradients of pressure generated by the VMP. For this reason, RFT may be false negative in case of VMP impairment [19,265].

## 2.4. Assessment Manoeuvres for Valve Competence and Shunts

*2.4.1. Valsalva's Manoeuvre (VM):* consists of forced systolic phase of the thoraco-abdominal pump (TAP) against a blocked expiration. The patient tries to expire with the glottis closed while contracting the thoracic muscles, diaphragm, and abdominal muscles all at once. Contemporaneously, venous flow is blocked and the abdominal veins are compressed, particularly the retro-hepatic cava vein, so that the pressure gradient is reversed. The transmission of this gradient involves a backward pressure wave in the entire venous network of the lower limbs and pelvis, stops the flow in competent veins, and involves reflux only in incompetent veins. VM is said to be negative when it blocks the flow, and positive when it induces reflux. As pointed out above, the reflux occurs at the escape point but may be antegrade, thus in the physiologic direction, in part or all of its superficial pathway. An example can be seen in the descending tributaries of the great saphenous arch when its antegrade flow is fed by a pelvic escape point during VM. Upon VM relaxation, normal flow is released in the normal direction (Figure 8.3a,b) [46,48,172,241].

*2.4.2. Manual Squeezing:* with proximal compression is used to test valve competence during squeezing, while distal compression is used to test valve competence when releasing. However, manual compression, particularly when intended to simulate the systoles and diastoles of the VMP, does not correspond accurately to normal or pathological behaviour. In fact, flow data depend on the location, duration, and force of manual compression [148,150,151]. In particular, flow duration and velocity may be underestimated, especially when the affected part of the VMP location is different from the compressed one. In addition, manual compression affects superficial veins, as opposed to VMP systole, which affects only deep veins. Lastly, manual compression may be not feasible in cases of large, stiff, wounded, or painful calf.

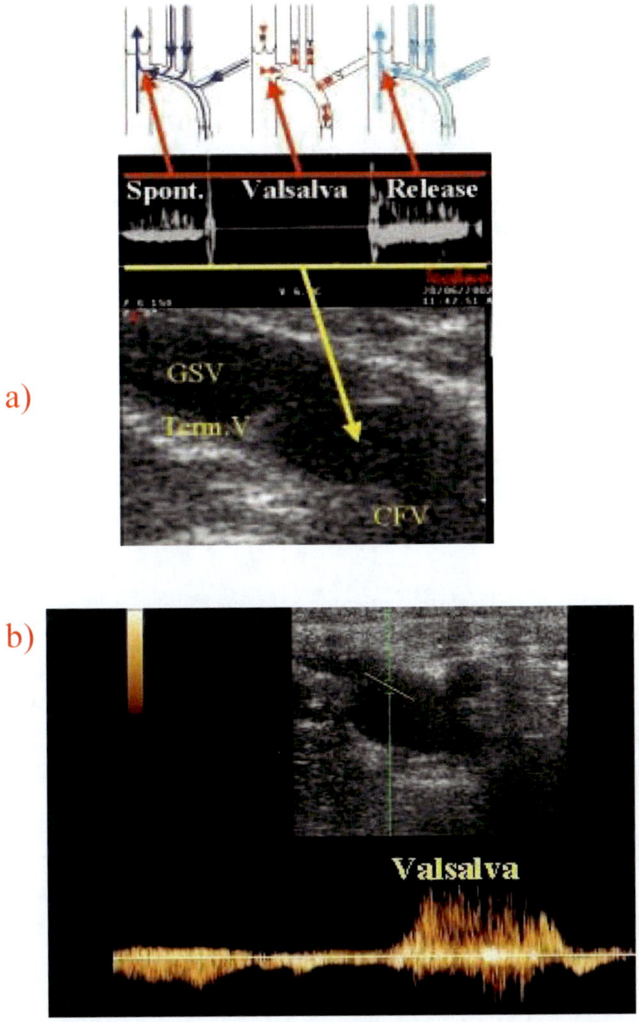


Figure 8.3. a) Valsalva negative manoeuvre b) Valsalva positive manoeuvre.

*2.4.3. Voluntary Muscular Contractions:* (walking, rising on tiptoes, etc.) and proprioceptive reflexes provide data that are preferable to those of manual compression because the former are physiological or pathophysiological.

***2.4.3.1. Paranà's maneuvre:*** consists of testing VMP-induced flows in subjects during immobile standing through use of the proprioceptive reflex. A slight push to the waistline triggers an isometric contraction of the leg muscles that activates the VMP and allows data recording. It induces VMP systole during the impulsion and diastole upon release. Thanks to the immobility, it is particularly interesting for Duplex-scan examination and is feasible as long as the patient can stand up [102].

***2.4.3.2. Oscillation manoeuvre:*** consists of simulating the first moment of plantar pressure of walking and is limited to it. The conditions of examination are similar to those of Parana's manoeuvre [257].

***2.4.3.3. Toe flexion manoeuvre:*** is performed voluntarily by the subject in the same position as Parana's manoeuvre with roughly the same meaning [151,179].

***2.4.3.4.* Active foot dorsi-flexion:** muscular systole is voluntarily provoked by the subject under this movement; muscular diastole corresponds to the subsequent rest position (the so called Wunstorf Manoeuvre).

***2.4.3.5. Rising on tiptoes manoeuvre:*** is performed in the immobile standing position. It is supposed to detect, in superficial veins, vicarious open shunts (VOS) due to dynamic and postural occlusions of deep veins.

***2.4.3.6. Walking*** is possible only with appropriate tests, such as plethysmography, but not with angiography or Doppler.

## 2.5. Assessment Manoeuvres for Physical Examination of CVD of the Lower Limbs

*2.5.1. Trendelenburg manoeuvre: (TM)* consists, according to the visible varices and making the patient standing up, in the application of a tourniquet. If the tourniquet presses at the level of, or immediately below an escape point, the reappearance of visible varices will not be immediate but delayed. This is related to the fractioning of hydrostatic pressure [14-17,238].

*2.5.2. Perthes manoeuvre: (PM)* also consists of applying a tourniquet at different levels of the leg, according to the location of visible varices. When the subject walks, the varices collapse if the deep veins are normal, but they do not if the deep veins are impaired. Like TM, this test involves fractioning the column of hydrostatic pressure and disconnecting superficial closed shunts simultaneously. For this reason, the varices collapse when the subject walks, due to the re-entry in an efficient valvulo-muscular pump (VMP). Varices do not collapse when the VMP is impaired, especially because of deep venous incompetence. This is also why Doppler cannot register any reflux flow in saphenas in cases of major deep venous incompetence, yet the saphenas are varicose, being dilated with incompetent valves [14-17].

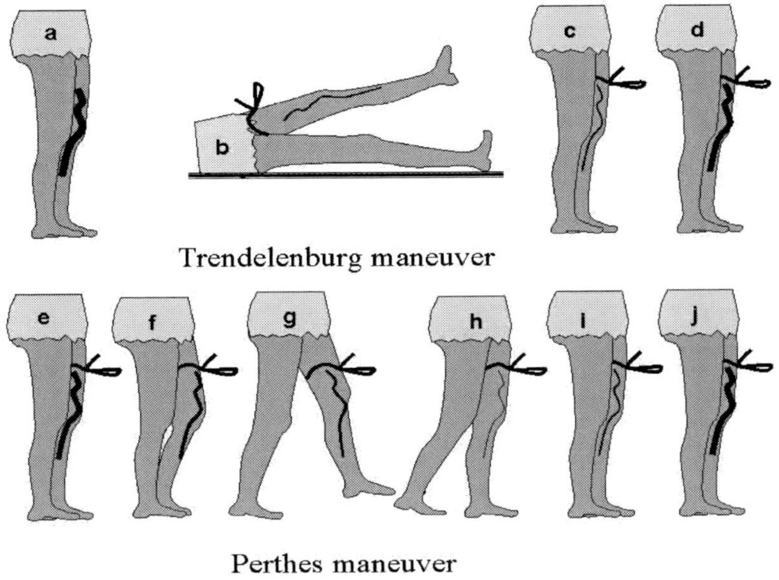


Figure 8.4. Trendelenburg and Perthes maneuvers. Trendelenburg maneuver: a: standing up varicose patient. Varice visible. b: in supine position varice reduces dramatically because Hydrostatic pressure due to gravity is close to 0. A tourniquet is placed at the root of the thigh. c:Then the patient stands up again but immobile . The reduction of the varice persists a while thanks to the fractionation of the hydrostatic pressure column but do not last because the valvulo-muscular pump is inactive and does not fractionate dynamically the deep column of hydrostatic pressure and refills the varice by connected vessels effect. If the maneuver is negative, that may mean that the tourniquet doesn't press properly the escape point of the CS or DOS or that the varicose is due to other causes as VOS or varices fed by an arterio-venous fistulae. e: If the maneuver is positive, the varice remains dilated again except if the patient walks. f,g,h: walking, the varices reduce their caliber because the valvulo-muscular pump is activated and fractionates dynamically the deep column of hydrostatic pressure, which pumps out the varice that cannot be overloaded anymore by the escape point of the shunt, thanks to well placed tourniquet. If walking is inefficient, that means that the valvulo-muscular pump cannot fractionate dynamically the hydrostatic pressure (DFHSP). The most frequent cause is a deep valvular incompetence.

Chapter 9

# HOW TO PERFORM A DUPLEX MAPPING

**Paolo Zamboni**
University of Ferrara, Italy

The next two chapters, due to their eminently practical objectives, are thought as an atlas text. We herein present several paradigmatic cases, choose among the more frequent situations in clinical practice, and adopting an educational technique defined Clinical Theatre. In the present chapter, by referring to the paradigmatic cases, we show as you can realize a complete venous mapping by reconstructing duplex findings found at different levels in the venous system of the lower extremities. Haemodynamic findings are drawn together in a pre-existent model of venous anatomy, subdivided in the different venous networks previously showed. The reader can easily learn a procedural duplex protocol in order to realize a complete venous mapping.

In the chapter 10, the same clinical cases undergo to a haemodynamic correction procedure (CHIVA) on the basis of the haemodynamic mapping showed in this chapter. The techniques will be demonstrated both by figures and operative pictures.

## CLINICAL CASE A: The lawyer.

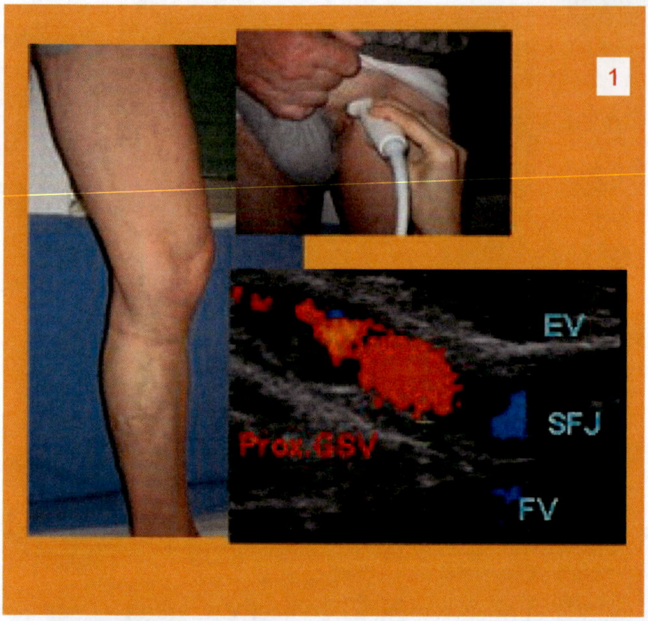


55 yo man, lawyer. Both parents affected by CVD. C2s (heaviness, ref. edema in the evening, in summer). Cosmetic complaints.

**Fig. 1:** Duplex mapping. Phase 1: investigation of the SFJ in standing. Rough analysis by the means of color Doppler and calf squeezing clearly shows reflux in the proximal GSV (red color) with normal emptying (blu color) at the level of the SFJ, epigastric vein EV and femoral vein FV.

## CLINICAL CASE A: assessment of the terminal valve

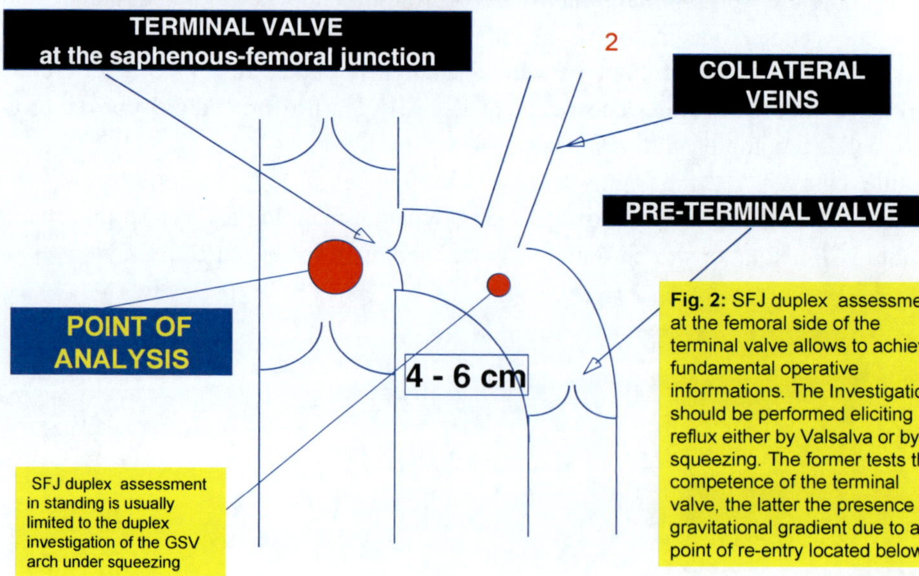


**Fig. 2:** SFJ duplex assessment at the femoral side of the terminal valve allows to achieve fundamental operative inforrmations. The Investigation should be performed eliciting reflux either by Valsalva or by squeezing. The former tests the competence of the terminal valve, the latter the presence of a gravitational gradient due to a point of re-entry located below.[46]

**Fig. 3:** Further analysis by placing the Doppler sample on the femoral side of the terminal valve demonstrate a competent valve at the Valsalva manoeuver. The correctness of the patient' s execution is proved by the re-appearance of the spontaneous forward flow at the Valsalva release.[46,241,245]

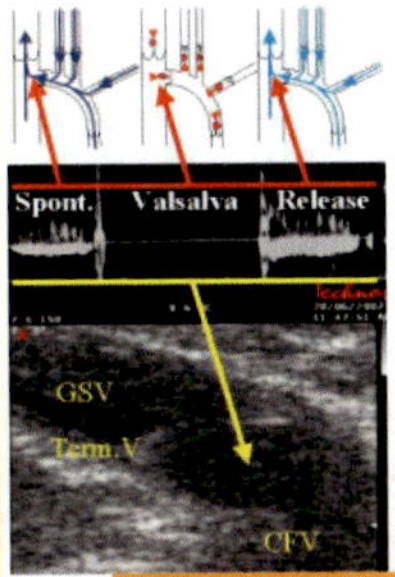


3

3a

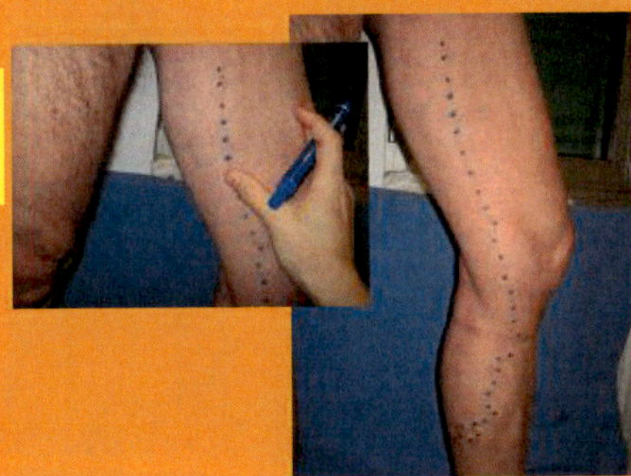

**Fig. 3a:** Any visible and palpable vein of the lower limb is then outlined by a waterproof pen.

# CLINICAL CASE A: SCANNING THE "EYE"

**Fig. 4:**

A. The saphenous eye sign, in the transverse access, allows to identify the GSV main trunk below the competent S-F terminal valve. GSV is insufficient when eliciting reflux by squeezing (Doppler PW trace: negative wave in compression-systole, positive wave at the release-diastole).

B. Localization of the junction between the GSV (N2) and the insufficient tributary T (N4). This is a reflux point N2-N4 (change of compartment from AC2 to AC3).

C. The escape point feed by reflux a tributary T, lying above the superficial fascia, whereas the GSV, markedly reduced in caliber, is now competent.

D. The long insufficient T re-enters into the N2 (GSV) for a short segment. This is the reason because the T is to be considered a N4 instead of a N3 (N2-N4-N2 circuit).

E. Again, through a second reflux point the blood changes compartment and flows from N2 to N3, feeding by reflux varicose veins of the medial and posterior aspect of the leg.

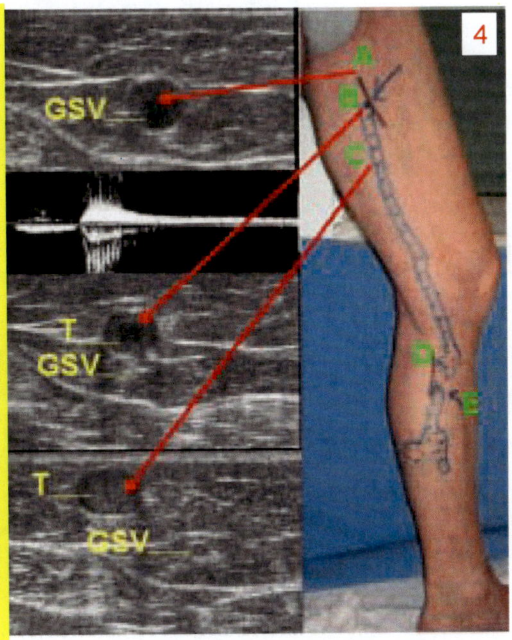


4

## CLINICAL CASE A:

## The concept of cartography.

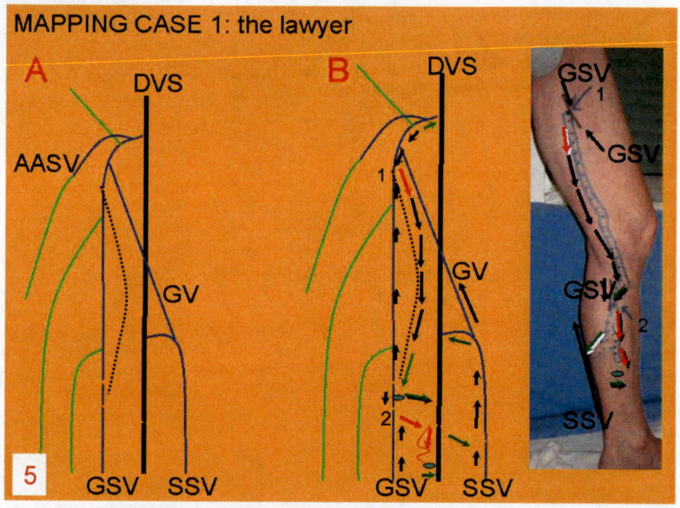


**Fig. 5:** Since duplex allows a perfect flow analysis but point by point, the investigator reports the findings on a model, depicted in panel A, in order to permit a coherent overview of the entire venous tree. Legenda: Black N1 segments, blue N2 segments, interrupted line N4 segments, green N3 segments. Downward arrows indicate reflux, while up-ward arrows competent segments. Red arrows depict points of reflux. Green arrows re-entry points. Green ovoid re-entry perforator.
B)1 Point of reflux N2-N4, 2 Point of reflux N2-N3.Green arrows re-entry points. Green ovoid re-entry perforator.

## CLINICAL CASE A: The lawyer. REFLUX ELIMINATION TEST

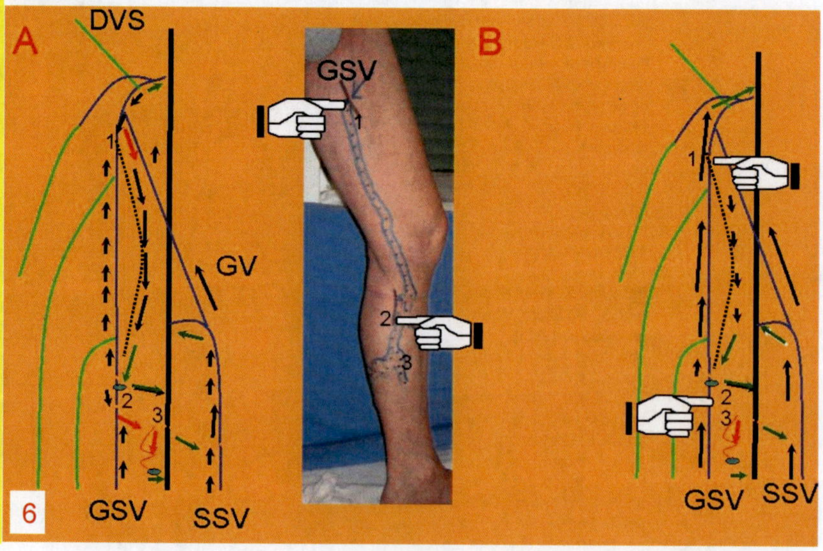


**Fig. 6:**
REFLUX ELIMINATION TEST. Simple finger compression of the origin of reflux in the tributaries allows to re-test the directional flow both in the GSV and in the N3-N4 tributaries, and to identify the shunt type, as well. In such case a type III shunt is showed (with competent terminal valve previously assessed).
In fact finger compression allows to completely eliminate reflux in the proximal GSV. This is the best demonstration that reflux in the GSV trunk is due to the antidromic gradient created by the long incompetent and valveless N4. [254]

# CLINICAL CASE B: The farmer

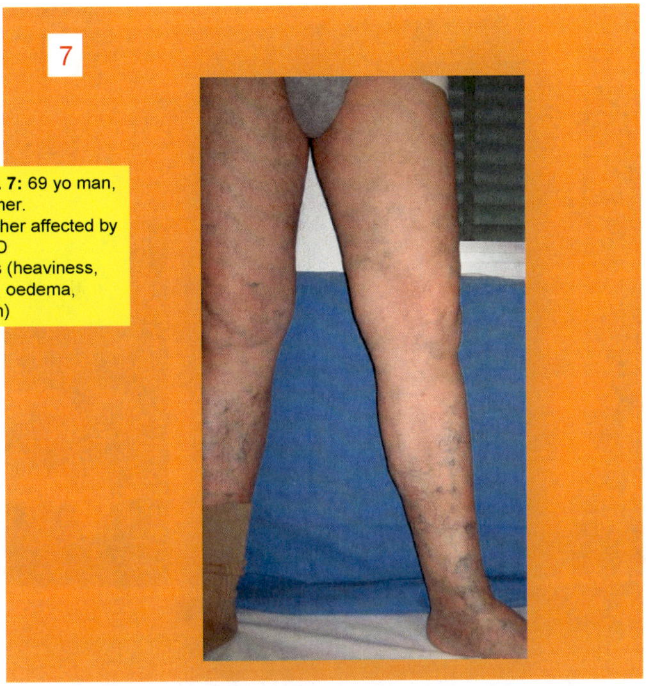


**Fig. 7:** 69 yo man, farmer.
Mother affected by CVD
C3s (heaviness, ref. oedema, pain)

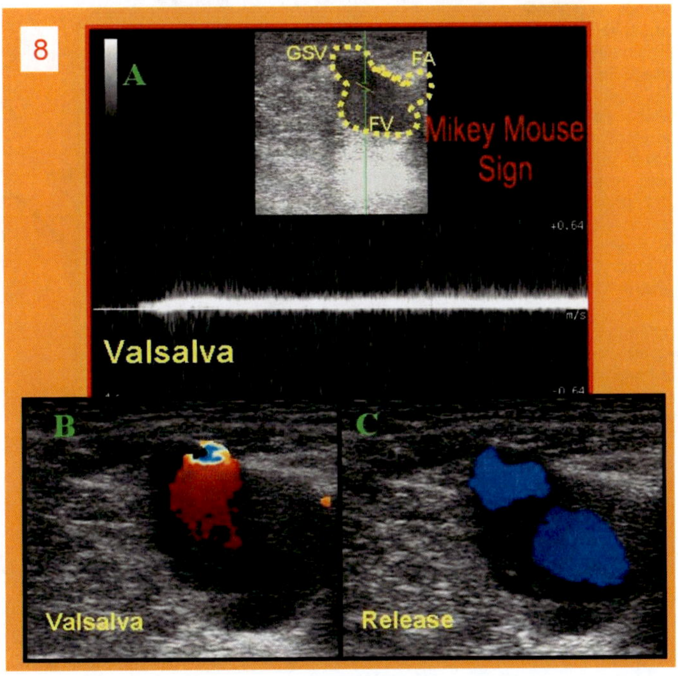


**Fig. 8:**
**Panel A:** SFJ is recognized by the so-called Mikey Mouse Sign, depicted in the transverse duplex access of the groin by the anatomical relationship of the FV, the head, with the 2 ears, GSV and FA, respectively. The Doppler PW sample placed on the femoral side of the terminal valve registers a SF reflux under Valsalva.
**Panel B:** Color Doppler mode confirms the incompetence of the terminal valve (red color through the junction).
**Panel C:** The correctness of the patient' s execution is proved by the re-appearance of the spontaneous forward flow at the Valsalva release, blu Color.

**Squeezing of the proximal GSV confirms reflux. Concordance of squeezing and Valsalva is the indication to the treatment of the SFJ.**

**Fig. 9:** Duplex findings are reported in a different cartographic model, which can be adopted by the reader in alternative to that proposed for the case A. It reports just N1 (deep) and N2 trunks (GSV, SSV, GiacV). It allows the reconstruction of the venous map step by step.

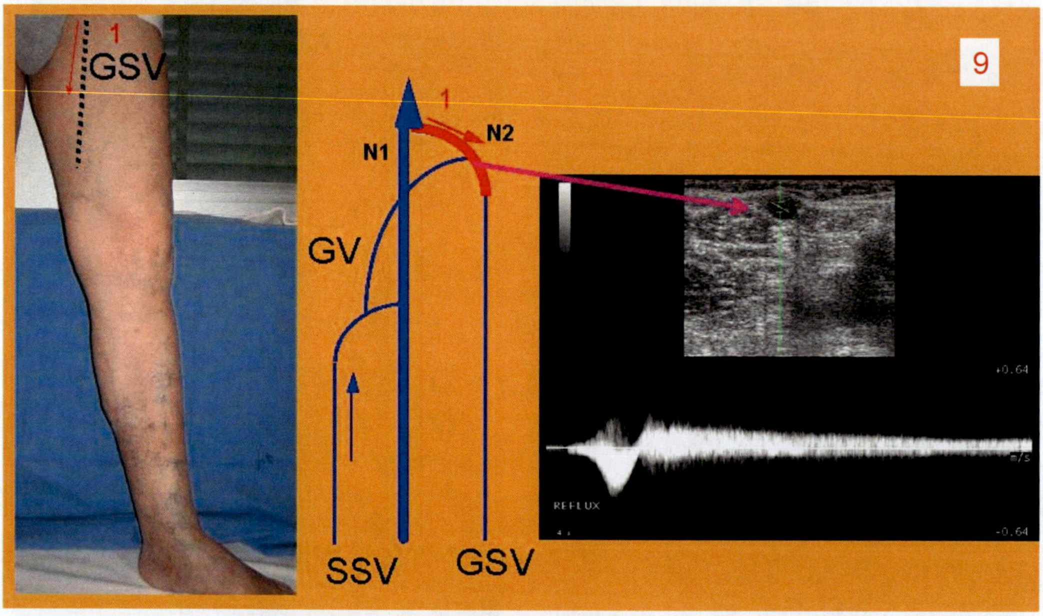


**Fig. 10:**
**Panel A:** thigh varicose vein originating from the GSV at point 2.
**Panel B:** Since it lies above the SF layer in the AC3, and re-enters in N1 through a re-entry perforator, it is a N3 tributary.
**Panel C:** Reflux N2-N3 with change of compartment is clearly documented by color Doppler and squeezing.

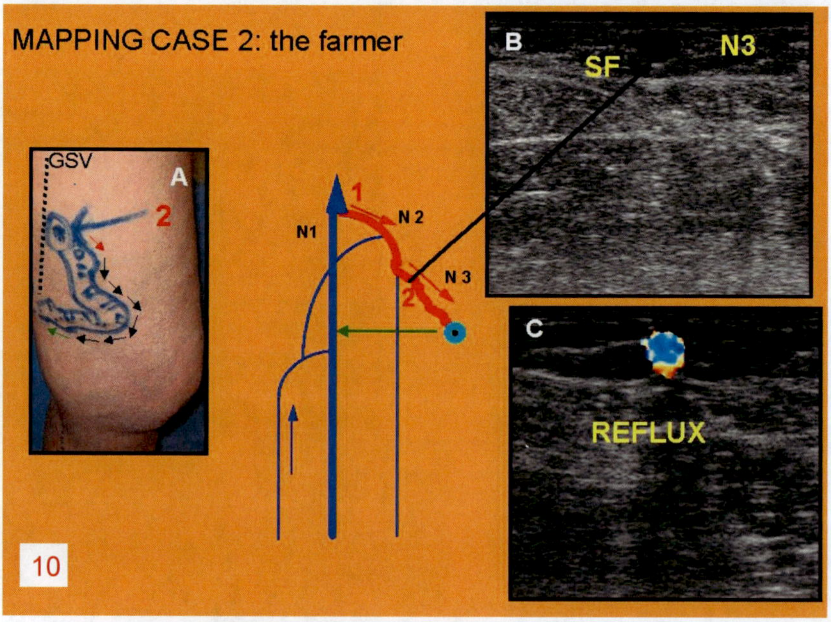

**Fig. 11:** Reflux is still present in GSV main trunk below the reflux point 2, N2-N3. This finding suggests the presence below of further re-entry points. " No reflux, no re-entry and viceversa".

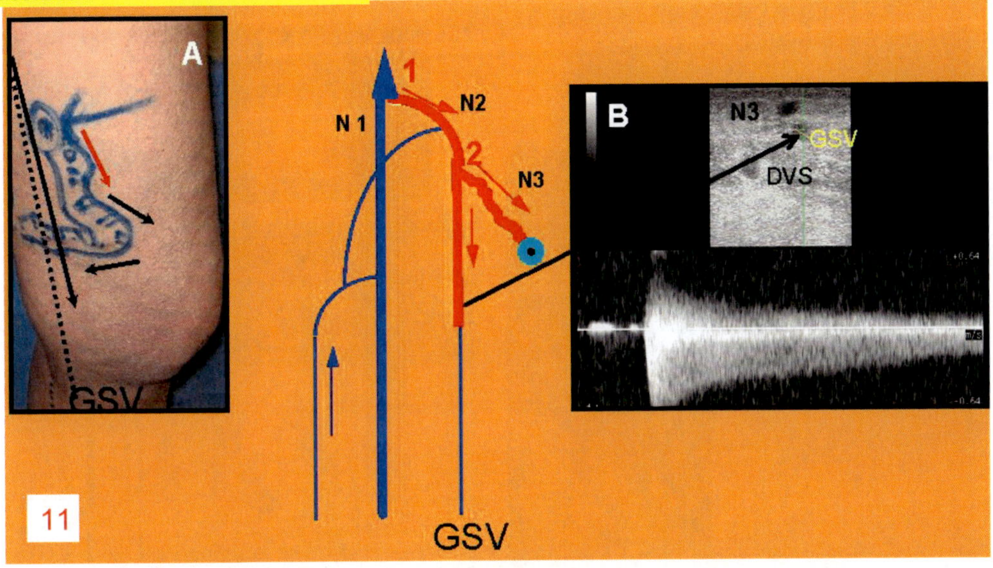


**Fig. 12:** Below the knee a new N2-N3 reflux point is detected at point 3. Again reflux in the GSV is detected below, suggesting the presence of a re-entry distally.

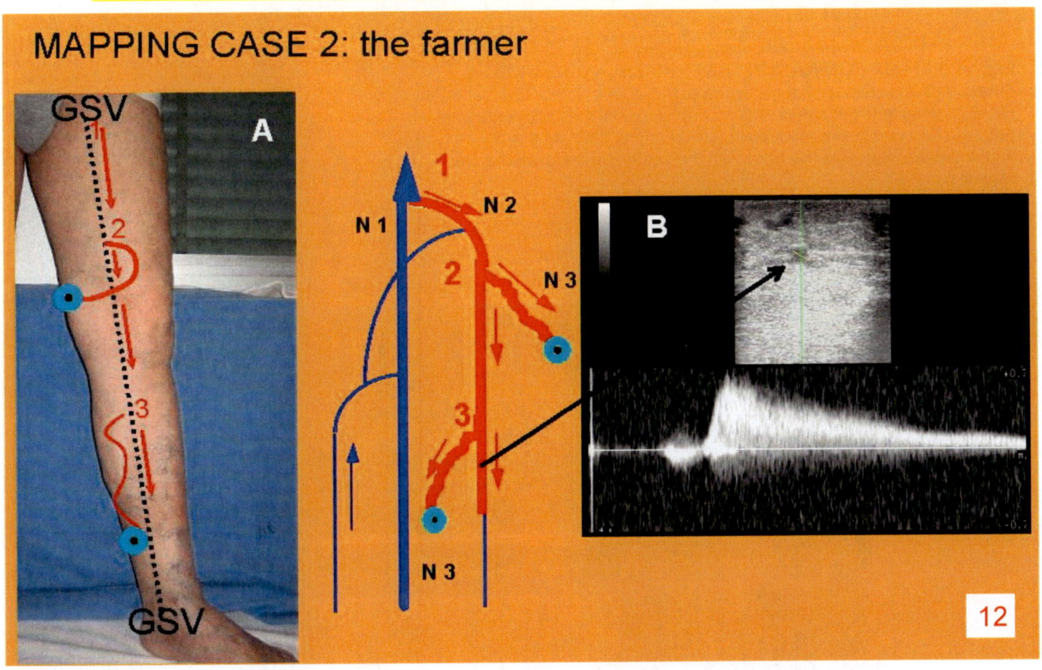

**Fig. 13:** Finally, few centimeters above the ankle a re-entry perforator located on the saphenous trunk is detected (A-B-C). Please, note the in ward flow demonstrated at the release-muscular diastole proved by the negative wave (D). Now the distal GSV is competent

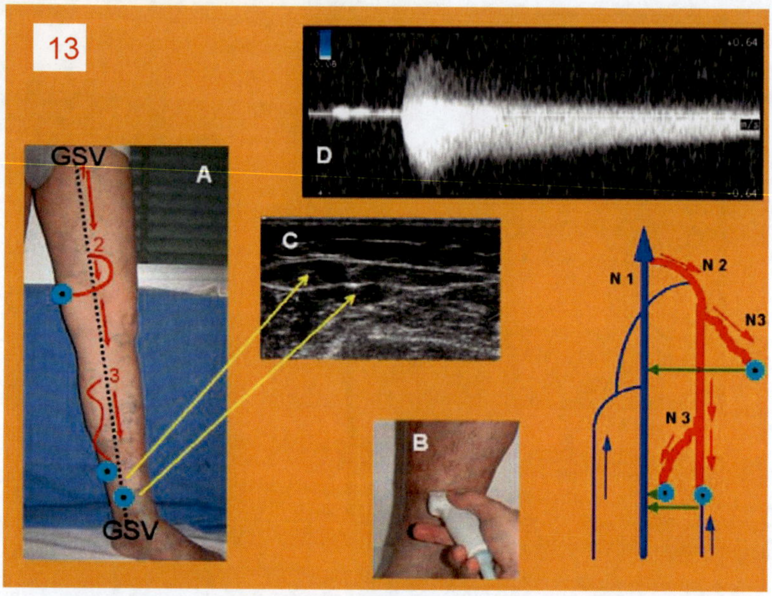


**Fig. 14: REFLUX ELIMINATION TEST AND SHUNT DEFINITION.** Finally, reflux is reduced but still active at the level of the GSV main trunk (B1-B2), despite finger compression of reflux points 2 and 3. A gradient between SFJ and the re-entry point (green arrow) maintains a closed type I shunt. Please, compare this case with the same test performed in the clinical case A.

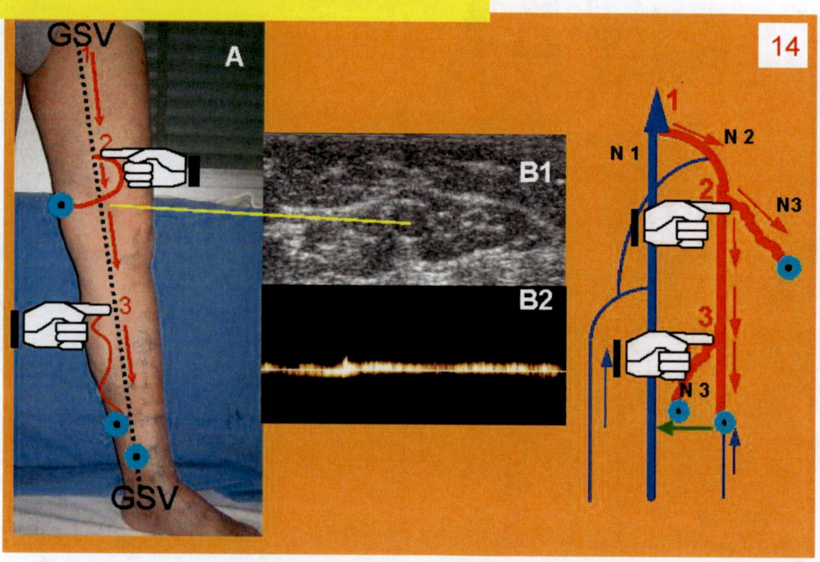

**Fig. 15:** Reflux elimination test permit to differentiate type III from type I shunt. Reflux elimination test in the case of the farmer was negative for the presence of a re-entry perforator on the GSV (persistent gravitational gradient). [254]

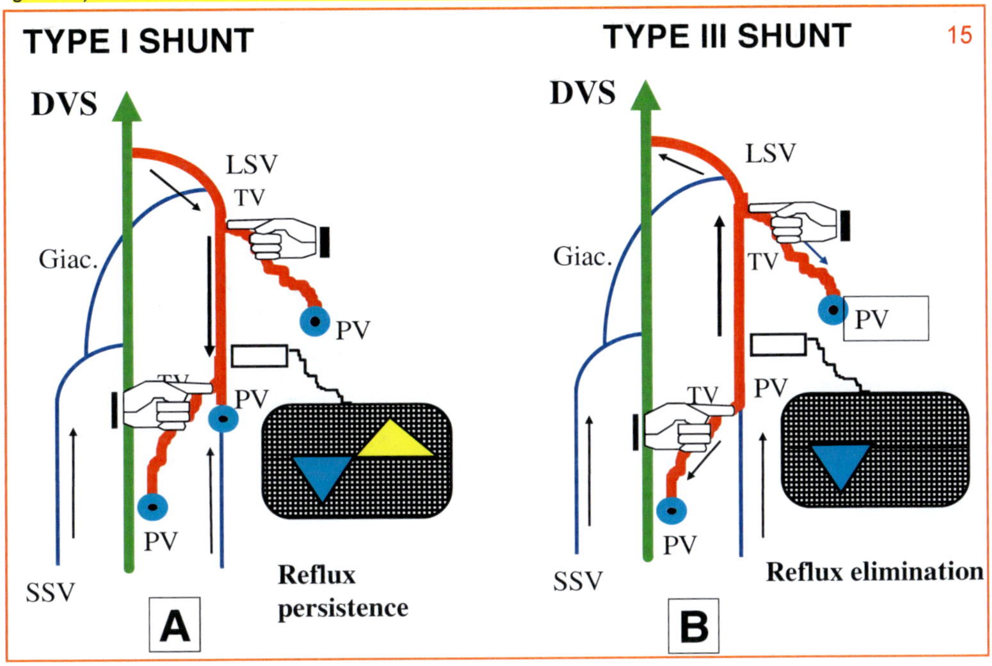


## Appendix To Clinical Cases A and B: absence of re-entry perforator on the saphenous trunk and incompetent terminal valve. The so-called type III shunt

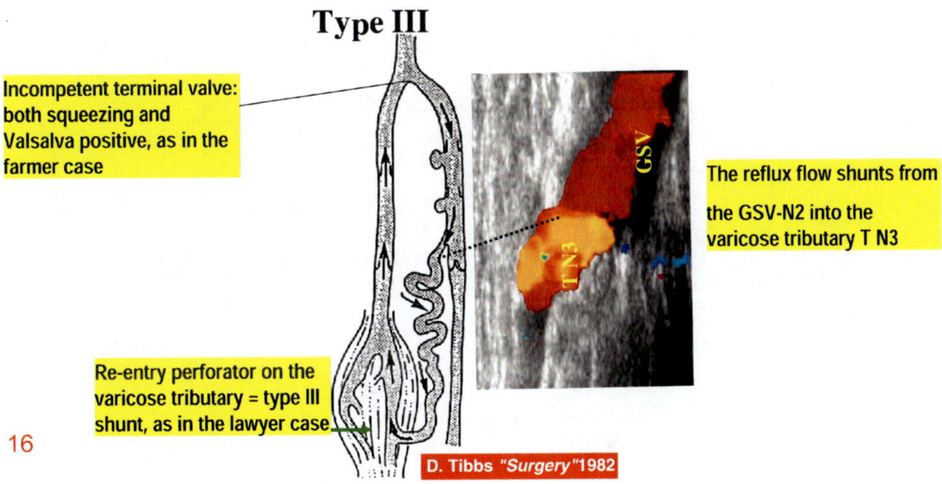

## The case of absence of re-entry perforator on the saphenous trunk and incompetent terminal valve.

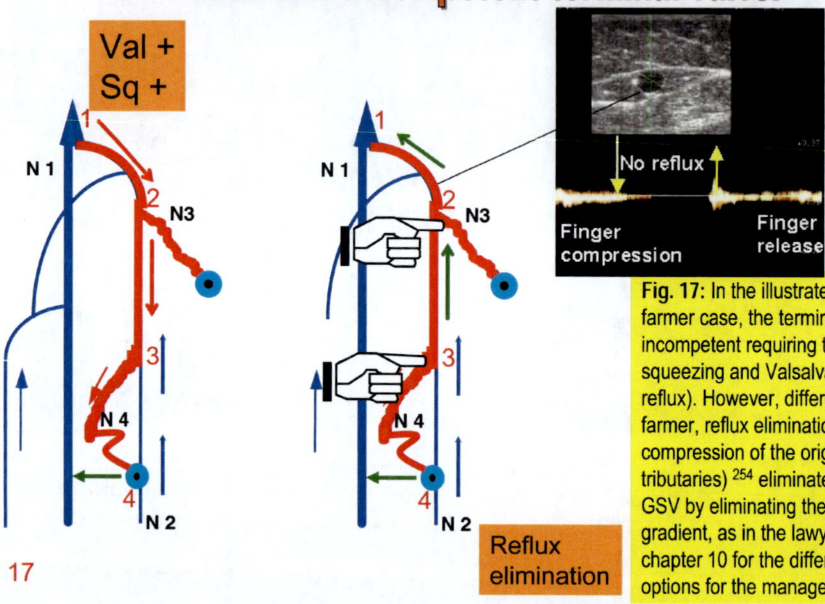


**Fig. 17:** In the illustrated case, as in the farmer case, the terminal valve is incompetent requiring treatment (both squeezing and Valsalva positive for reflux). However, differently from the farmer, reflux elimination test (finger compression of the origin of the tributaries) [254] eliminates reflux in the GSV by eliminating the gravitational gradient, as in the lawyer case. See chapter 10 for the different CHIVA options for the management of this case.

## CLINICAL CASE C: woman in child birth

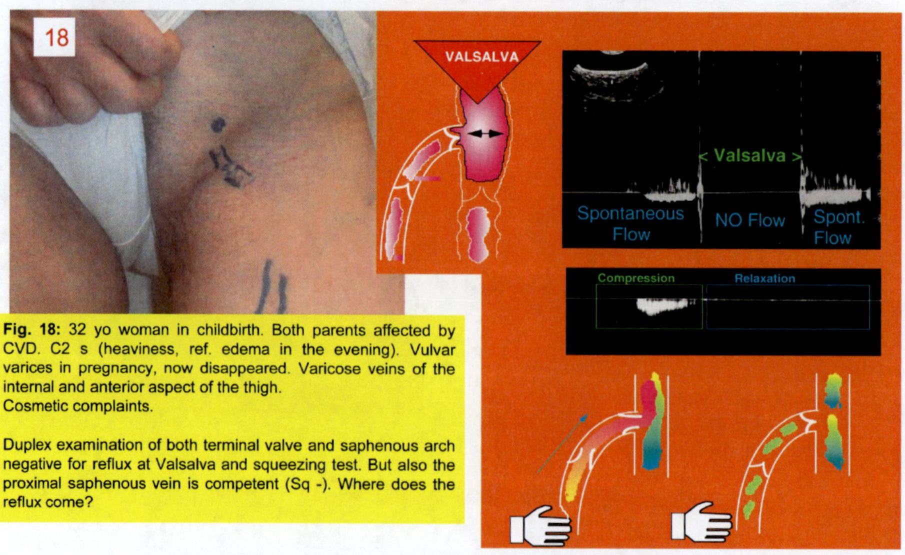


**Fig. 18:** 32 yo woman in childbirth. Both parents affected by CVD. C2 s (heaviness, ref. edema in the evening). Vulvar varices in pregnancy, now disappeared. Varicose veins of the internal and anterior aspect of the thigh.
Cosmetic complaints.

Duplex examination of both terminal valve and saphenous arch negative for reflux at Valsalva and squeezing test. But also the proximal saphenous vein is competent (Sq -). Where does the reflux come?

# CLINICAL CASE C: pelvic shunts

**Fig. 19:**

A. As previously stated duplex investigation in standing demonstrates at the SFJ level (Minnie sign in woman) a competent terminal valve with no reflux in the proximal GSV. This finding is reported in map 1.

B. Following by the duplex probe the outlined varicose veins clinically manifest at the groin level (C), we find out a reflux of the round ligament vein at the level of the inguinal canal. It fed a N3 vein of the thigh through the so-called I point (see chapter 7), corresponding to the external opening of the inguinal canal (C).

2. Corresponding duplex map shows the above described findings, and the re-entry of the insufficient N3(red tortuos line) in the GSV 30 cm below the SFJ.

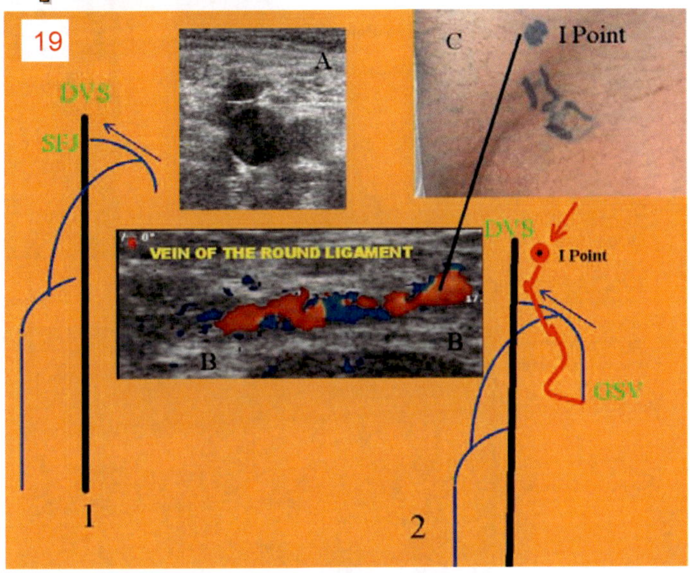


**Fig. 20:**
Careful observation of the patient demonstrates varicose veins also in the upper internal aspect of the thigh, corresponding to the P point described at chapter 7, blue circle. The corresponding ultrasonography is given in A.
In B, reflux through the P point, via the vein of the Alcock canal, into the insufficient N3 is well demonstrated.

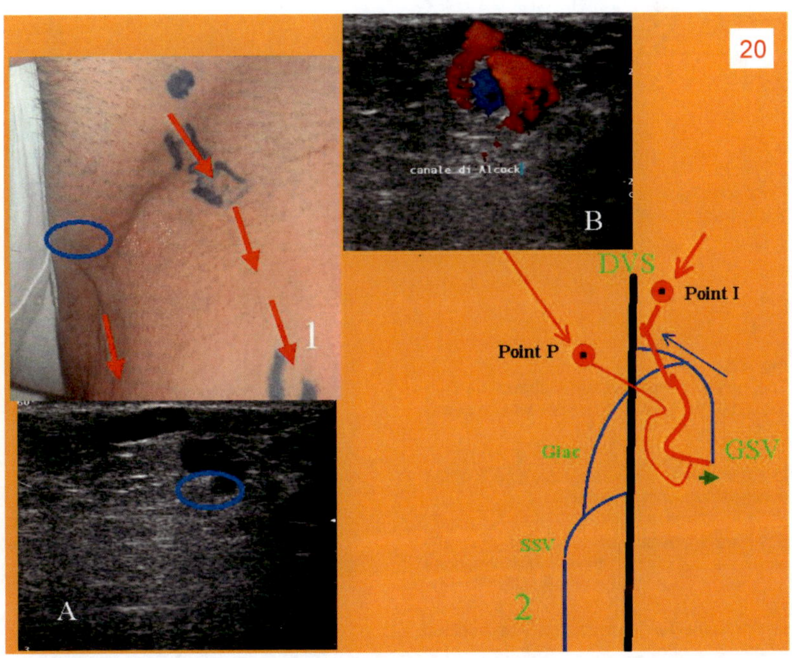

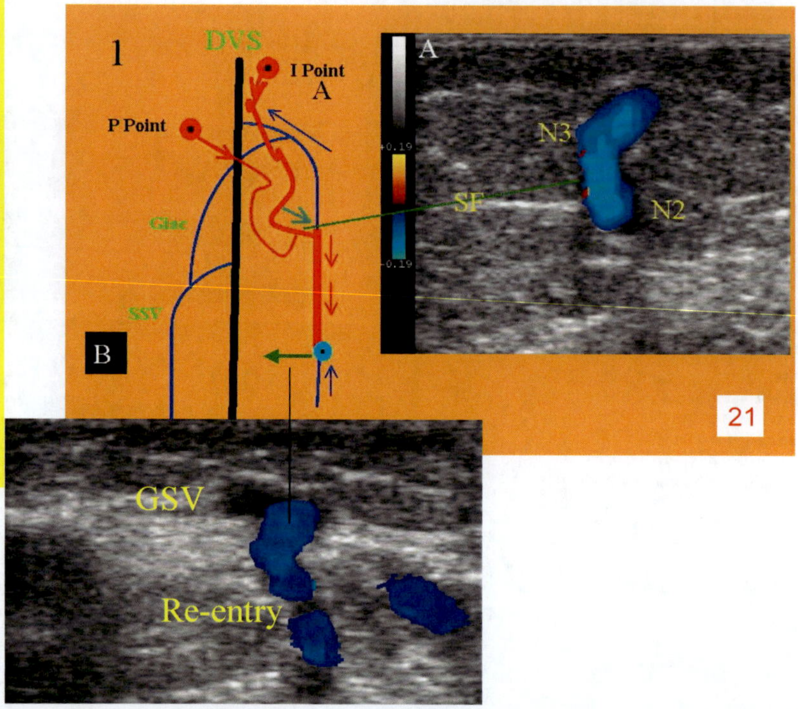


**Fig. 21:** The corresponding map indicates that the second insufficient N3 joins the first one, and re-enters the GSV through a common segment, in A. The GSV, fed by both pelvic refluxes is incompetent below the re-entry point. In turn, the GSV re-enters through a paratibial perforator into the competent N1.

# SOME THOUGHTS ON CLINICAL CASE C

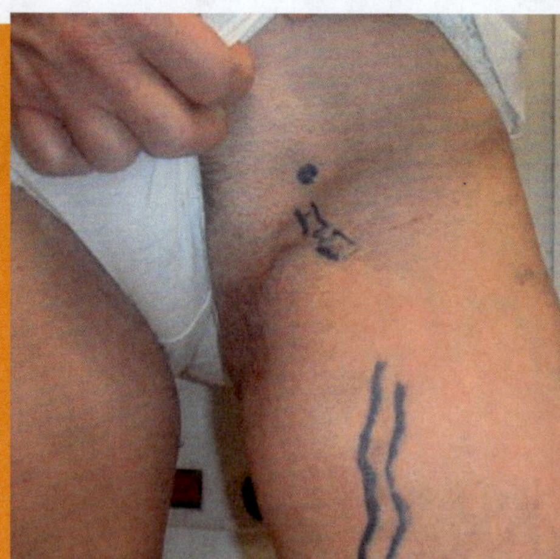

**Fig. 22:**
The herein presented case shows CVD in the GSV territory with competent proximal GSV.

In our survey this case represents 8% of the varicose networks in females.

Standard\endovascular surgery should eliminate the main outflow route and does not treat the real source of reflux.[2,63.64]

In this case we cannot use standardized ablative\ endovascular procedures but surgery tailored and guided by duplex findings (see chapter 10, 20-22).

22

# CLINICAL CASE D: the hairdresser

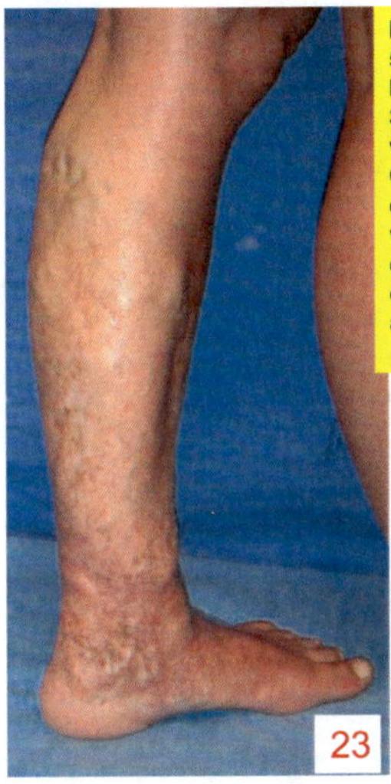


**Fig. 23:** 52 yo woman, hairdresser. Symptomatic varicose veins 8 years ago. C5 s (heaviness, pain, edema, recurrent varicose ulcers despite elastic stocking exerting 20-30 mmHg at the ankle). Low QoL

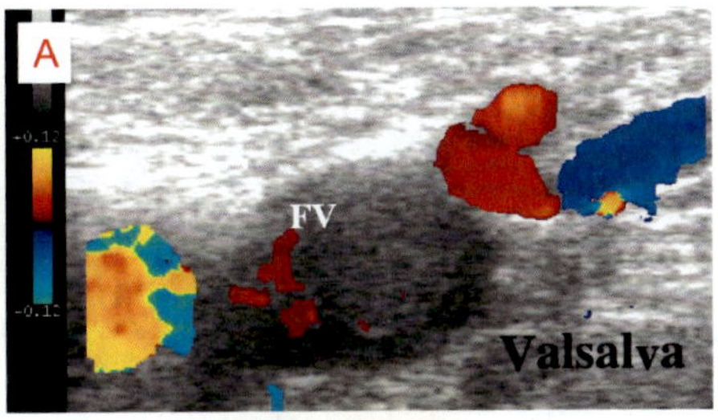


**A:** Duplex investigation in standing of the GSV territory is completely negative. However, physical examination indicates CVD from reflux in the SSV territory. No DVS incompetence.

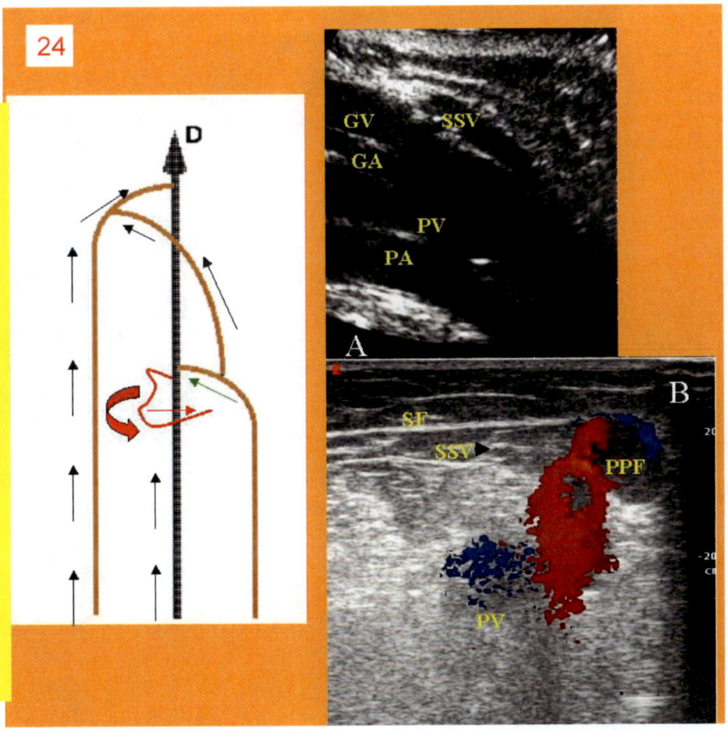


**Fig. 24:**
A) Further duplex investigation of the popliteal fossa in the longitudinal access reveal no reflux either under squeezing or Valsalva at the level of the SSV, popliteal vein (PV), gastrocnemius vein (GV). PA and GA are referred to popliteal artery and gastrocnemius artery, respectively.

B) ColorDoppler investigation in the transversal access of the popliteal fossa demonstrates a huge reflux starting on the lateral side of the competent PV. Note the little diameter of the competent SSV, which proximally is not involved in the reflux (saphenous eye sign, where SF indicates the superficial fascia). The reflux goes outward through a vein called perforator of the popliteal fossa (PPF). Such vein is also named Dodd or Thiery perforating vein from the name of the Authors who described it.

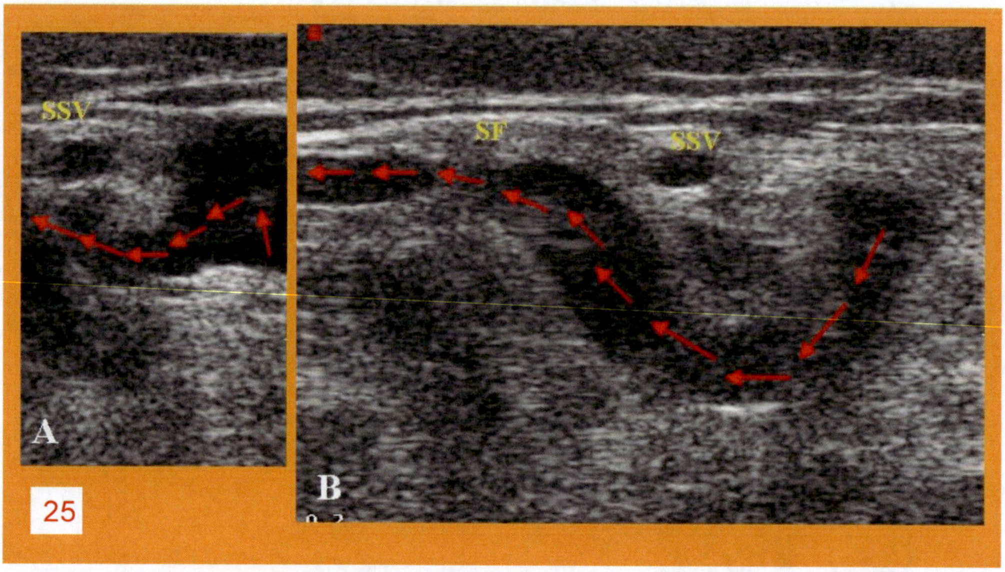


**Fig. 25:**
**A. B.** Following the route of the PPF it easy to demonstrate the absence of contact with proximal SSV (eye sign, SF superficial fascia). The route of the PPF from its origin on the lateral side of the PV is really very tortuos.

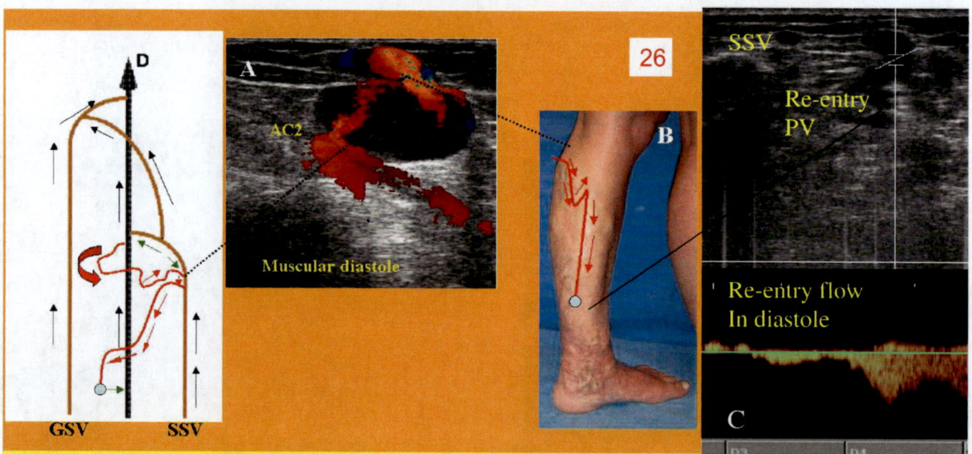


**Fig. 26:**
A) After a long subfascial pathway, previously shown, the PPF enter in the AC2 compartment and feed by reflux the SSV, which becomes incompetent for a very short segment. Note the enlargement of the SSV after connection with the refluxing PPF (non terminal perforator, reflux outward flow in muscular diastole). Immediately below such connection, the reflux shunts from the AC2 compartment to the AC3 compartment (reflux N2-N3).

B) The N2-N3 reflux makes apparent a varicose vein located really distally from the reflux point in the popliteal fossa.

C) The N3 goes downward and runs medially toward the re-entry perforating veins, where the reflux re-entries into the N1. Inward flow in muscular diastole

The map reports all the above described duplex findings.

# SOME THOUGHTS ON CLINICAL CASE D

**Fig. 27:** The herein presented case shows severe CVD, CEAP C5, related to varicose veins of the SSV territory. However, duplex mapping demonstrates that reflux was detected in SSV main trunk just in a segment of few centimeters. In addition, the SPJ as well as the rest of the trunk are completely competent.

In this case we cannot use standardized ablative procedures but surgery tailored and guided by duplex findings (see chapter 10).[63-65, 76, 83, 88, 109, 190, 198]

Finally, the closed shunt is a circuit between two perforators: In the popliteal fossa the reflux point is a non terminal perforator (reflux in diastole, see chapter 12), at the ankle the re-entry point is a terminal perforator (correct flow in-ward in muscular diastole).

The re-entry perforator is located close to the scar of the healed ulcer and such a topography is enough for indicating its ablation, despite the correct haemodynamic function. To the contrary, its flow is insufficient respect to the reflux flow transported through the PPF. The haemodynamic overload should be corrected by the treatment of the latter.

The preoperative assessment of the flow direction at muscular relaxation in perforators is the key for giving or not the surgical indication to their treatment (chapter 12).

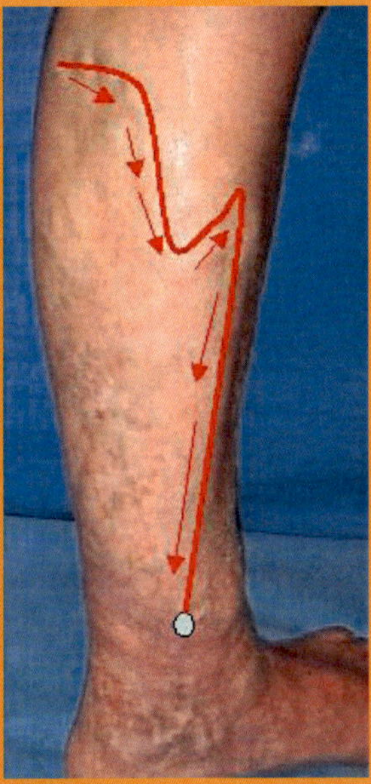

27

# CLINICAL CASE E:saleswoman

**Fig. 28:** 46 yo man, saleswoman.
Varicose veins in the left calf heaviness, pain, edema, hitching confined to the left leg C2S
Working disability

Duplex investigation in standing of the GSV territory is completely negative. Truncular varicose veins are visible and palpable at the left calf, according to referred symptoms.

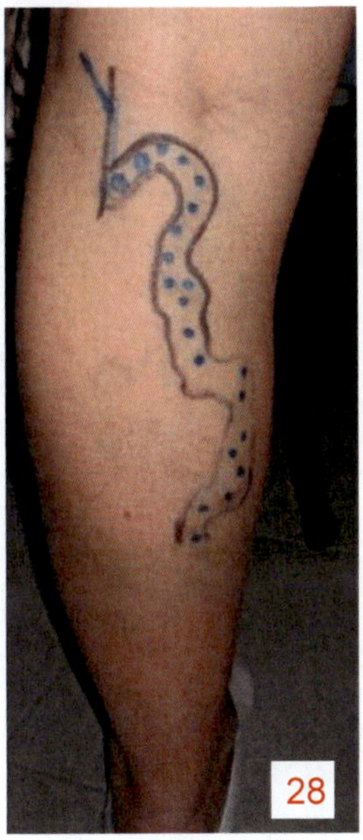

28

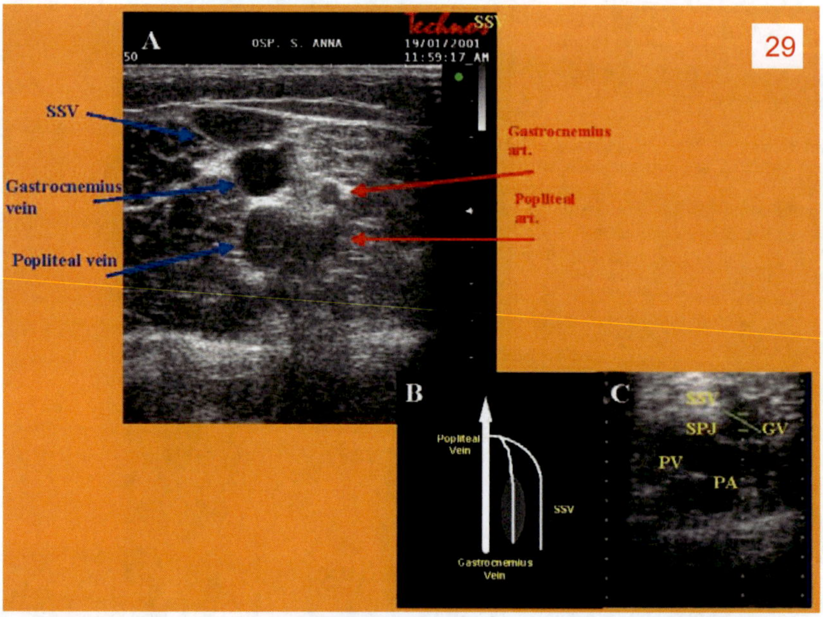


**Fig. 29:**
A.Duplex exploration of the popliteal fossa shows a dilated SSV and gastrocnemius vein (GV) at the level of the poplitel fossa.

B-C
SPJ is a common trunk with the terminal GV
The common outlet of both SSV and GV is showed in relative map and B-Mode image

**Fig. 30:**
A.Both Paranà and squeezing manouver demonstrates reflux at the SPJ and in the SSV main trunk. Valsalva is positive at the confluence between SSV and GV , indicating the incompetence of such valve.

B.We document reflux also in the GV, elicited by active manouvers and not by Valsalva, indicating the competence of the common trunk terminal valve. From the common outlet in the PV, reflux is extensively propagated along the entire muscle in the AC1, while PV is competent below the SPJ.

C.The above reported findings are reported in the map under construction.

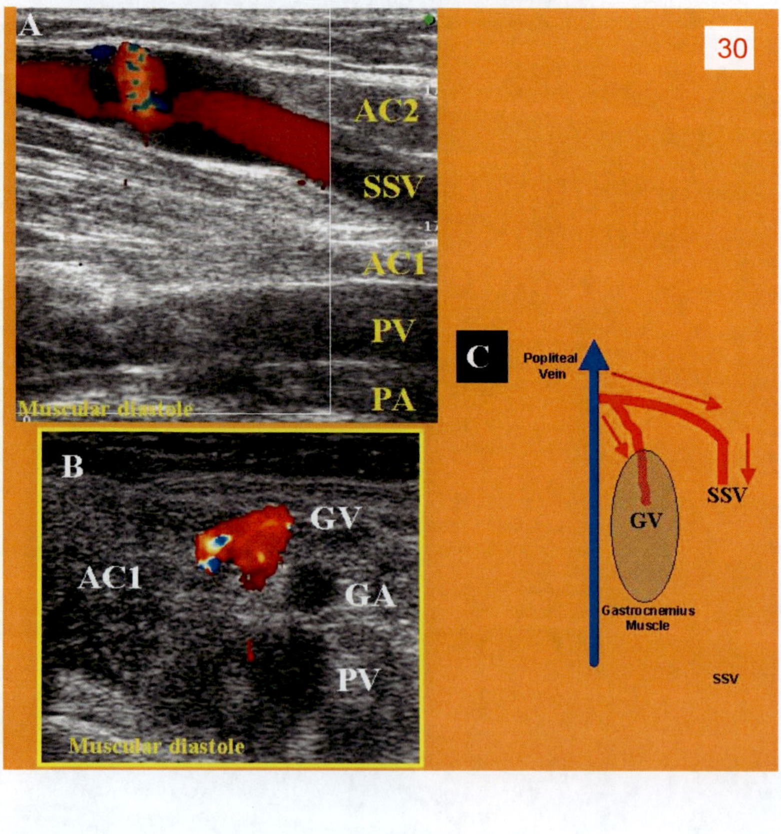

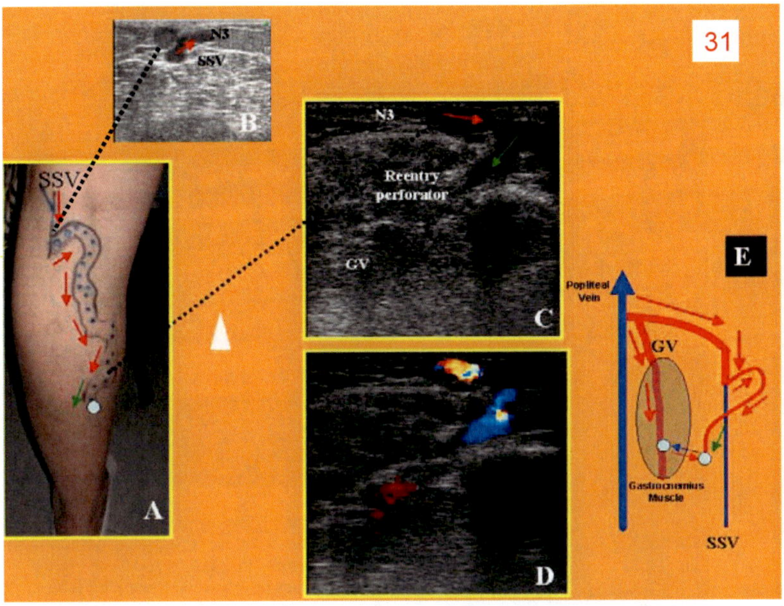


**Fig. 31:**
A. Reflux from the SSV shunts to N3, and feed a gross varicose tributary of the posterior aspect of the calf.

B. The corresponding B-mode image of the N2-N3 reflux.

C. The long N3 reenters in a calf perforator connected with the GV.

D. The corresponding colorDoppler of C demonstrates the reflux in the N3 (red), the reentry in the N1 (blue), and the propagation of reflux in the distal GV (red).

E. The corresponding map of the above reported findings.

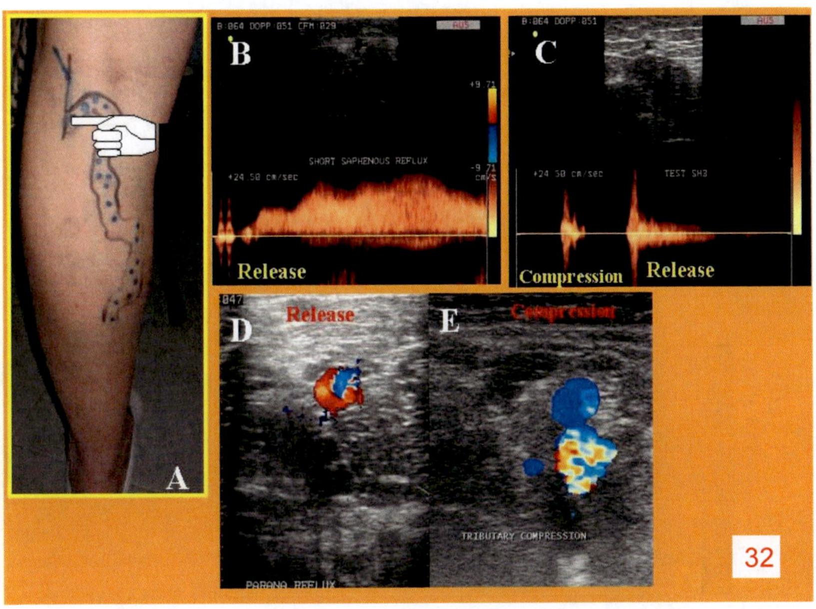


**Fig. 32:**
A. Modification of the haemodynamic pattern by elimination of the gravitational gradient created by the incompetent N3, obtained by finger compression of its origin on the SSV trunk.

B. Pattern of reflux in the SSV main trunk.

C. Disappereance of SSV reflux by finger compression, and re-appearance at finger release.

D. Reflux in the Gastrocnemius vein.

E. Reflux elimination in the Gastrocnemius vein by simple finger compression of the N3 which aspirates blood flow from N1.

# Clinical Case E: haemodynamics of the Giacomini' vein

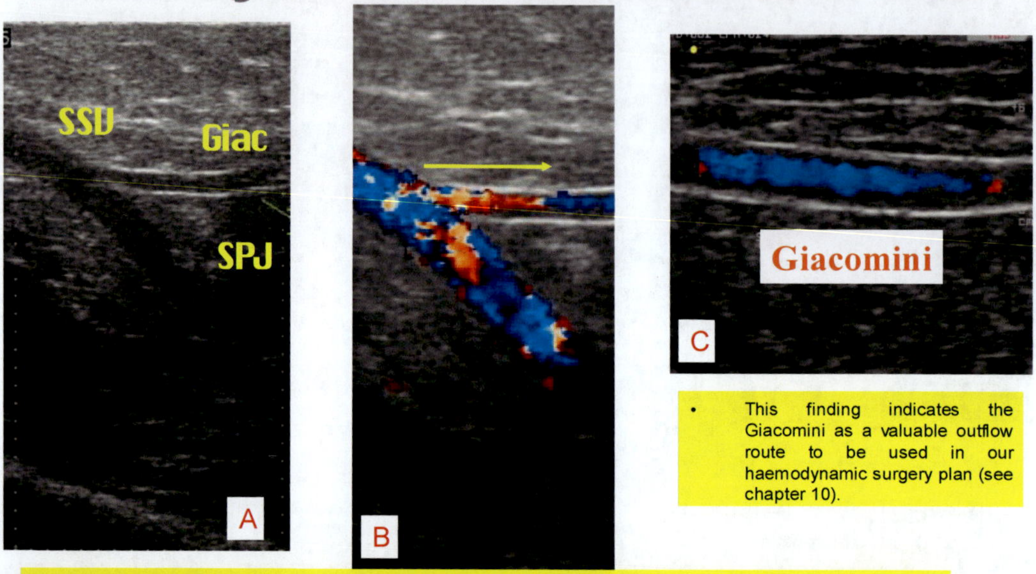


• This finding indicates the Giacomini as a valuable outflow route to be used in our haemodynamic surgery plan (see chapter 10).

**Fig. 33:**
A. B-mode study of the Giacomini vein.
B. Emptying under Paranà manouvre also through the Giacomini' vein.
C. Forward flow along the Giacomini' vein during muscular systole.

33

## COMMENT ON CLINICAL CASE E: saleswoman

34

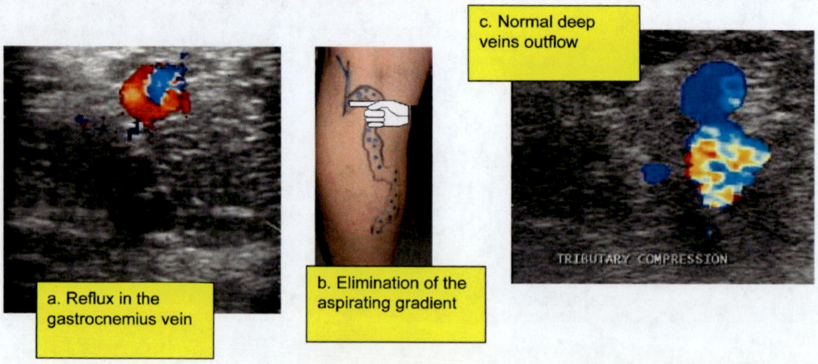


**Fig. 34:** We learn from this case the followings:

•A deep reflux could be the haemodynamic effect of blood aspiration from a refluxing superficial vein. [133,210,247]

•A primary deep reflux is not always synonymous of a disease of the deep veins

•It could be managed by simple superficial surgery, avoiding either unsatisfactory conservative treatment or useless aggressive surgical procedures.

# CLINICAL CASE F:the molecular biologist

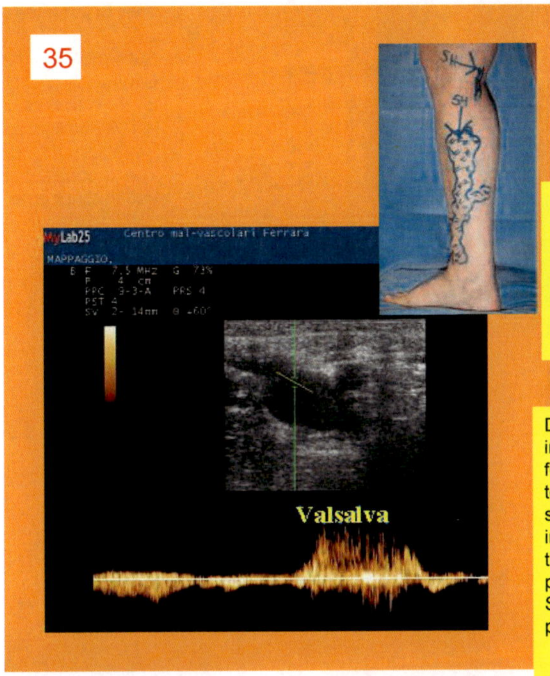


**Fig. 35:** 45 yo woman, molecular biologist. Varicose veins, heaviness, pain, oedema, hitching confined to the the right leg. C2S

Duplex investigation at the femoral side of the terminal valve shows clearly the incompetence of the valve (Valsalva positive). Squeezing is even positive.

# CLINICAL CASE F: Lambda SFJ

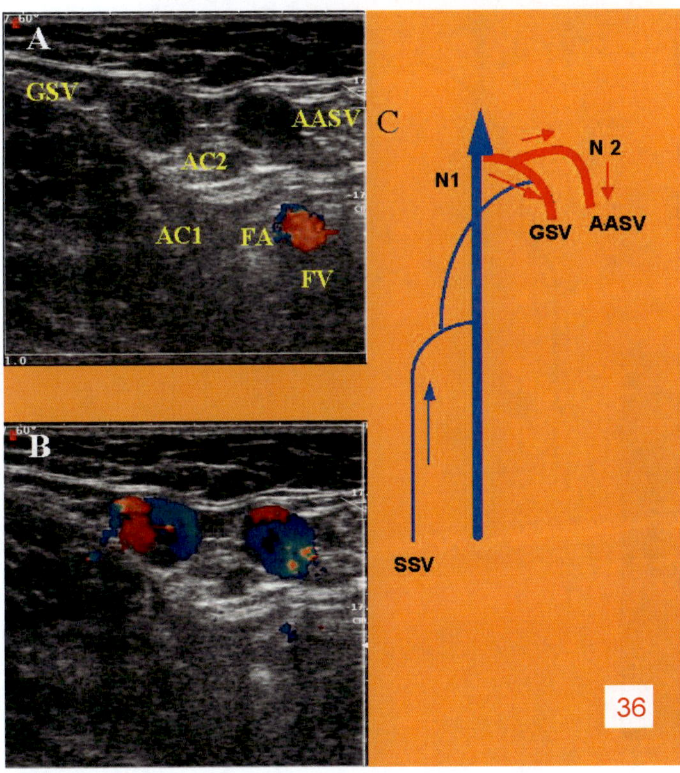


**Fig. 36:** Immediately below the junction the saphenous trunk is split into two veins, both of the AC2. The alignment sign indicates the anterior accessory saphenous vein (AASV) as the vein on the right, while the vein not aligned with the femoral vessels (FA, FV) is the GSV (Fig. A). Both the GSV and the AASV appear insufficient at squeezing manouvre (Fig. B). The map under construction shows the so called lambda presentation of the sapheno femoral junction.

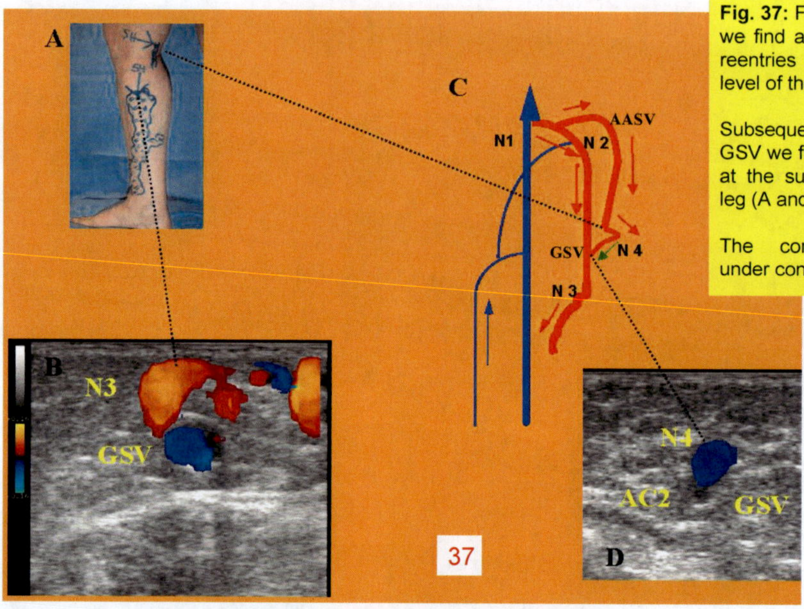


**Fig. 37:** Following the AASV we find a N2-N4 reflux that reentries in the GSV at the level of the knee (D).

Subsequently, following the GSV we find a N2-N3 reflux at the superior third of the leg (A and B).

The corresponding map under construction

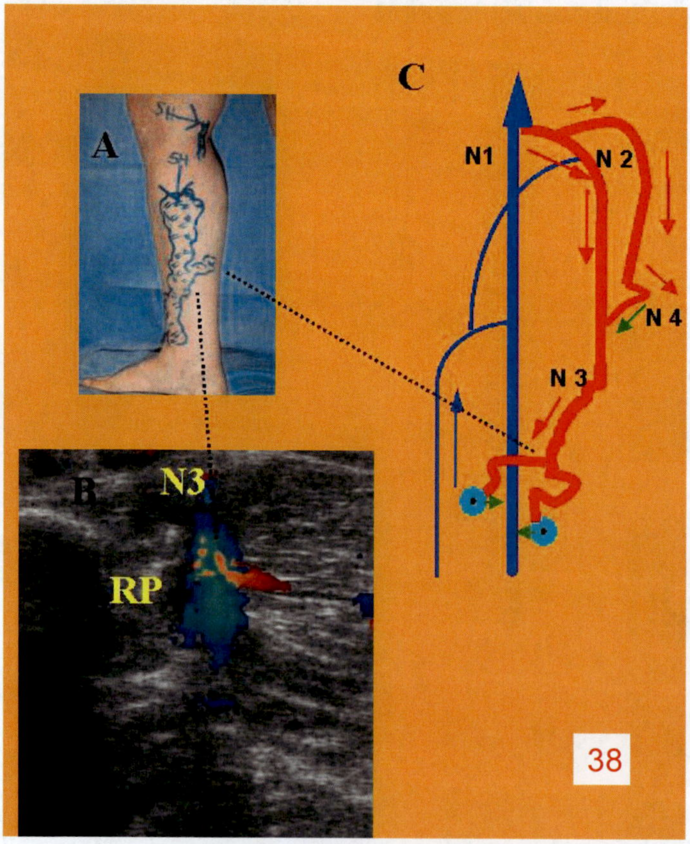


**Fig. 38:** Following the N3, it feeds by reflux large varicose veins. The main circuit reenters in a Cockett perforator (B), while a secondary circuit lies posteriorly where in turn reentries.

B)Reentry through a Cockett perforator in muscular diastole of the main N3 circiut (blue color indicates the inward flow).

The corresponding map is given in C.

**Fig. 39:** Finally, following the GSV reflux by duplex scan we identify its re-entry through a perforator (Fig. A) in muscular diastole. As we can see in Fig. B It is placed on the GSV trunk at the level of the middle third of the leg.

The corresponding map is now totally constructed.

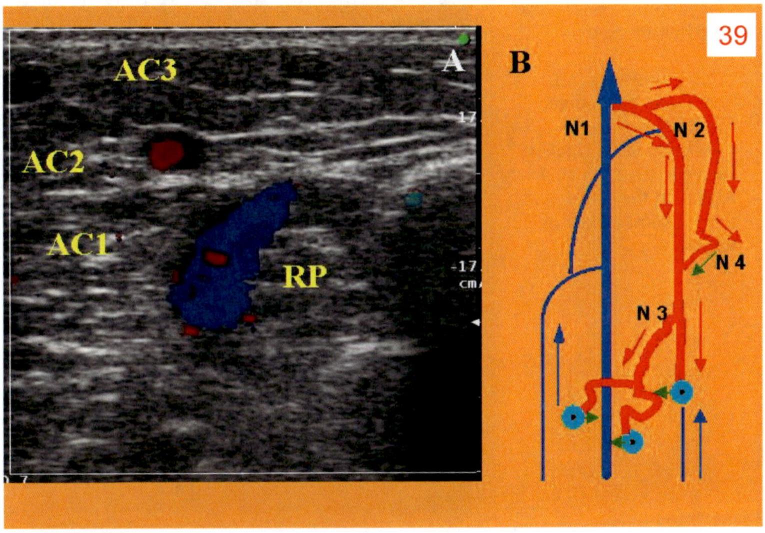


# CLINICAL CASE F: lesson learned from the molecular biologist

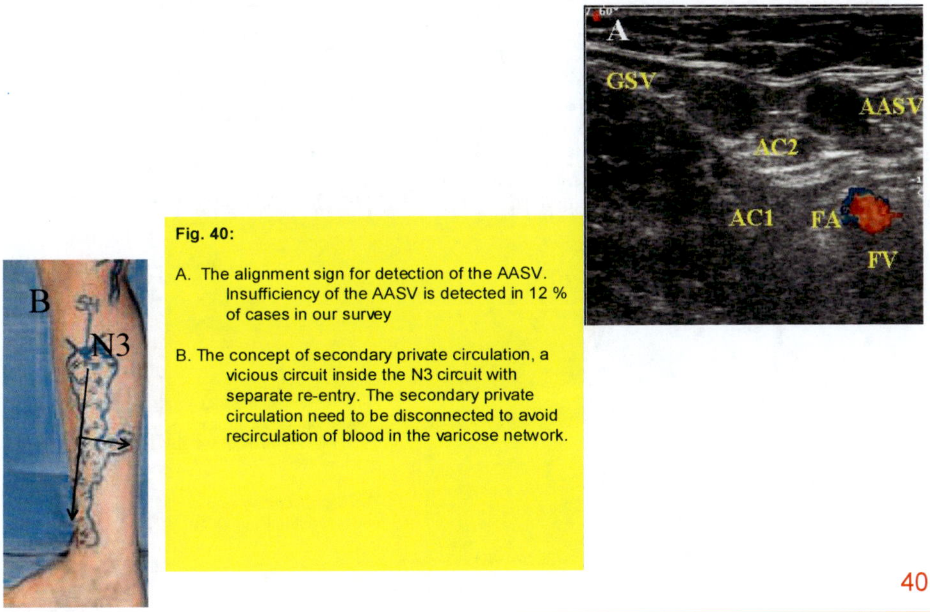


**Fig. 40:**

A. The alignment sign for detection of the AASV. Insufficiency of the AASV is detected in 12 % of cases in our survey

B. The concept of secondary private circulation, a vicious circuit inside the N3 circuit with separate re-entry. The secondary private circulation need to be disconnected to avoid recirculation of blood in the varicose network.

# CLINICAL CASE G: the tobacconist

**Fig. 41:**
- 56 yo man, tobacconist.
- Mother affected by CVD.
- C2s (heaviness, ref. oedema in the evening, in summer).
- Varicose veins clinically visible in the para-tibial region, at the knee, and in the lateral aspect of the leg.

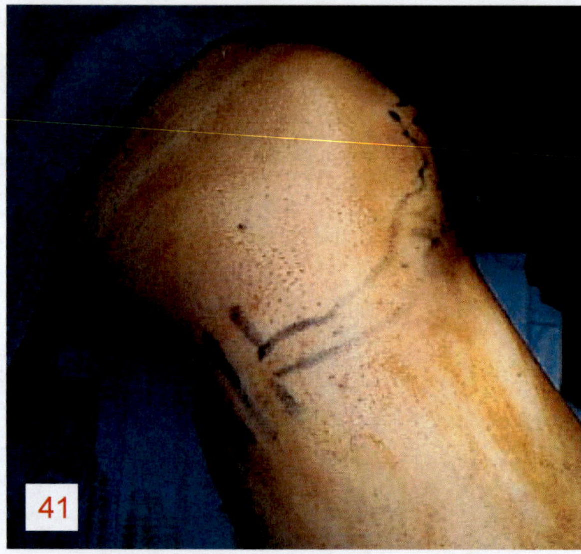


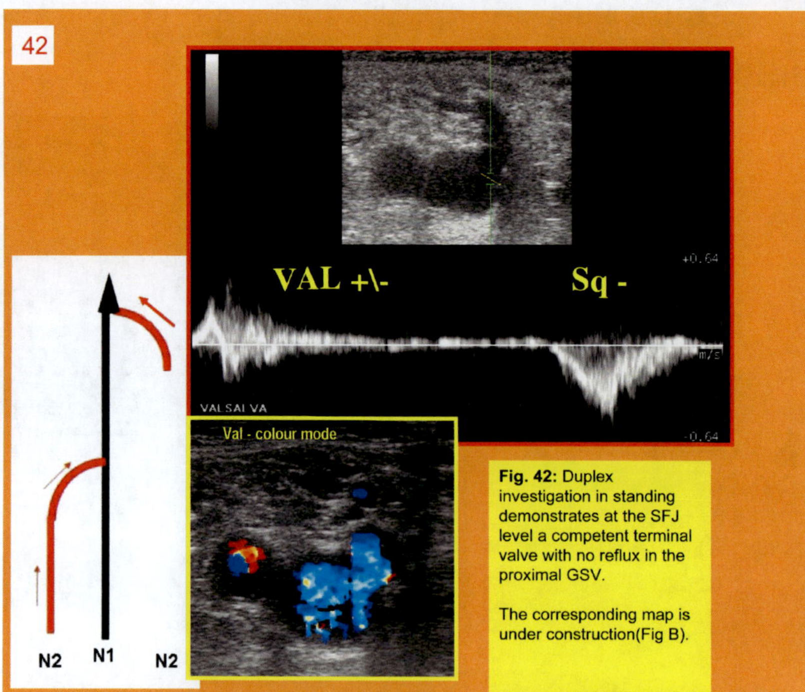


**Fig. 42:** Duplex investigation in standing demonstrates at the SFJ level a competent terminal valve with no reflux in the proximal GSV.

The corresponding map is under construction(Fig B).

43

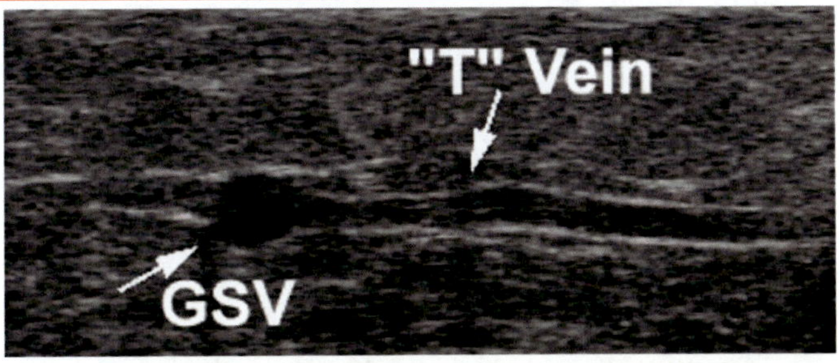


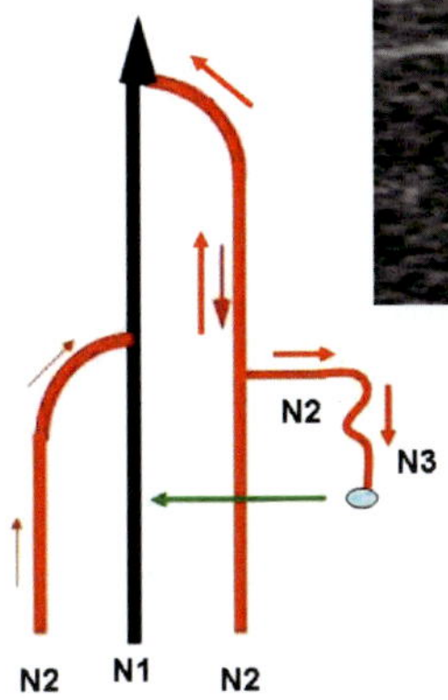


**Fig. 43:** Following by the duplex probe the outlined varicose veins, clinically manifest at the para-tibial region and at the lateral aspect of the leg, we find out a tributary of the saphenous vein with the origin in the saphenous compartment of the medial aspect of the upper third of the leg and with its re-entry focused in the N3 compartment.
It runs inside the compartment AC2 with a transversal direction from the medial aspect of the leg to the antero-lateral one for at least 5 cm (Fig. A).
Its deep position makes often impossible its inspection and palpation.
The same tributary feeds the visible varicosities mentioned above.
For the peculiarity of its anatomical shape as well as duplex appearance we defined it as the "T" vein.[253]

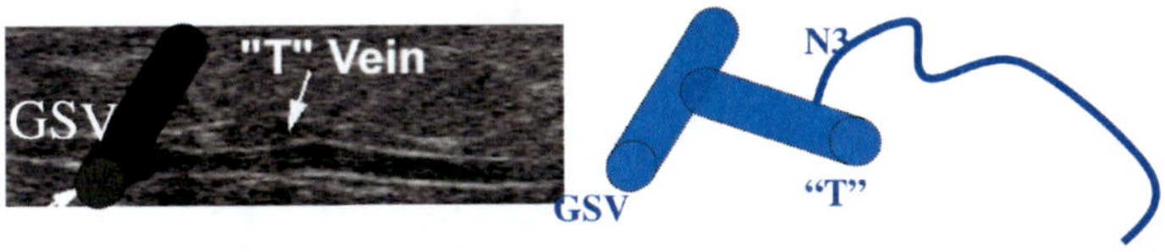


## Lesson from the tobacconist

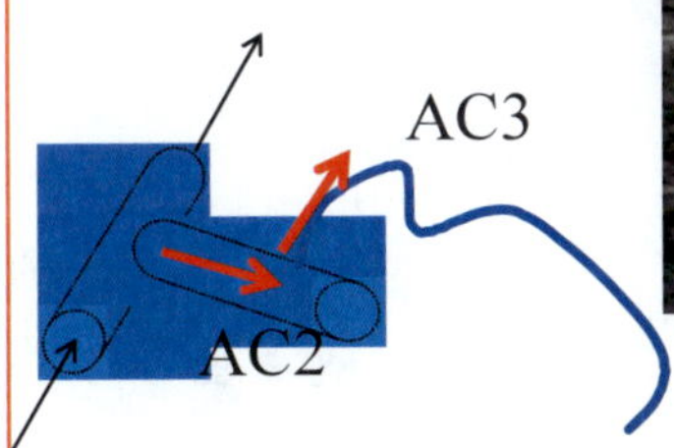


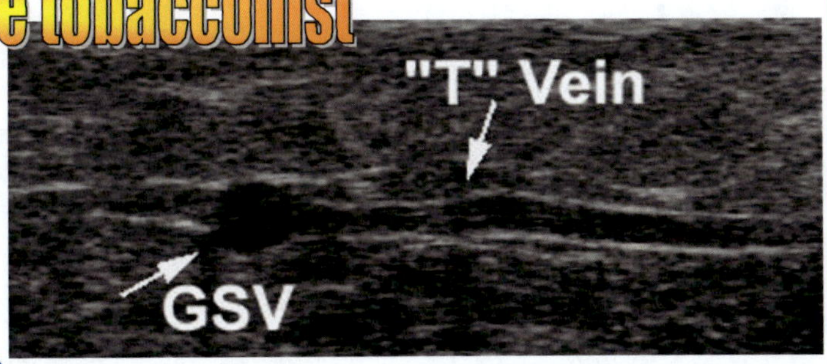


**Fig. 44:**

•Varicose veins occurs in the GSV territory with a competent GSV trunk. [152]

•This contributes to overcome the old concept that superficial reflux means saphenous reflux.

•N2-N3 reflux points and change of hierarchical order of emptying from AC2 to AC3 play a major role in CVD

44

Chapter 10

# FROM THE MAP TO CHIVA PROCEDURE

*Paolo Zamboni*
University of Ferrara, Italy.

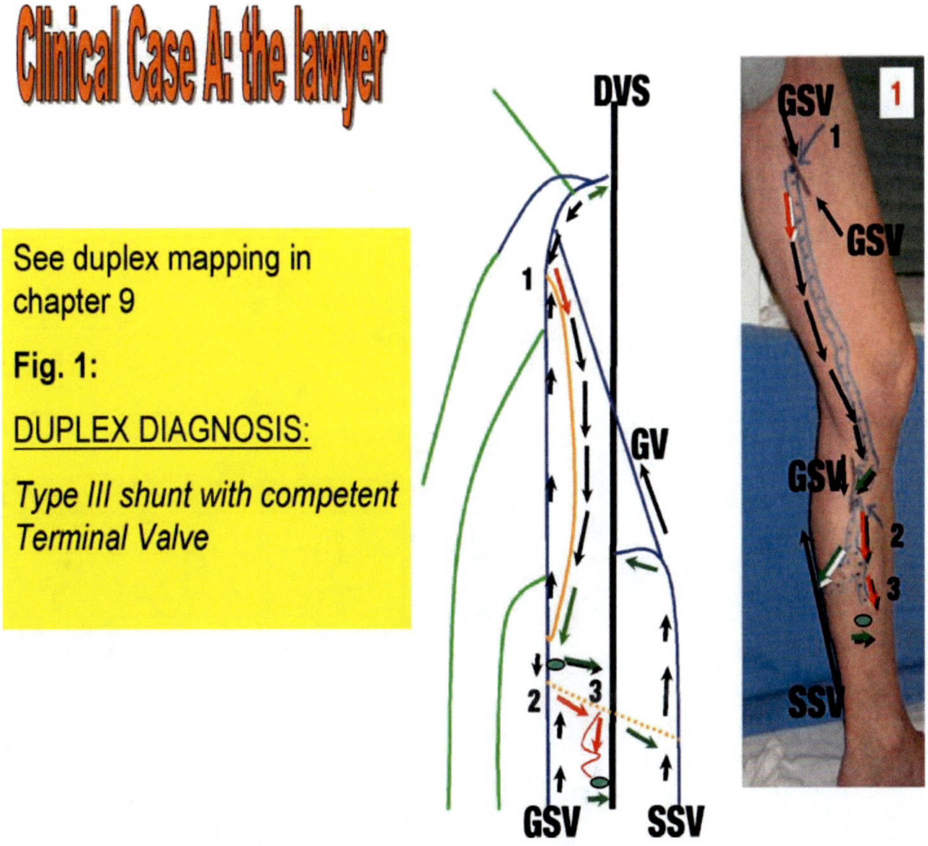

**Fig. 2:** Disconnection of the tributary from the GSV (N2-N3 disconnection)

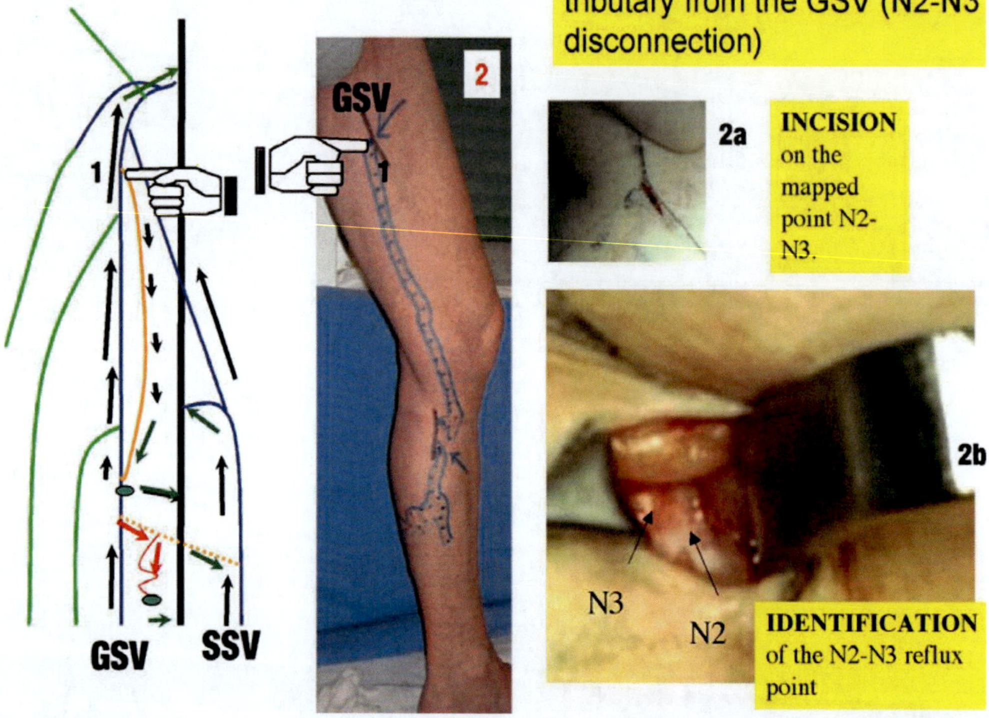


**Fig.3:** flush ligation and disconnection of the tributary (T) (N3) from the GSV trunk (N2).

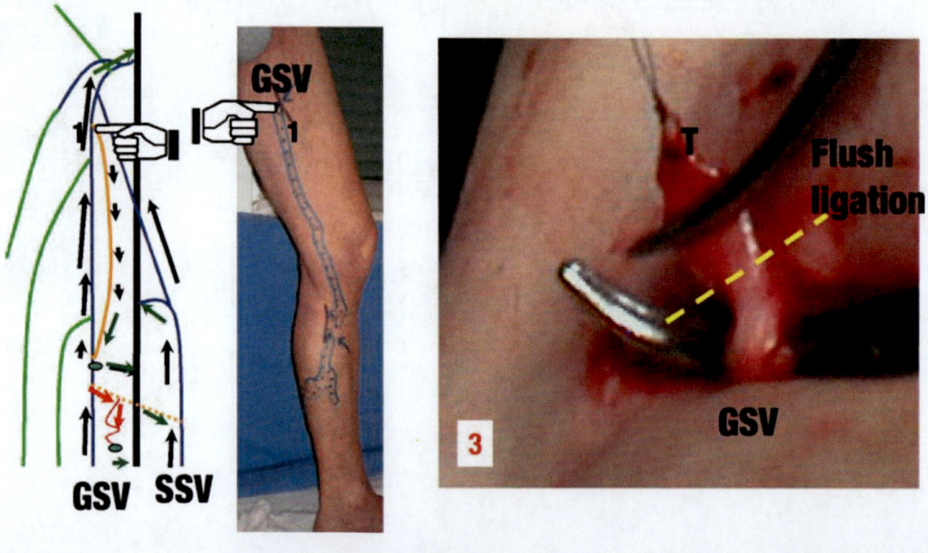

**Fig.4:** Muller phlebectomy of the proximal segment of the T.

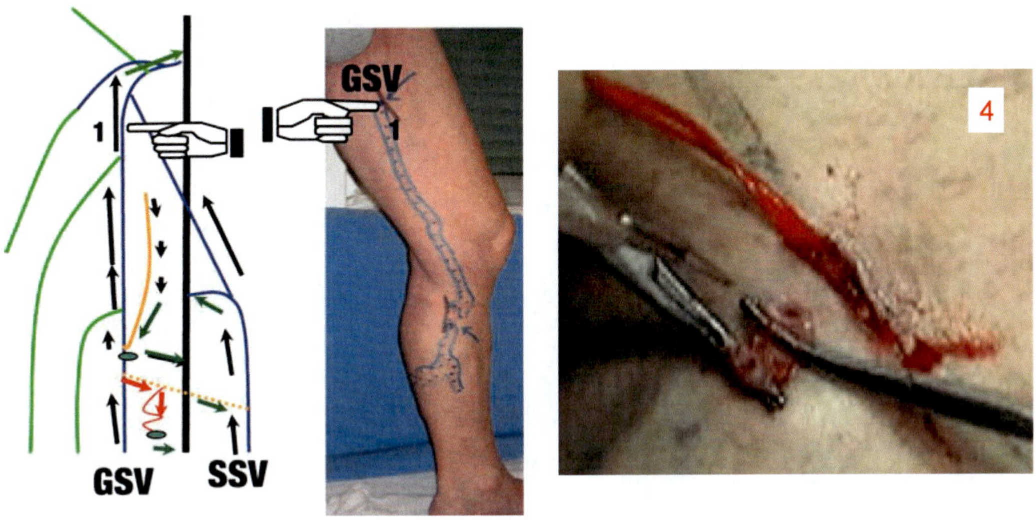


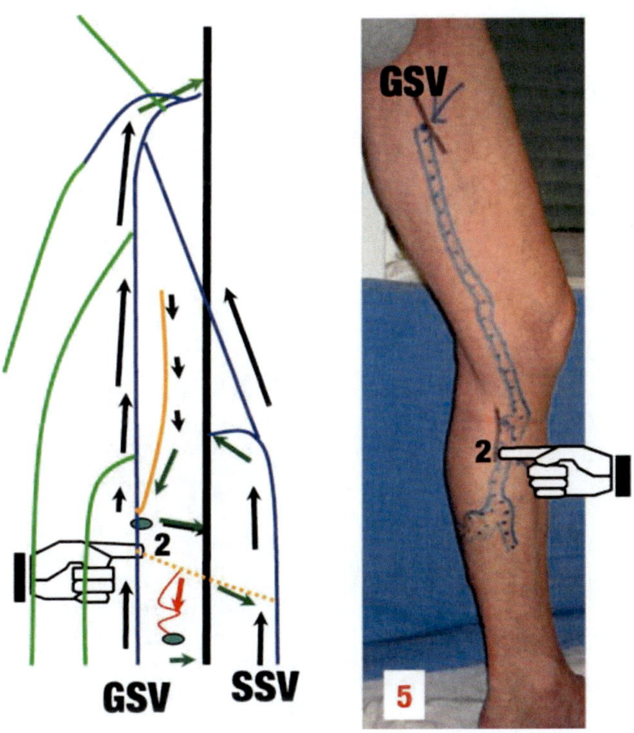


**Fig. 5:** Again, at the level of the subsequent N2-N3 reflux point we perform the same procedure described in figure 3 (flush ligation and disconnection of the T from the GSV)

**6a:** Incision at the level of the secondary private circulation

**6b-6c:** Hook phlebectomy of the secondary private circulation

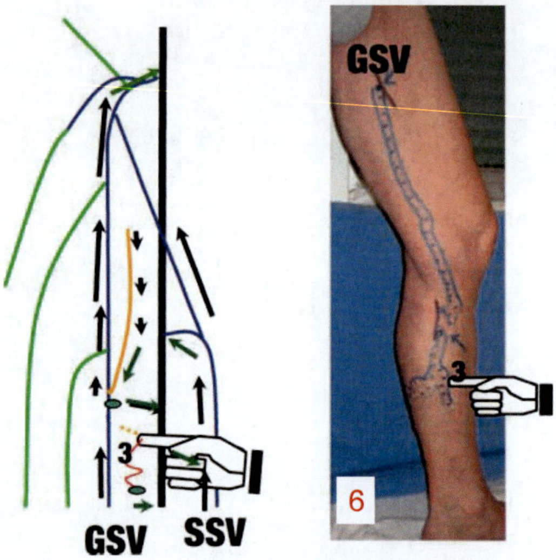


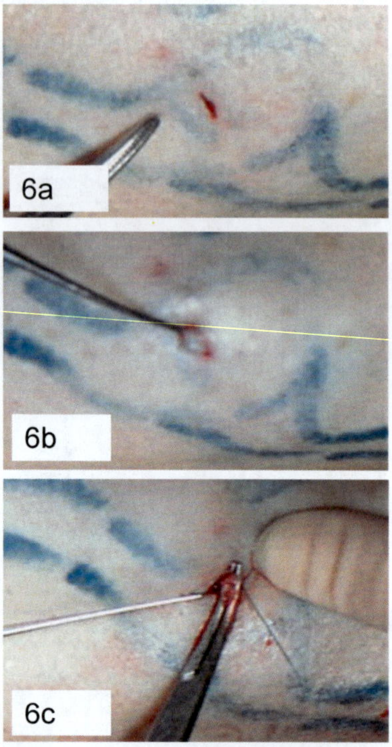


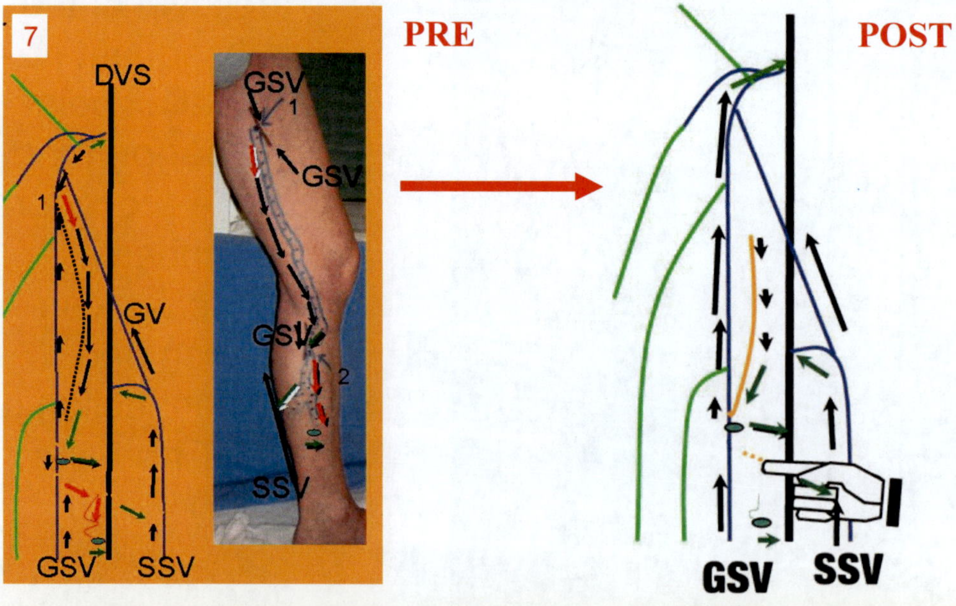


**Fig. 7:** Haemodynamic correction CHIVA from pre to post:

- Upward flow in the entire GSV trunk
- Restored hierarchical order of drainage (N2-N1, N3-N1or N2)
- Cosmetic compliant

**Fig. 8:**
**INCOMPETENT GSV ARCH WITH COMPETENT TERMINAL VALVE**

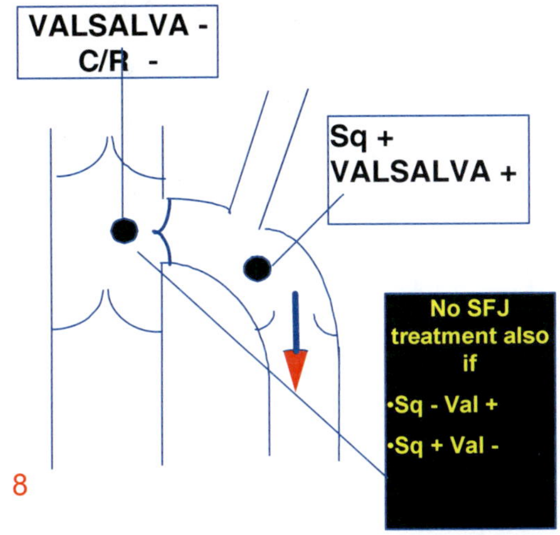


## The lesson learned from Clinical Case A

THIS MEANS:

- A CAREFUL INVESTIGATION OF THE JUNCTION AVOIDS APPROXIMATELY IN ALMOST THE HALF OF CASES, THE ABUSIVE LIGATION\ OBLITERATION OF THE SFJ

- CONSEQUENTLY, IT AVOIDS THE CRITICAL STEP OF VARICOSE VEINS TREATMENT REDUCING RECURRENCE 44,71,97,110,114,130,163.191,211,248

- TREATMENT BECOMES CHEAPER, MINIMALLY INVASIVE AND EFFECTIVE (FLUSH LIGATION AND TRIBUTARY AVULSION)

- IT RESTORES THE PHYSIOLOGIC FLOW DIRECTION IN THE GSV TRUNK

## Clinical Case B: the farmer

**Fig. 9:**

DUPLEX DIAGNOSIS:

*Type I+N3 with incompetent Terminal Valve*

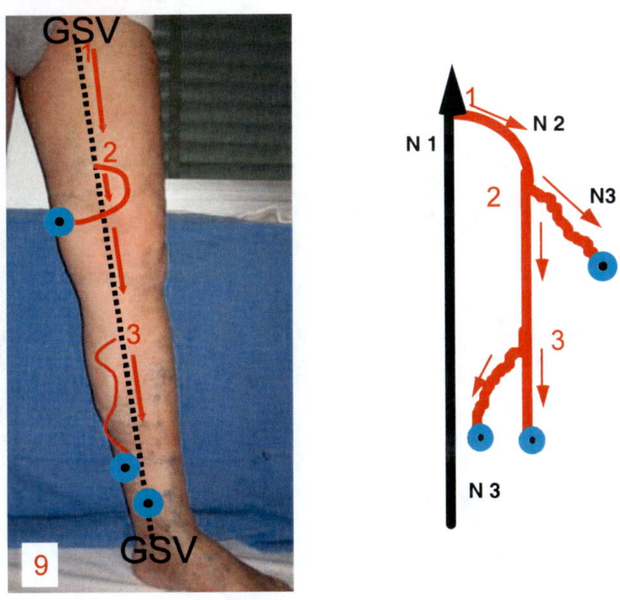

***SAPHENO-FEMORAL HIGH LIGATION:***

**Fig.10a:** Groin incision at the level of the SF junction outlined over the skin by the means of B-mode imaging. Progressive compartments dissection, in order to identify AC2 and the Saphenous trunk lying into it.

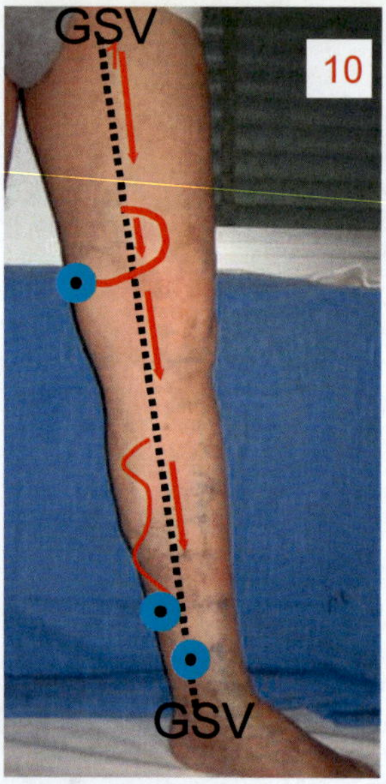


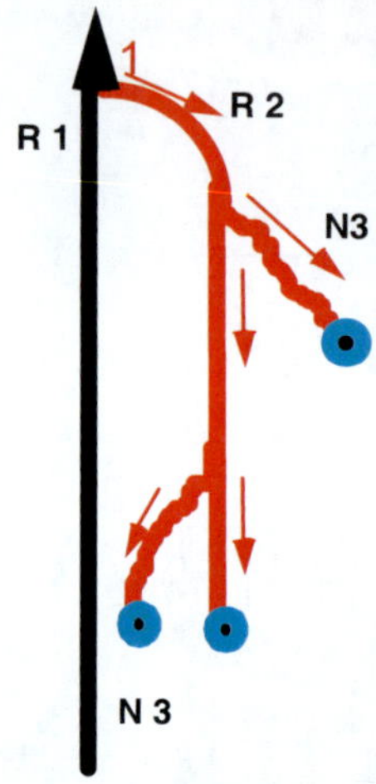


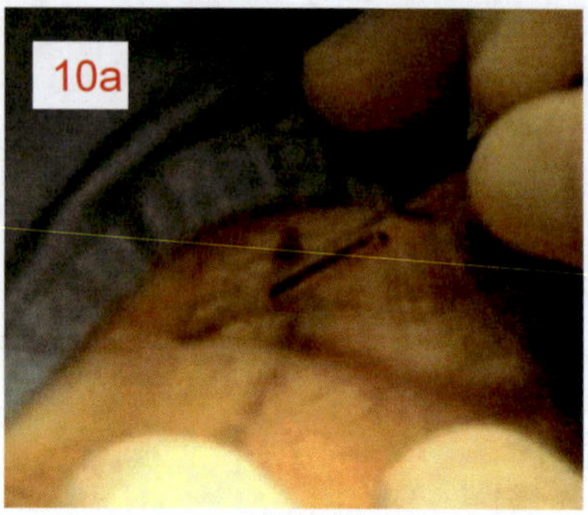


**Fig. 11:** Opening of the superficial fascia and exposure of the GSV trunk, SFJ and of the tributaries. The latter are encircled by a rubber loop in order to spare them (when possible).

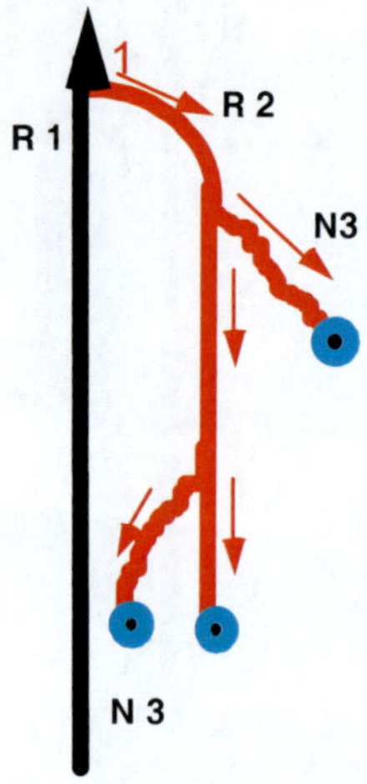


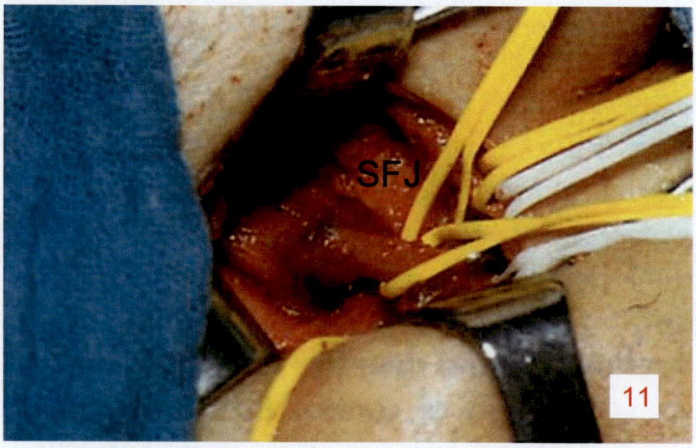

**Fig.12:** Right angle under the SFJ before high tie.

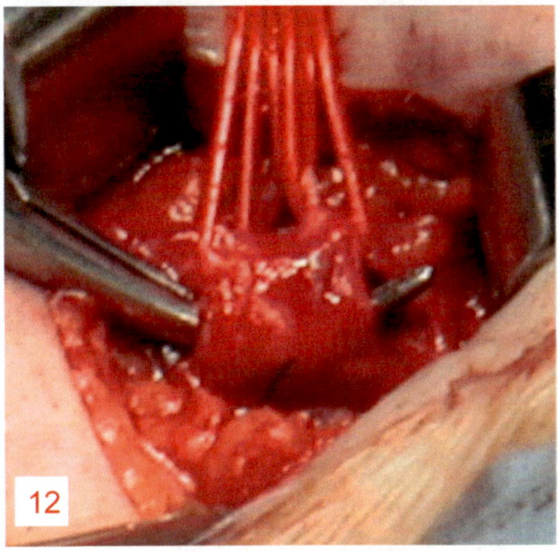

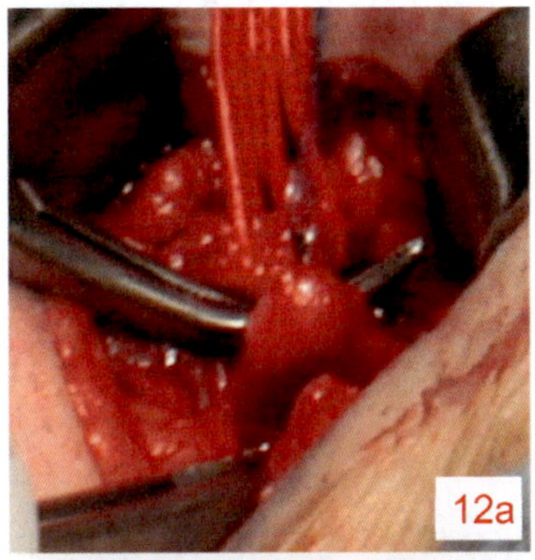

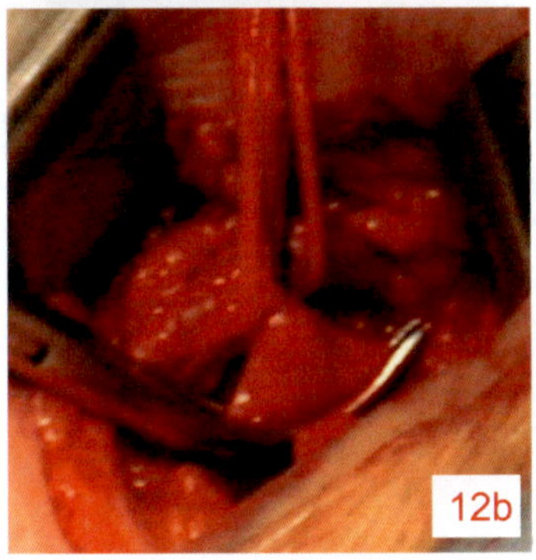

**Fig.12a:** Ligation of the distal part of the junction stump of the saphenous trunk.
**Fig.12b:** Clamping of the SFJ.

**Fig.13:** After ligation also of the proximal side, further clipping and disconnection of the SFJ.

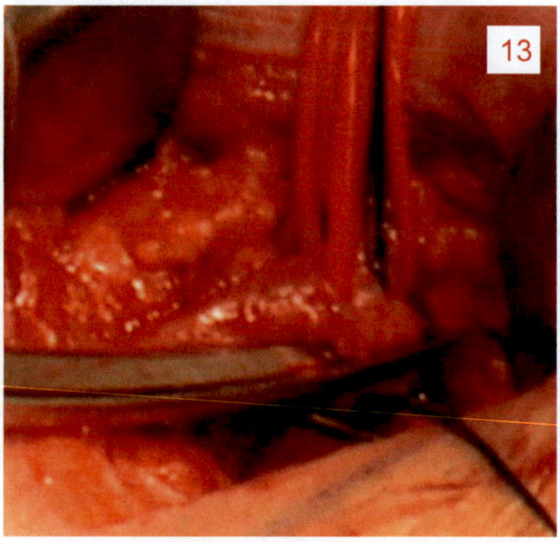


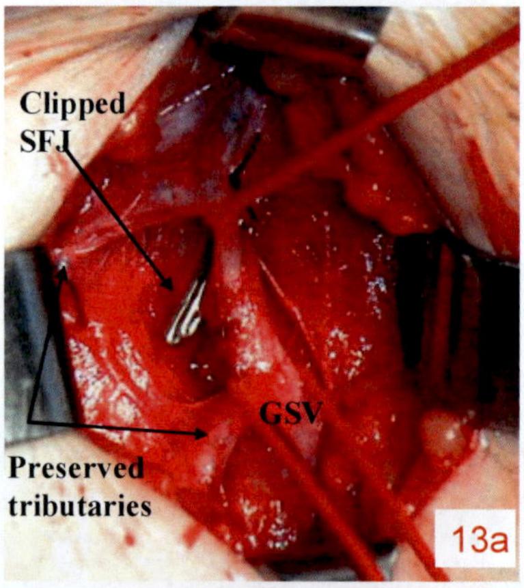


**Fig.13a:** In alternative, the picture shows double clipping of the SFJ without interruption. Tributaries preservation allows to mantain pelvic drainage into the GSV. The concept is to avoid interruption because could favourite the development of vicariant circulation and recurrence from neo-vascularization.

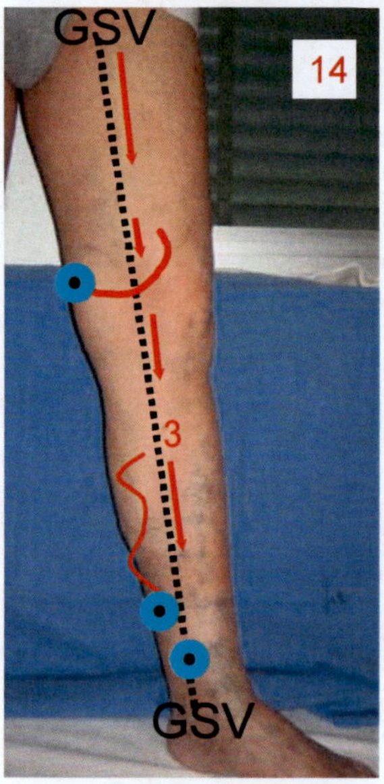


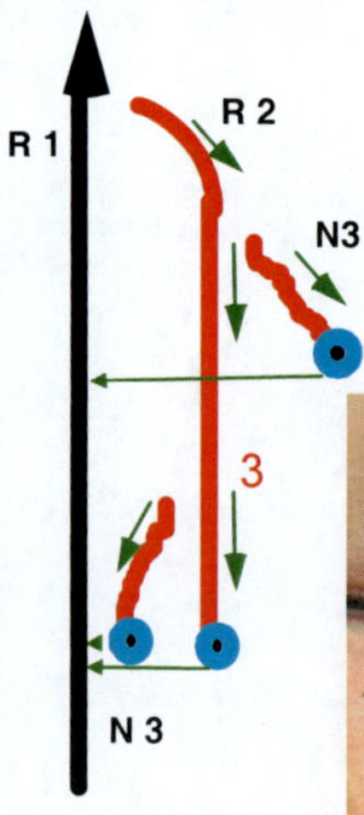


**Fig. 14:** Disconnection of the proximal and distal refluxing tributaries (N3) from the Saphenous trunk by the same technical procedure described in case A.

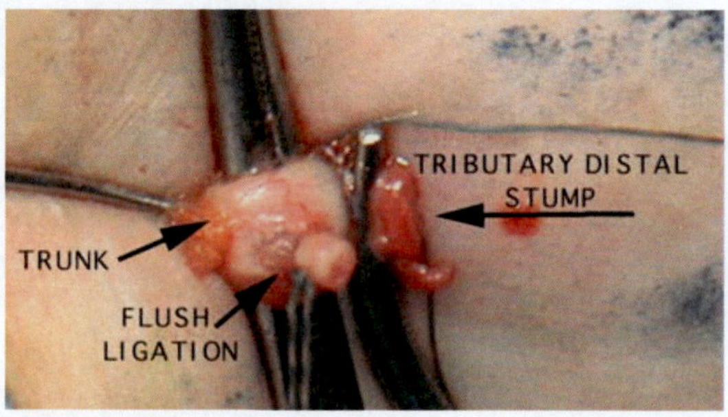

## Appendix to Clinical Cases A and B: Type III Shunt with Incompetent Terminal Valve

**Fig. 15: Incompetent terminal valve: both squeezing and Valsalva positive**

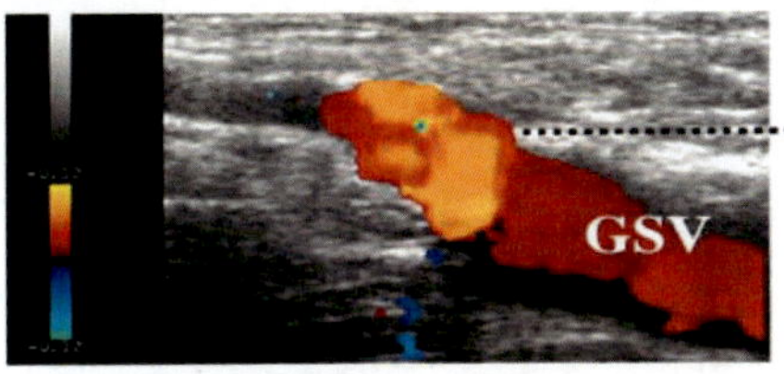


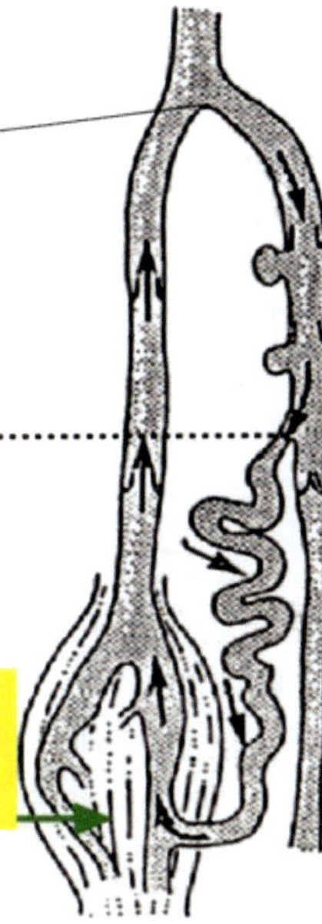

**Re-entry perforator on the varicose tributaries = type III shunt**

15

**SHUNT III**

**Fig. 16:** One shot solution with high tie determines a high rate of GSV thrombosis for creation of a non draining system. It was abandoned. [9, 47, 255]

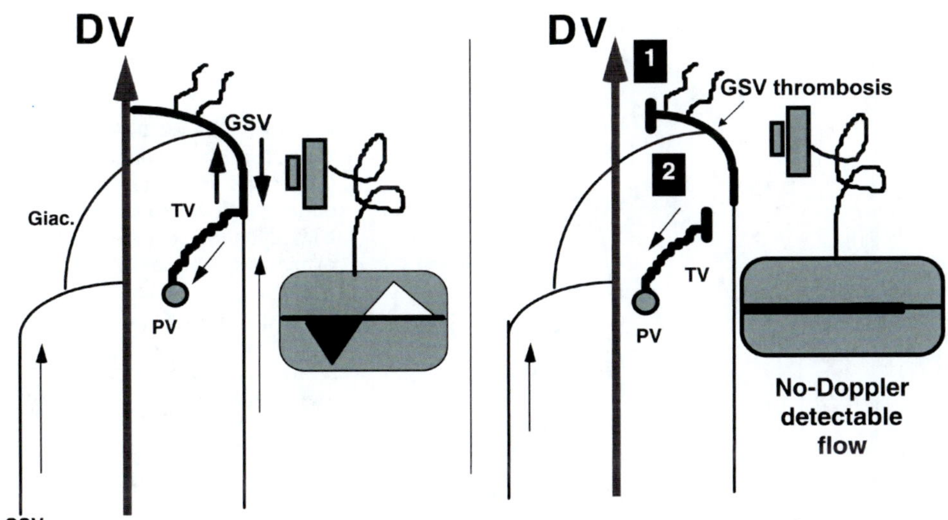


**Conservative but not hemodynamic treatment**

16

**Fig. 17:** One shot solution with high tie in a draining system was even abandoned. In fact the maintenance of the N2-N3 reflux determines an unsatisfactory cosmetic result . [9, 47, 255]

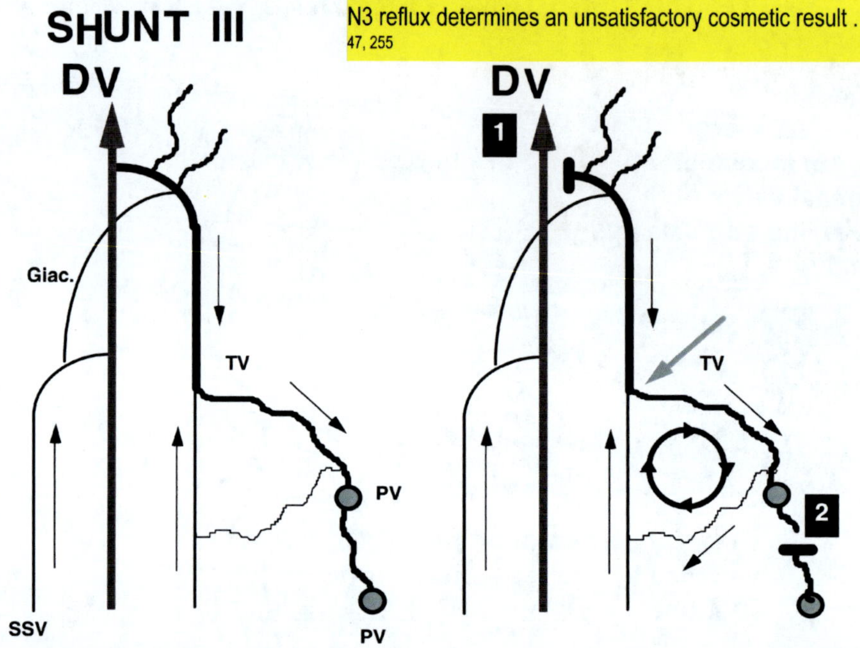


17

## The case of absence of re-entry perforator on the saphenous trunk and incompetent terminal valve.

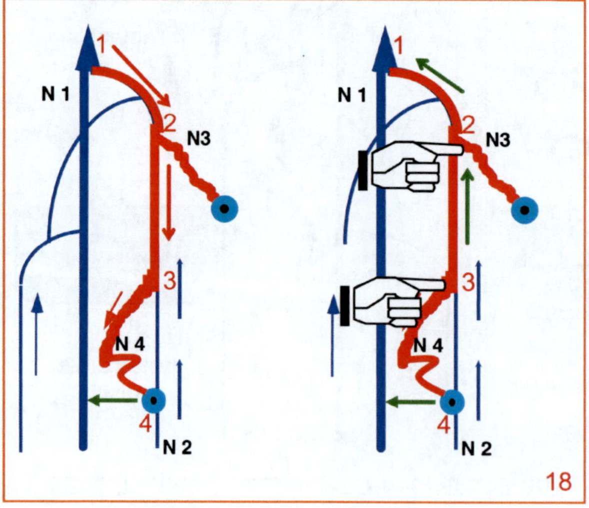


18

**Fig. 18:** In the illustrated case, the reflux elimination test (finger compression of the origin of the tributaries) [254] eliminates reflux in the GSV by eliminating the gravitational gradient. The logical consequence is to perform flush ligation of the origin of the tributaries (the so called 1st step of the CHIVA 2 procedure). [9, 47,90, 252, 255] This operation restores the physiological saphenous outflow in all cases.

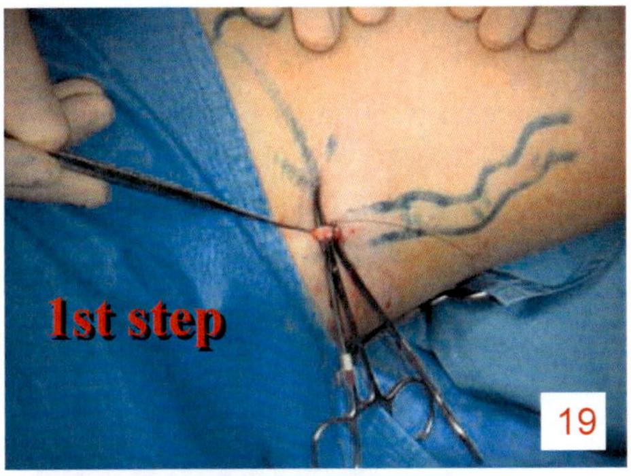


**Fig. 19:** However, after the 1st step a re-entry perforator along the GSV trunk could develop in a variable number of cases.[9, 47,90, 252, 255] This leads to re-appearance of reflux (type III shunt transformed in type I).

Such eventuality often occurs in case of incompetent terminal valve, and is managed by sapheno-femoral disconnection in a second session (the so called 2nd step of the CHIVA 2 procedure).[92]

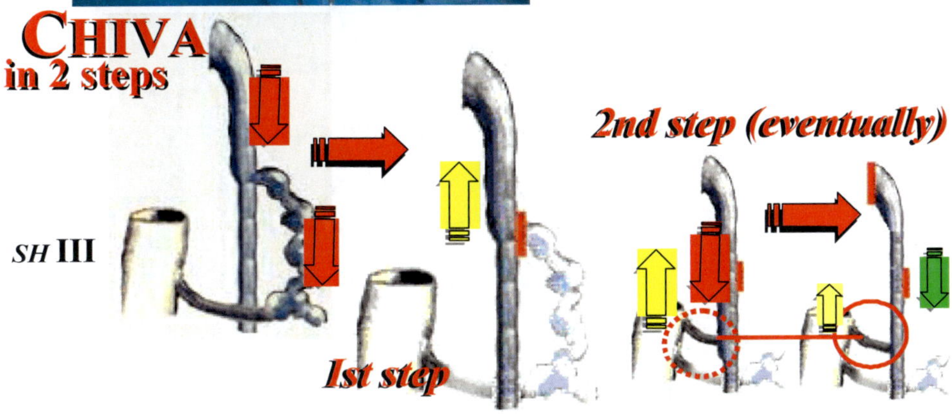


# One shot solution for type III shunt with associated incompetence of the terminal valve

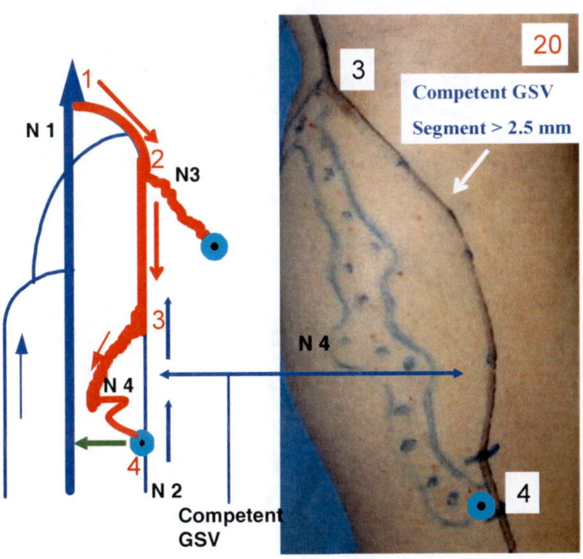


**Fig. 20:** Type III shunt with incompetent terminal valve, but with a re-entry perforator located in a competent segment of the GSV (from point 3 to point 4). Unfortunately the retrograde flow after high ligation cannot reach the re-entry at point 4 permitting a one shot solution.

If the competent segment of the GSV should be greater than 2.5 mm diameter, it should be possible to perform a "single shot" operation by using a valvulotomy in the competent GVS segment. The aim is to allow a retrograde flow along the trunk toward the selected re-entry perforator.

## Valvulotomy for type III shunt with associated incompetence of the terminal valve

**Fig.21a:** After careful exposure at point 4 of the saphenous trunk at its confluence with the perforator and the N4, GSV transversal venotomy and introduction of the valvulotomy is performed.
**Fig.21b:** Progressive introduction of the valvulotomy from point 4 to point 3 part of GSV.

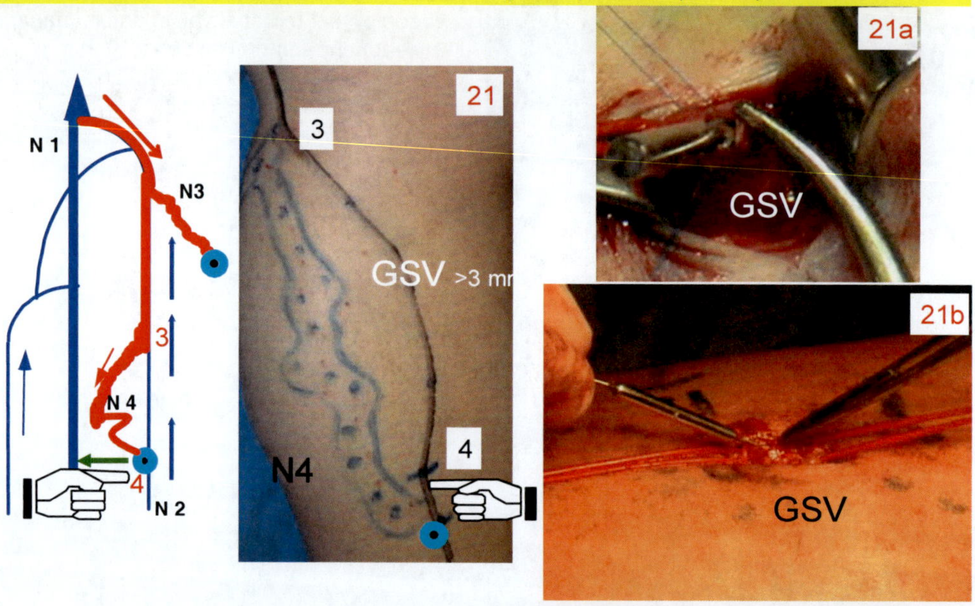


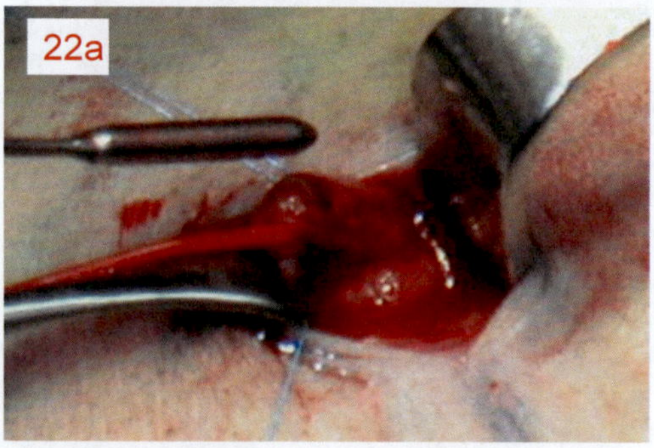


**Fig. 22a:** In alternative recanalization of the GSV segment can be achieved by gently and progressive veno-dilation, using rigid cylinder-tipped dilators of increased size.

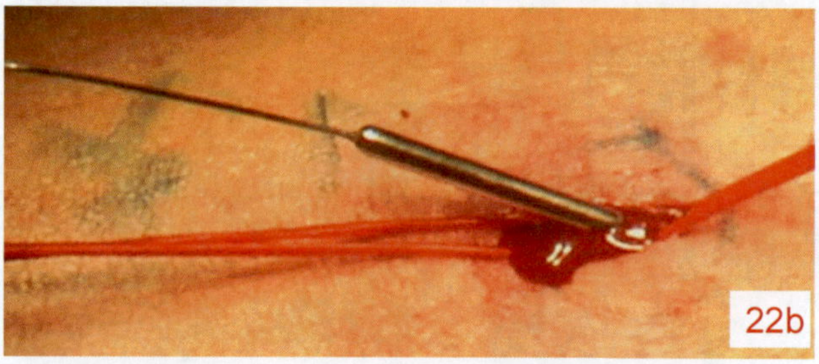


**Fig. 22b:** Removal of the valvulotomy

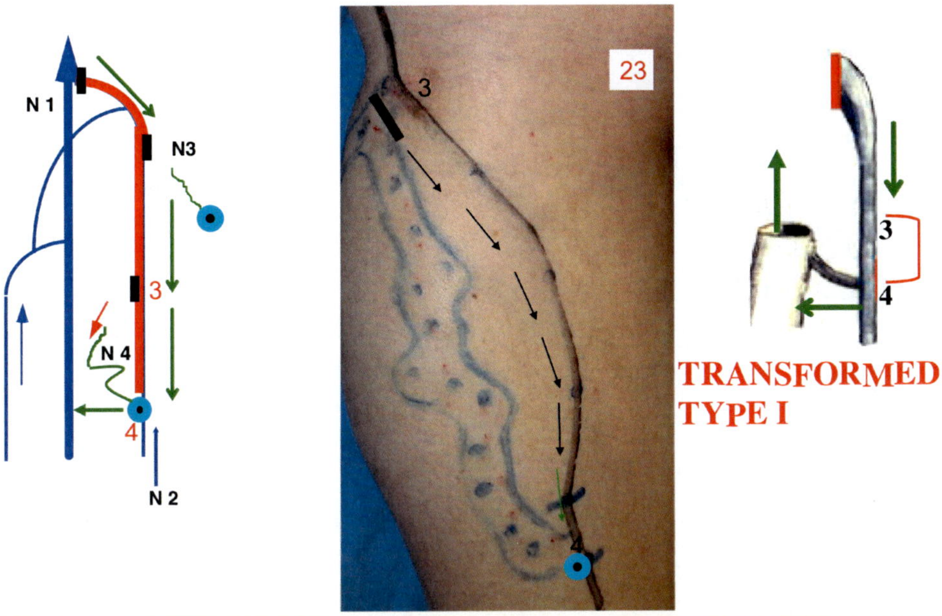


**Fig. 23:** This leads to the transformation of a type III shunt into a type I shunt on the operatory table.
The operation can be completed as a CHIVA I procedure (high tie plus disconnection and Muller avulsion of the proximal varicose tributaries), as showed in the map.

24

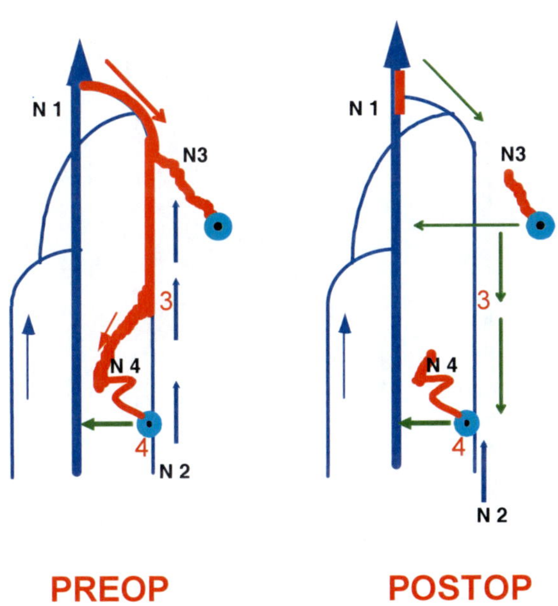


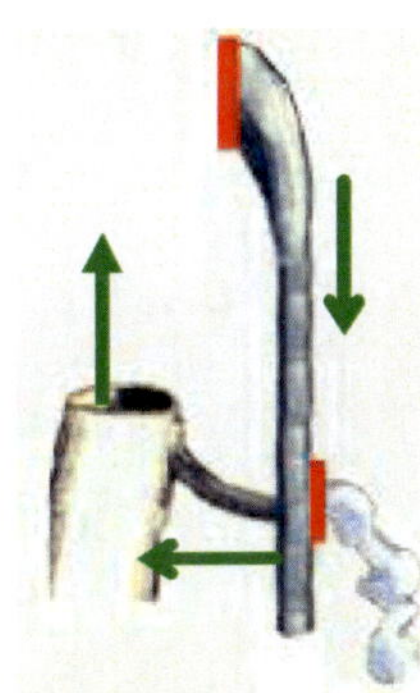

**Fig. 24:** The Saphenous drainage is restored and the reflux with changes of compartment eliminated in one shot procedure.
The hierarchical order of empting is even restored, from N2 to N1, from N3 to N1, and from N4 to N1.

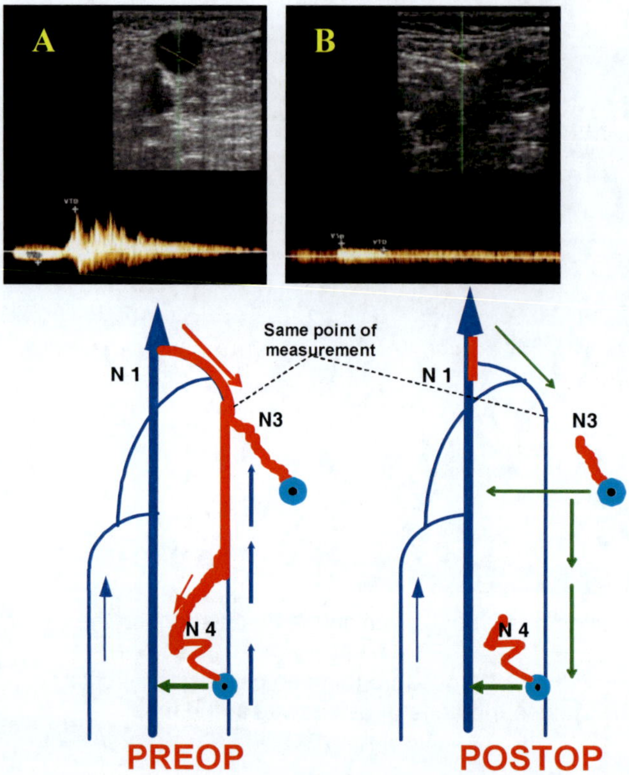


**Fig. 25:** A draining reverse flow is induced in the GSV either after one shot CHIVA 1 procedure, or after the second session of the CHIVA in 2 step procedure. Such reverse flow is a monodirectional low velocity flow (B), significantly different in the haemodynamic parameters from reflux with change of compartment assessed preoperatively (A) (see chapter 11). In addition, by comparing the preoperative cross sectional area of the GSV visible in the B-mode of the panel A with that depicted in panel B, a dramatic reduction of the saphenous vein dilatation is absolutely apparent postoperatively. This testifies the significant reduction of the GSV volume overload.

25

# Clinical Case C:woman in child birth

**Fig. 26:**

<u>DUPLEX DIAGNOSIS:</u>

*Shunt type IV (Pelvic shunts).*

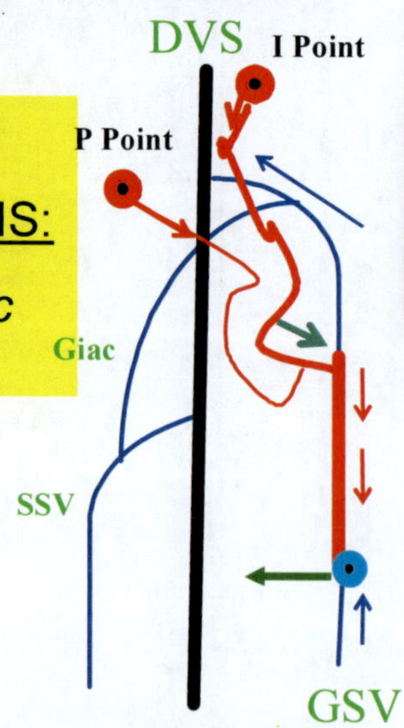


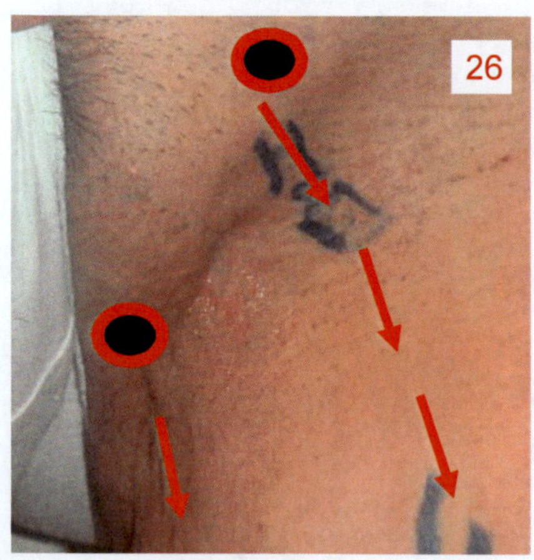

26

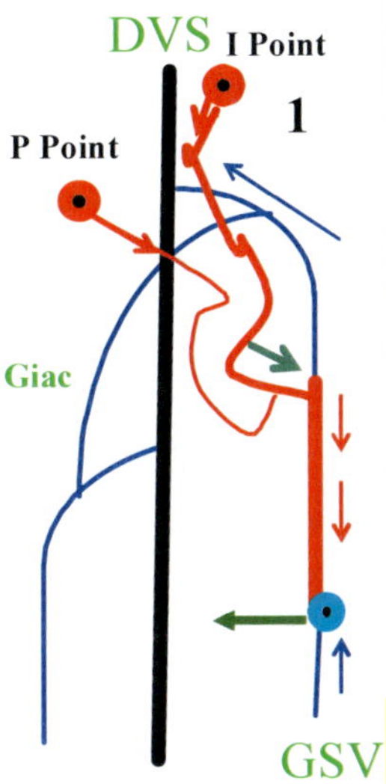


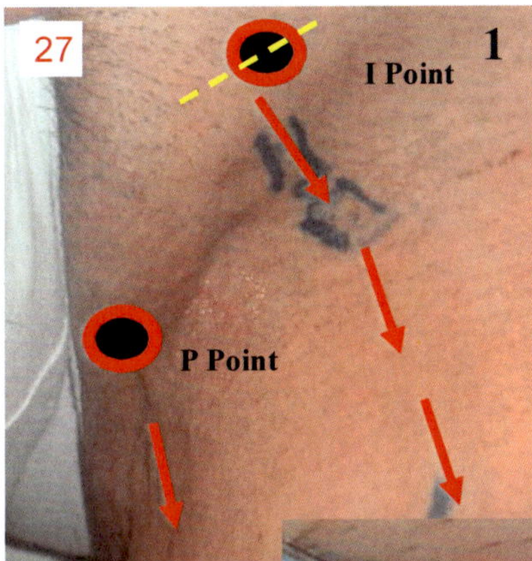


**Fig. 27**: Site of the incision corresponds to the external orifice of the inguinal canal (I Point).

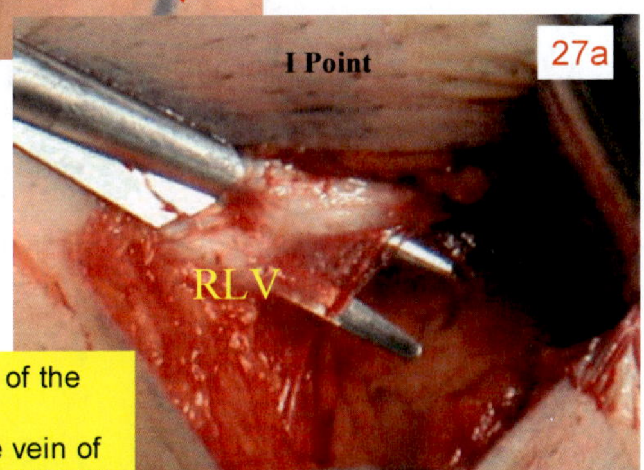


**Fig. 27a:** Opening of the inguinal canal and identification of the vein of the Round Ligament (RLV).

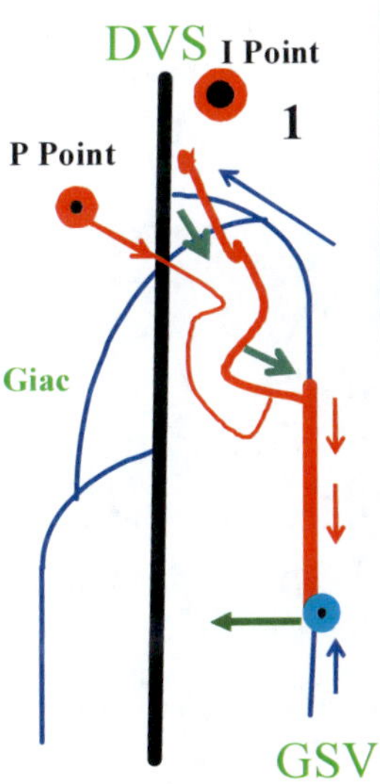


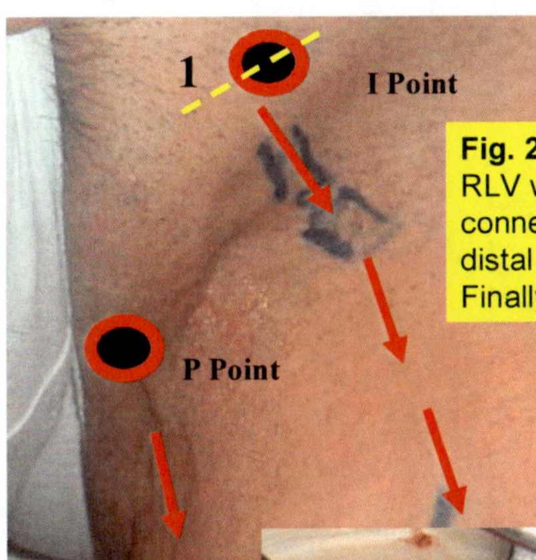


**Fig. 28**: Completed exposure of the RLV with the proximal stump connected with the pelvic area, the distal stump draining labium major. Finally the pelvic shunt is interrupted.

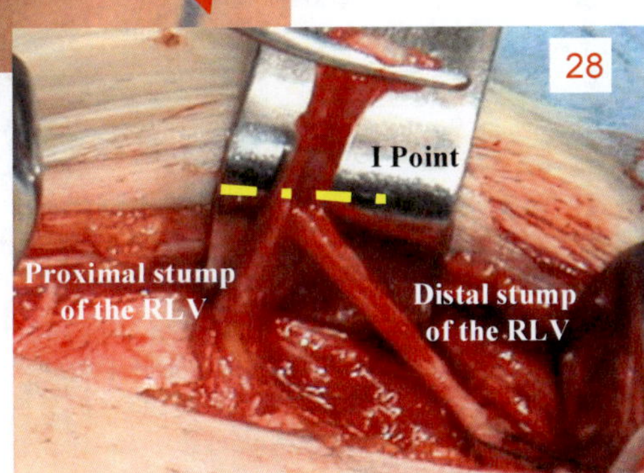

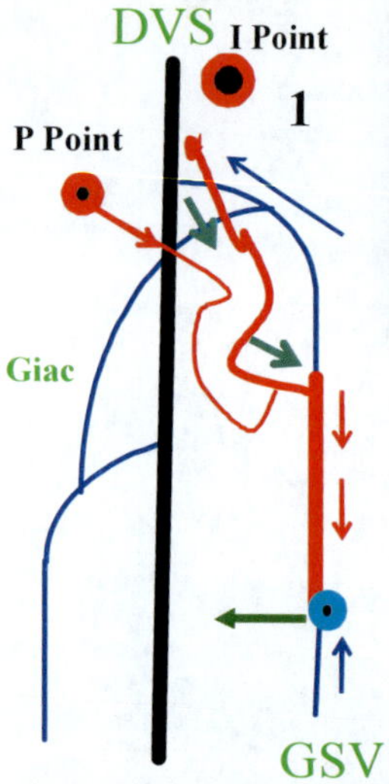


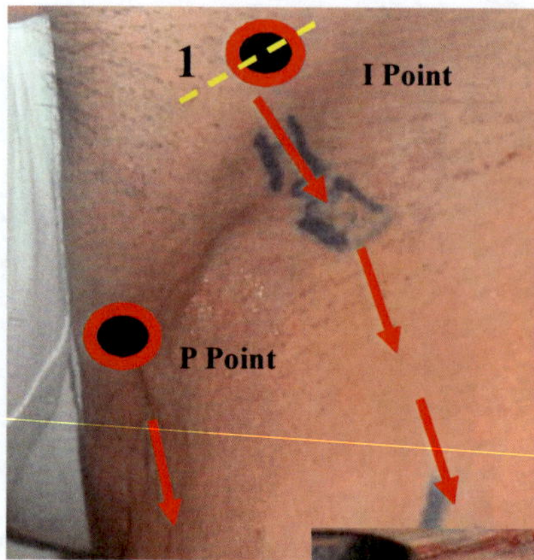


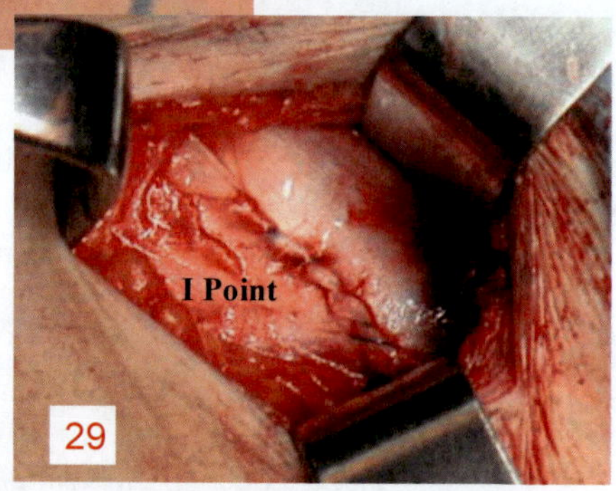


**Fig. 29:** Suture of the external inguinal orifice and of the roof of the inguinal canal.

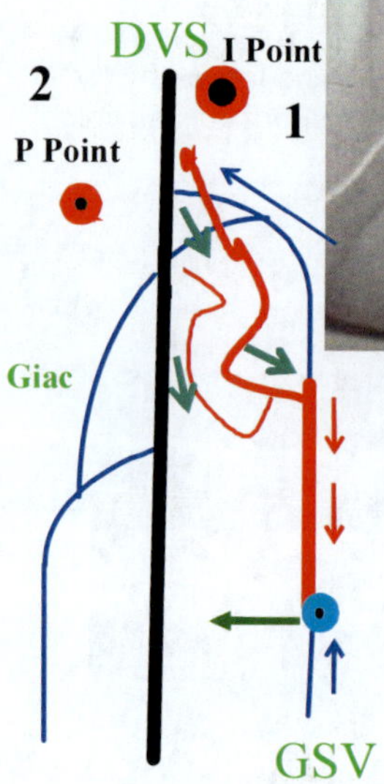


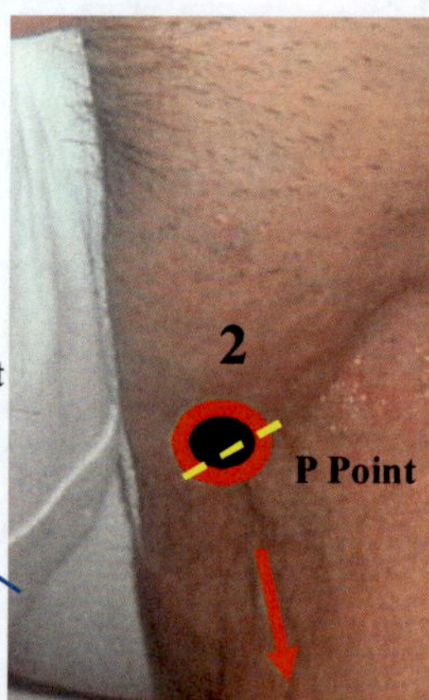


Exposure of the vein of the Alcock canal. This will be interrupted at the level of the fasciae, with further suture at the superficial orifice of the Alcock canal.

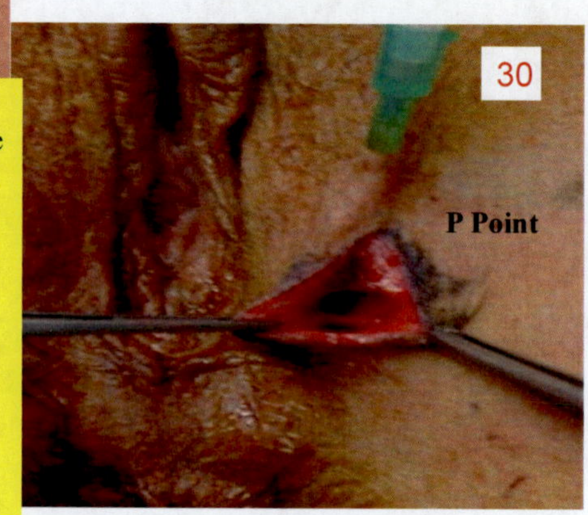


**Fig. 30**: Incision of the superficial opening of the Alcock canal, better identified by using a echo-guided needle *reperage* of the vein. This because in supine posture this vein collapses and its identification could become a challenge.

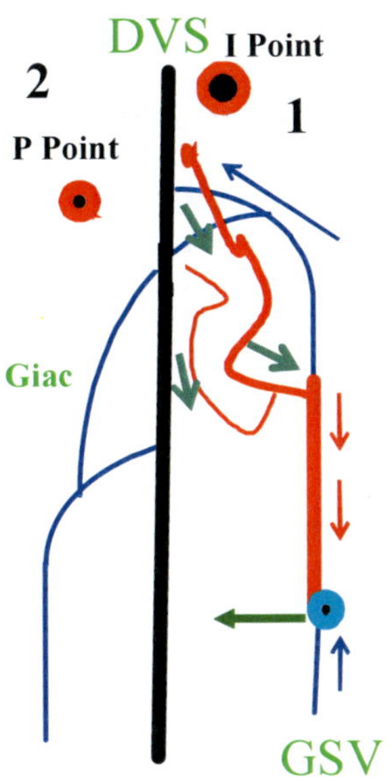


**Fig. 31:** The procedure is completed by multiple stab avulsion of the proximal varicose veins.

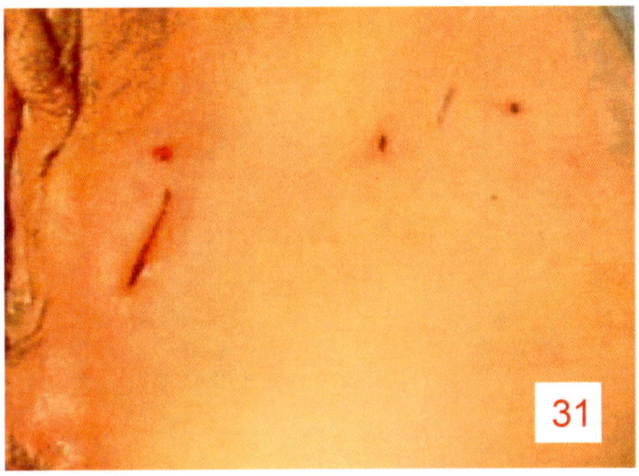


# Clinical Case D:the hairdresser

**Fig. 32:**

DUPLEX DIAGNOSIS:

*Shunt type III with* perforator of the popliteal fossa (PPF, the so defined Thiery or Dodd perforator) as primary reflux point and competent SPJ. [65-67]

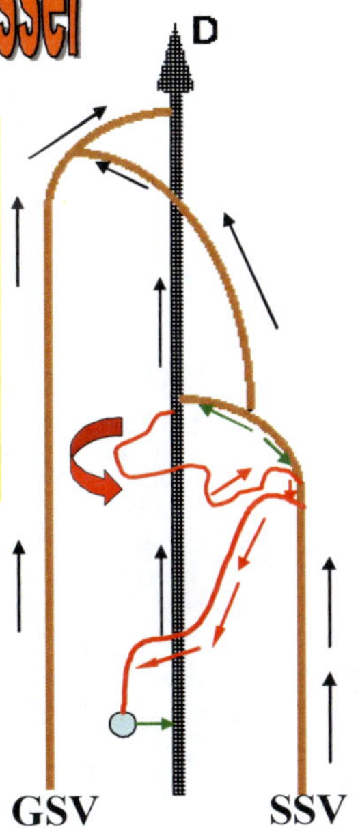


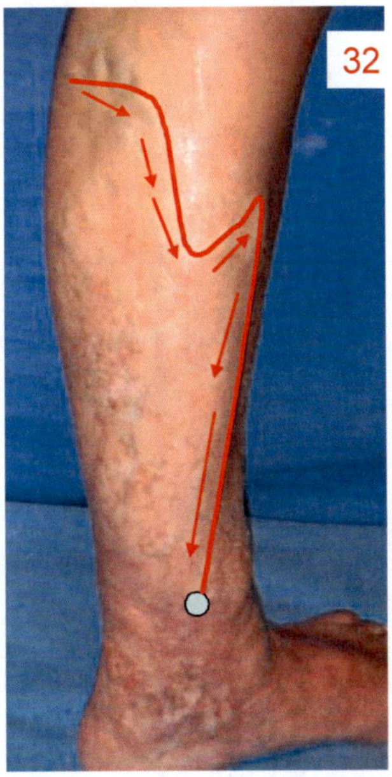

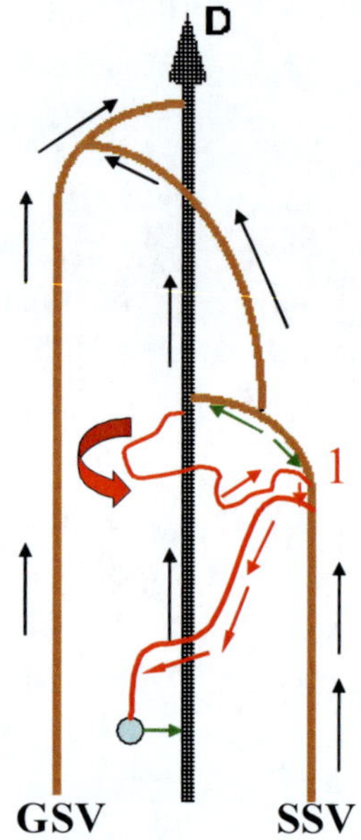


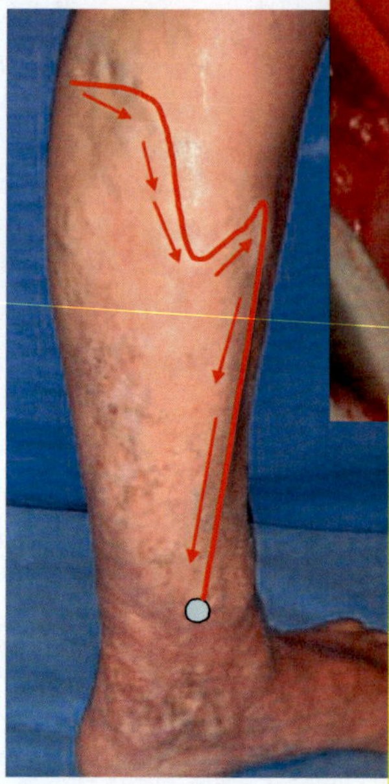

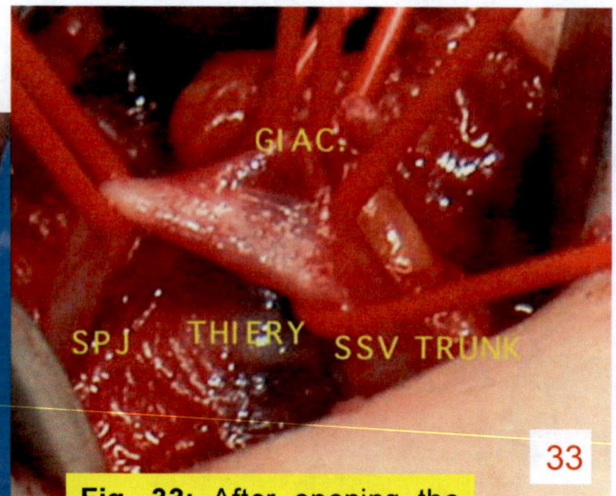


**Fig. 33:** After opening the popliteal fossa, below the superficial fasciae the SSV trunk is carefully exposed. Subsequently, the competent SPJ, the Giacomini's vein are both encircled by a rubber loop. Gently traction allows to identify under the SSV trunk the PPF.

**Fig. 34:** Disconnection of the PPF from the SSV trunk. The stump is clamped for making easier the dissection toward the popliteal vein. The procedure is then completed by flush ligation of the PPF on the popliteal wall.

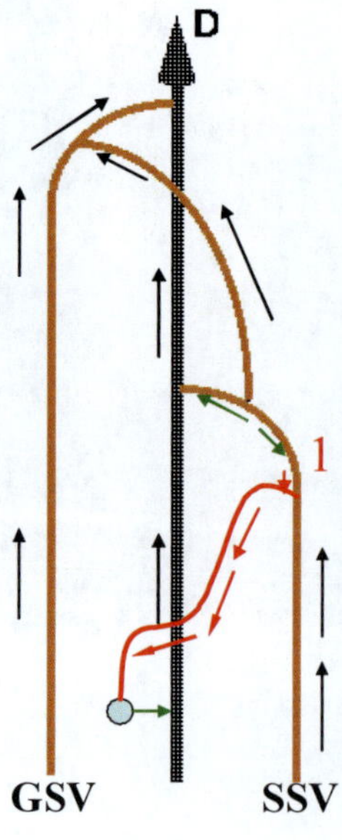


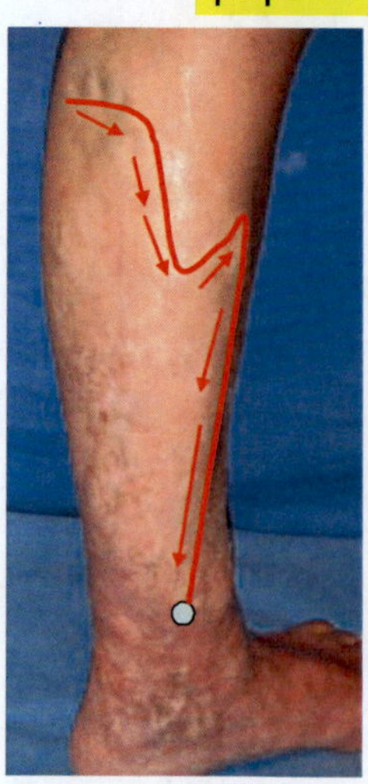

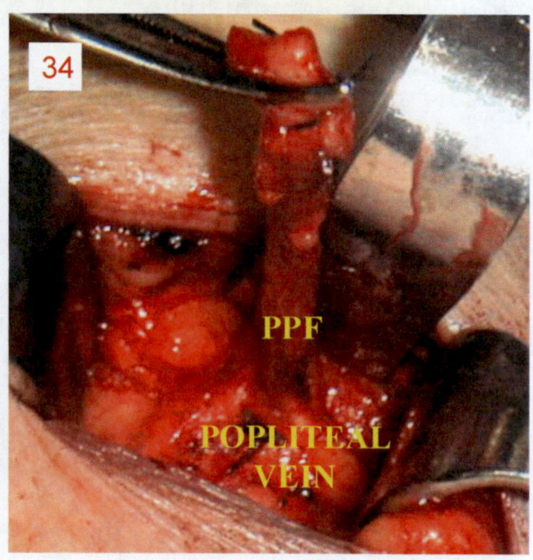

35

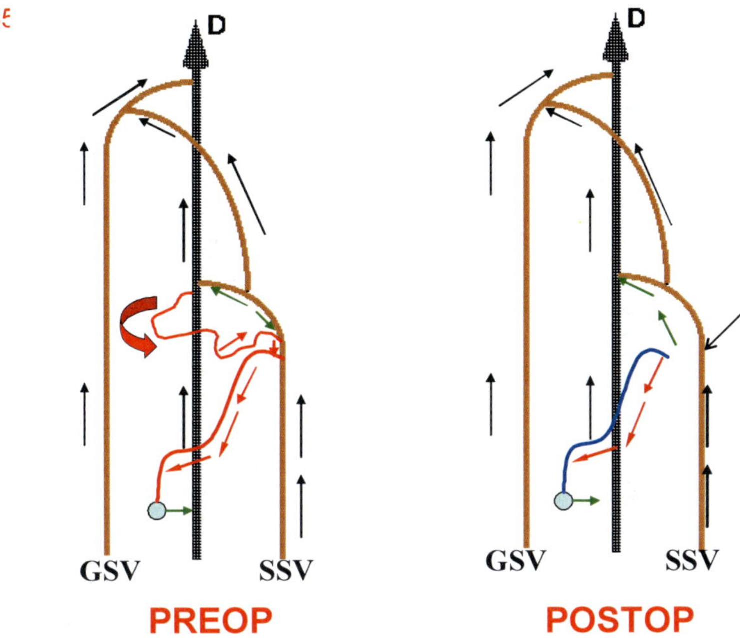


**Fig. 35:** Finally, N2-N3 flush ligation of the further N2-N3 completes the haemodynamic correction. We obtain a physiologic outflow in the SSV.

# Clinical Case E: saleswoman

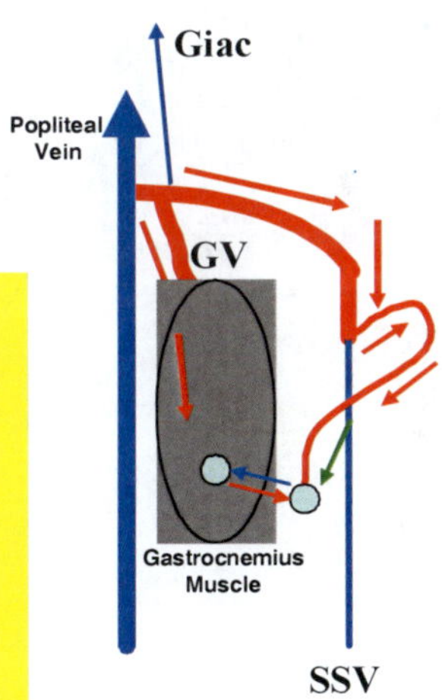


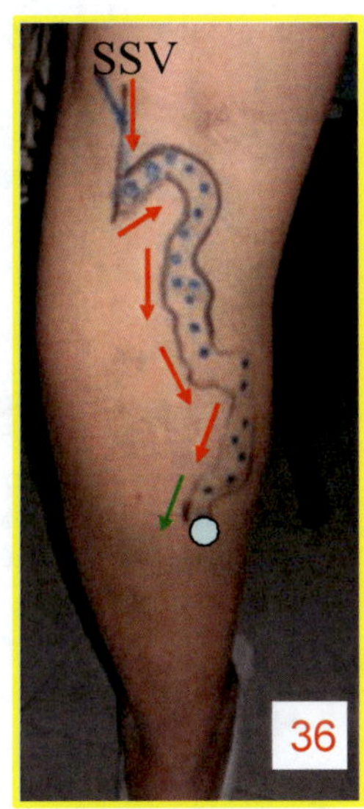


**Fig. 36:**

DUPLEX DIAGNOSIS:

Type III shunt of the SSV with concomitant GV reflux. GV and SSV outlet is a common trunk. Competent terminal valve of the SPJ.

Tested outflow route through the Giacomini'.

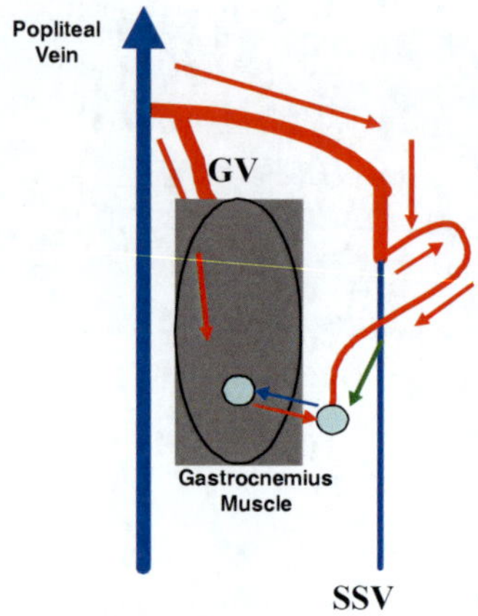


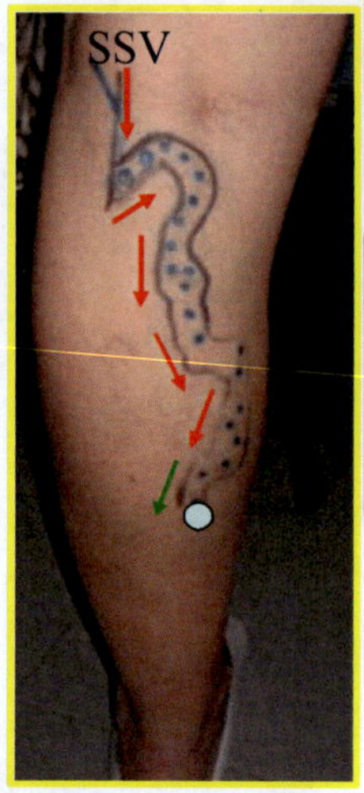


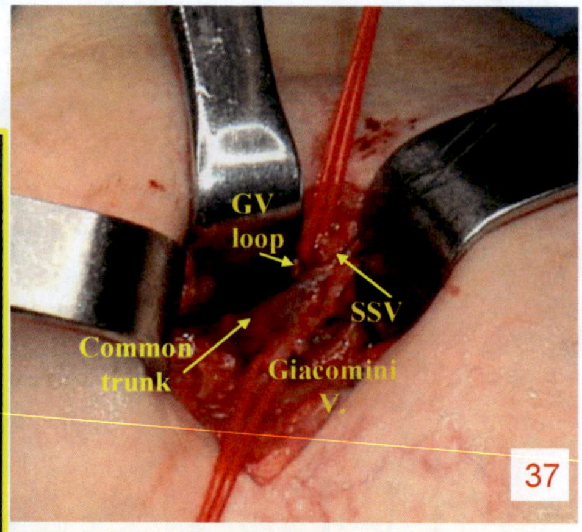


**Fig. 37:** Exposure of the veins of the popliteal fossa. The common trunk into the popliteal vein is well apparent.

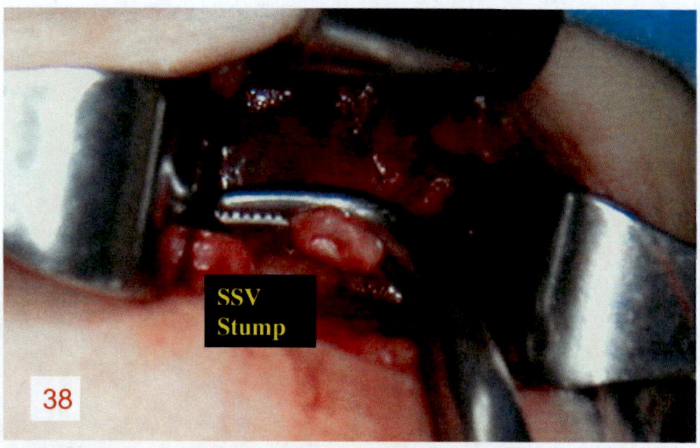


**Fig. 38:** Disconnection of the SSV at the level of the common trunk maintaining the gastrocnemius vein opening into the popliteal vein, as well as the continuity of the SSV into the Giacomini's vein.

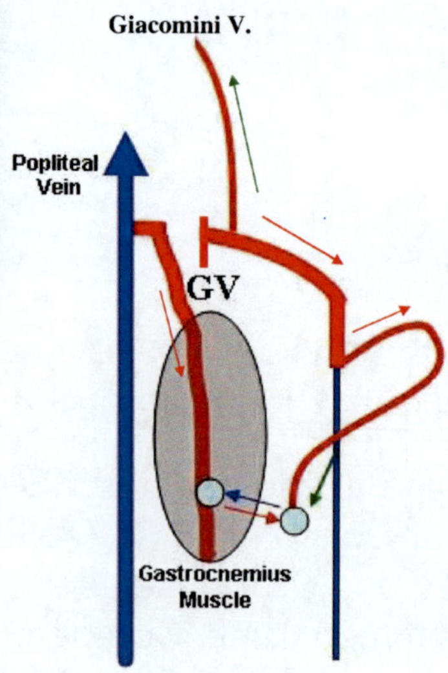

39

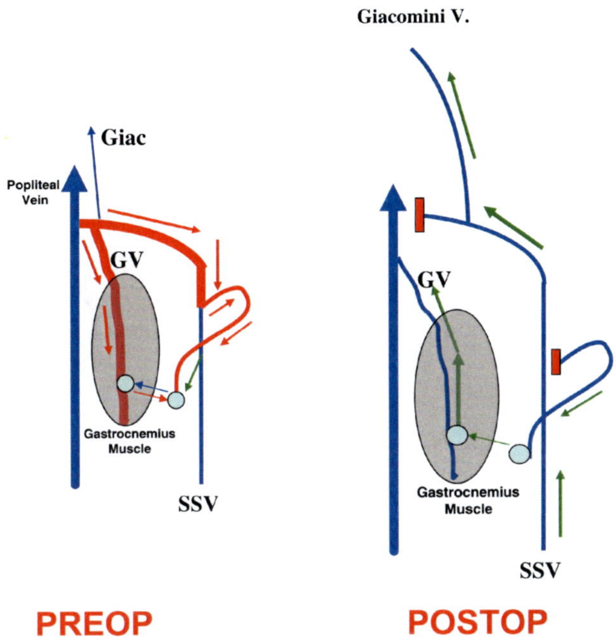


**Fig. 39:**
Disconnection of the refluxing N3 from the Saphenous trunk. Finally, we obtain the elimination of reflux both in the SSV and in the GV, with restoration of a physiological upward flow. In the former through the Giacomini's vein; in the latter toward the popliteal vein thanks to the elimination of the hydrostatic gradient. This is an example of indirect correction of deep reflux in the GV, acting on a superficial reflux.

Haemodynamic achievements:

- Reflux with change of compartment elimination in the SSV, GV, and N3.
- Physiologic forward flow in both SSV and GV
- Flow direction hierarchically correct N3-N1 in the tributary.

# Clinical Case F: the molecular biologist

**Fig. 40:**

<u>DUPLEX DIAGNOSIS:</u>

Combined Type I Shunt of GSV and Type III Shunt of AASV

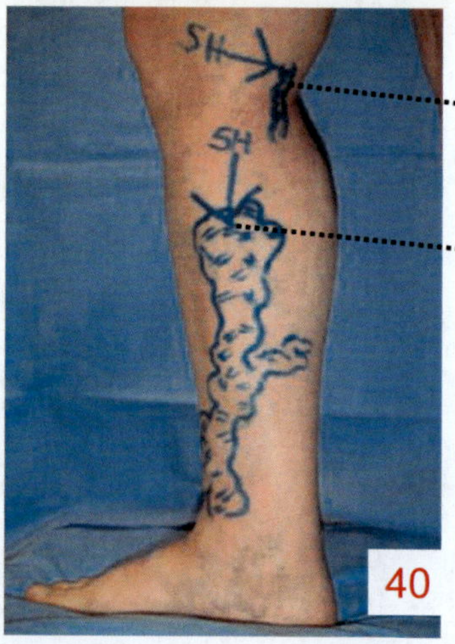


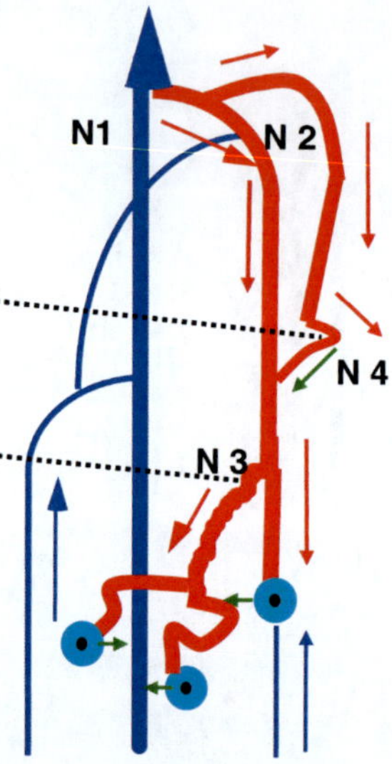

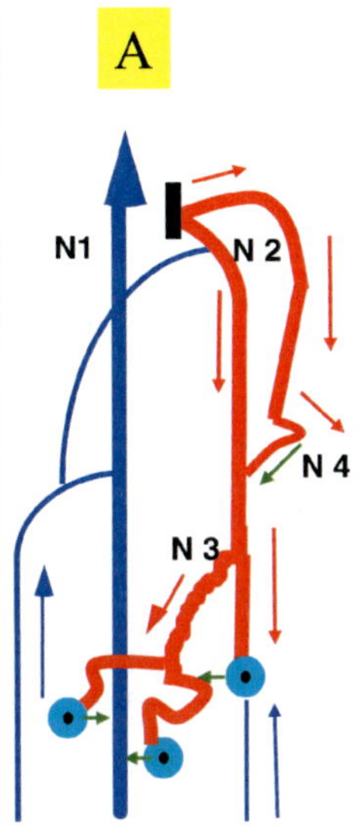


41

**Fig. 41:**
•The case depicted in fig. B is defined lambda SFJ, for the particular shape of the AASV and GSV outlet. A typical high ligation is performed, preserving the outlet of the AASV into the GSV, as clearly seen in Fig. C.
•This allows the drainage of the AASV into the GSV and the re-entry of both down-ward to the re-entry perforator, as depicted in Fig. A.

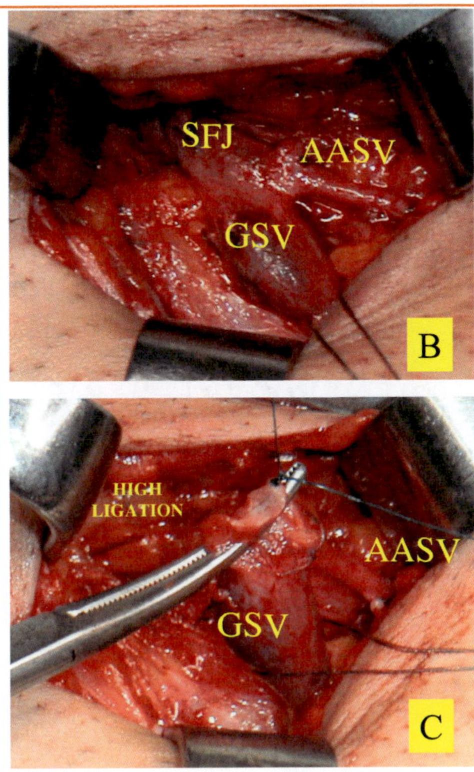


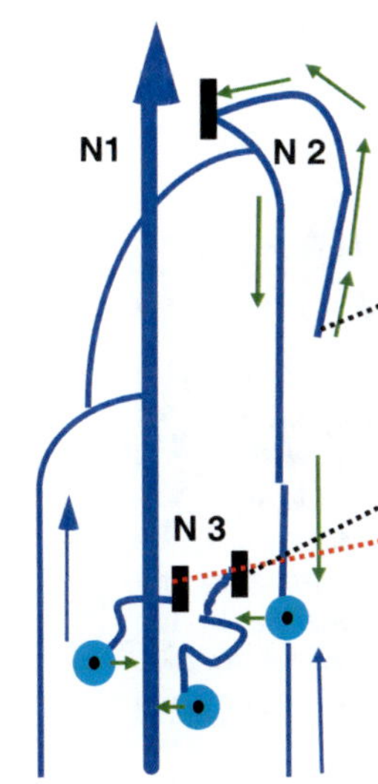


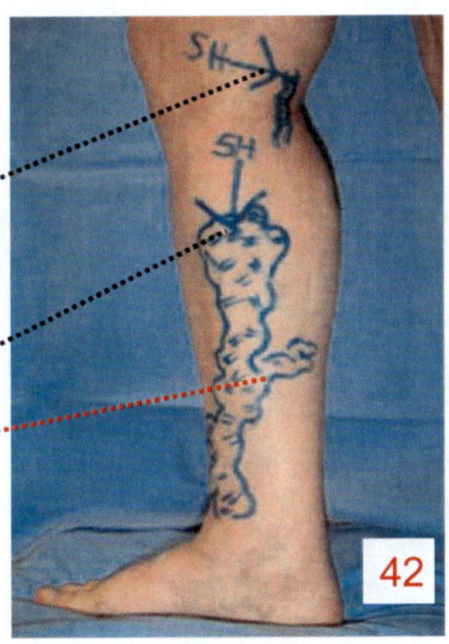


42

**Fig. 42:**
•The procedure is completed by double N2-N3 disconnection, multiple stab avulsion of the proximal varices, and disconnection of the secondary private circulations.

## Anatomical variation of the so called LAMBDA SFJ

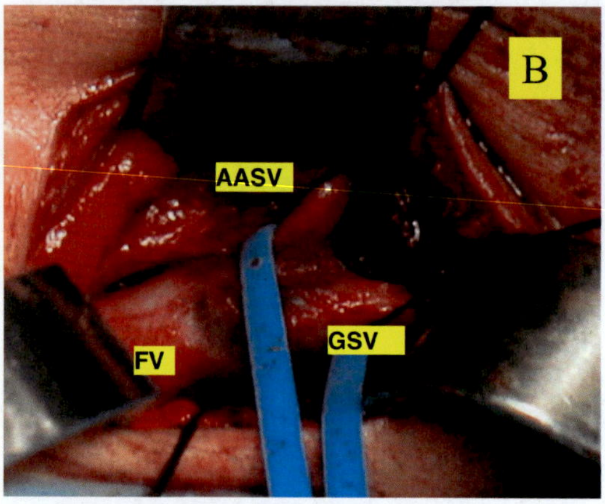


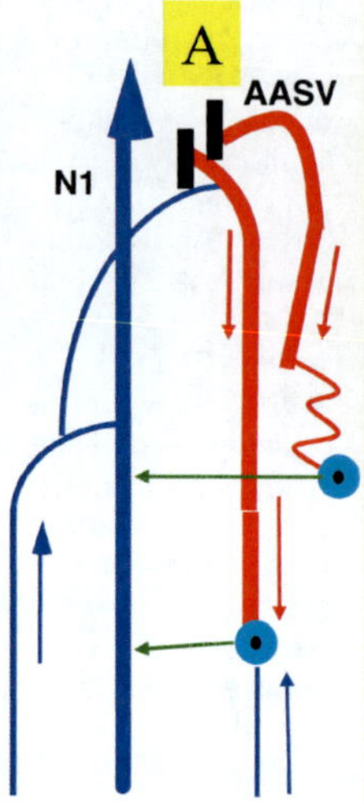


43

**Fig. 43:** If unfortunately the AASV outlet is too close to the SFJ (Fig B), usually surgeons perform disconnection of both the saphenous veins, as depicted in Fig. A. However, such a surgical solution isn't a haemodynamic one, because provokes a flow reversal from its physiological direction in the AASV. The lack of anatomic pathways located along the AASV for re-entering flow in-ward, it is more likely to feed by reflux a tributary. Along time the latter will become varicose, leading to recurrences (red line depicted in Fig. A). [249]

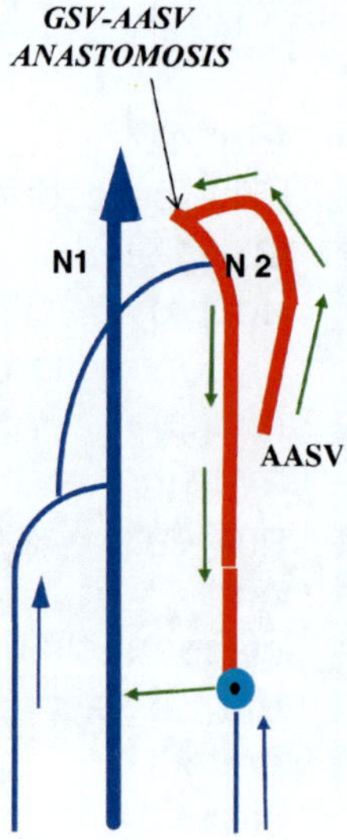


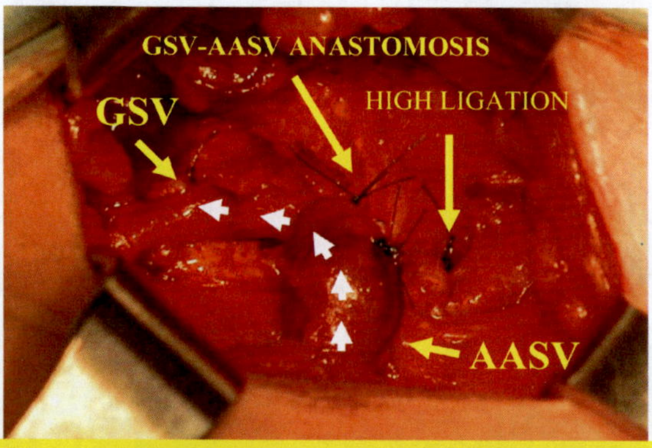


44

**Fig. 44:** In the case showed in the previous slide the haemodynamic alternative is aimed to preserve the outlet between the AASV and the GSV, despite the too close AASV to the SFJ. So far we performed end to end venous anastomosis in order to allow the drainage of the AASV into the GSV. This certainly is the most skilled but also effective surgical strategy, allowing AASV to drain into the GSV in muscular systole, and in turn the GSV to drain down-ward to the re-entry perforator in muscular diastole.

# CLINICAL CASE G:the tobacconist

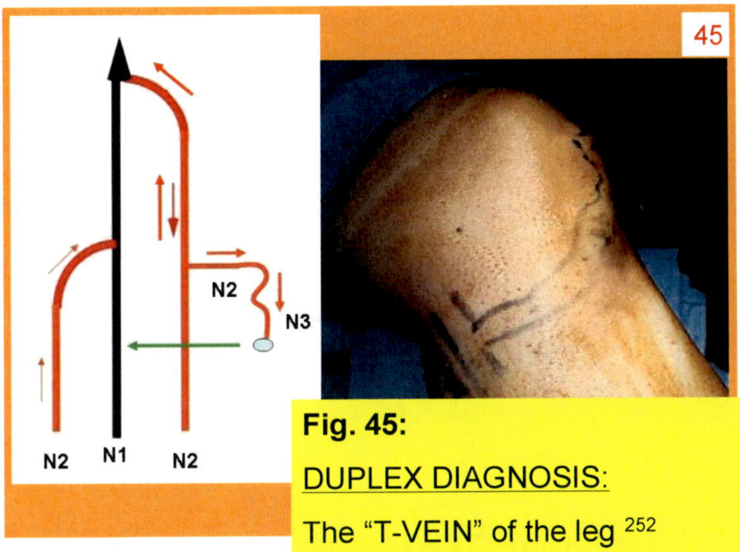


**Fig. 45:**

DUPLEX DIAGNOSIS:

The “T-VEIN” of the leg [252]

Type II shunt

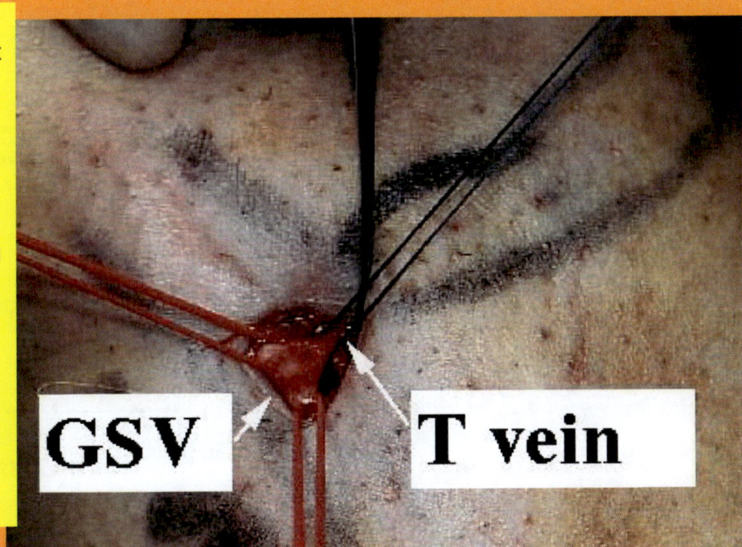


**Fig. 46:** As far as surgery is concerned it is impossible to treat properly such clinical case through a traditional phlebectomy micro-incision.
Due to the overlapping of the fascial layer and the T termination a flush ligation is possible only through a larger incision (1,5-2 cm), that allows a careful exposure of both saphenous vein and AC2.

46

## CONCLUSIONS

At the conclusion of chapters 9 and 10, we would like to emphasize how pathological venous networks are extremely variable, and how standardized surgery cannot be adequate to all variants. We herein presented several paradigmatic cases, choose among the more frequent situations in clinical practice, and demonstrated how venous surgery could be tailored and coherent with preoperative duplex haemodynamics. The concept of Doppler guided surgery is set against that of standardized classic or endovascular ablative surgery.

CHIVA aim is to restore venous drainage by restoring the hierarchical order of emptying of the venous networks and suppressing points of reflux.

However, despite the variability of shunts presentation, CHIVA procedures can be standardized taking into account the haemodynamic findings and their relative incidence as follows:

### CHIVA-TAILORED SURGERY

| DUPLEX INDICATION | PROCEDURE |
|---|---|
| • ANY SHUNT TYPE, COMPETENT TERMINAL VALVE | CHIVA1 shot without high tie: T flush ligation-avulsion (case A, E, G). 45% in clinical practice |
| • TYPE I SHUNT, INCOMPETENT TERMINAL VALVE | CHIVA1 shot: high tie and T flush ligation-avulsion (case B, F). 25% in clinical practice |
| • TYPE III SHUNT INCOMPETENT TERMINAL VALVE | CHIVA2 steps: T flush ligation-avulsion, followed by high tie 6-18 months later; or, if technically feasible CHIVA 1 shot with valvulotomy (case B appendix) . 25% of cases |
| • OTHER HAEMODYNAMIC PRESENTATIONS | SINGLE SHOT CORRECTION *a la carte* Case C, D |

Chapter 11

# THE CHIVA RESULTS

***Paolo Zamboni***
University of Ferrara, Italy.

Probably, a new method of treating varicose veins and CVD was never fully and longer studied than the CHIVA strategy. Pathophysiologic changes induced by CHIVA procedures are extremely interesting models of either venous haemodynamics or patho-physiology.

We can divide results of haemodynamic correction CHIVA in functional and clinical one.

## A. FUNCTIONAL RESULTS

Venous function can be assessed invasively, by the means of duplex, ambulatory venous pressure (AVP), and non invasively, by the means of photoplethysmography (PPG)-light reflection reography (LRR), or air plethysmography (APG) (see chapter 8).

### 1. Duplex Scanning

One of the most debated point of the so called CHIVA 1 procedure is the reverse flow downward the re-entry perforator obtained after high ligation (see chapter 10). Many investigators considered it a reflux [108,211]. Postoperative duplex investigation in CHIVA 1 procedure demonstrates significantly different haemodynamic parameters of the reverse flow without change of compartment as compared to preoperative reflux.

Particularly, peak systolic velocity (PSV), peak diastolic velocity (PDV) and resistance index (RI) as an impedance parameter derived from the formula

RI = PSV/PSV-PDV are significantly different (G. Tacconi, E. Menegatti personal communication EVF Annual Meeting Barcellona 2008). Furthermore draining reverse flow corresponds to significant reduction of the cross sectional area of the GSV, which is in turn correlated to reduction of venous volume (Figure 11.1).

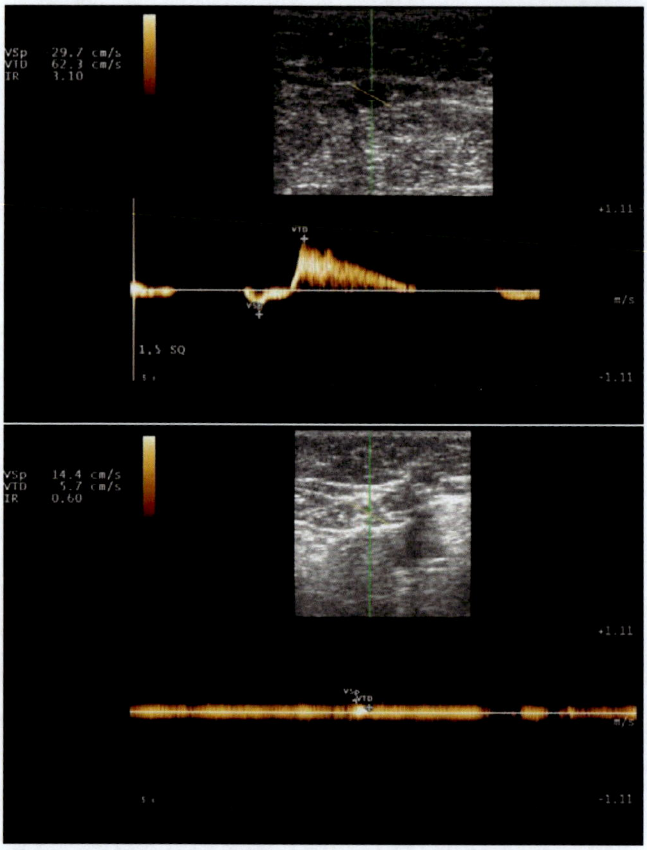


Figure 11.1. Top panel: preoperative reflux wave assessed 15 cm below the SFJ in type I shunt. Bottom panel: draining reverse flow assessed in the same position 6 months after CHIVA 1 procedure. The significant change in PSV PDV and RI are indicated as Vsp, VTD, and IR respectively on the left side of the Doppler trace of the top and bottom panel. Particularly, RI passed from 3.10 to 0.60 clearly indicating the modification of flow impedance obtained by CHIVA 1 procedure. In addition the dramatic reduction of the cross sectional area of the GSV are apparent by comparing the preoperative saphenous eye image with that obtained postoperatively.

Therefore, reverse flow of drainage without change of compartment is observed also in human physiology and is classified as shunt 0 (see chapter 5). In addition, the significance of the draining reverse flow is testified by the relationship between it and the improvement of functional parameters like AVP and APG described in the next paragraphs.

## 2. AVP (Ambulatory Venous Pressure)

The fall of venous pressure occurring with exercise represents the functional reserve of the venous system of the lower limbs and closely correlates with the clinical class of CVD [23,183,184]. It can be measured by the means of a needle transducer inserted into a foot vein, assessing the pressure at rest in standing (hydrostatic pressure), and after exercise (usually 10 tip-toe movements). In addition, it permits to assess the refilling time RT, i.e. the time to return from the minimal pressure value reached stopping the exercise to the initial value in standing position (Figure 11.1). Parameters can be assessed also excluding the superficial reflux by encircling the thigh with a tourniquet. Although some overlap exists between AVP values obtained in either healthy or insufficient veins of the lower limbs, such a measure is widely considered the gold standard in the evaluation of venous function.

Seventythree patients underwent preoperatively and 6 months postoperatively AVP assessment by the means of classic puncture with a needle transducer of a foot vein, after a CHIVA I procedure. CHIVA I contemplated SF disconnection plus flush ligation of the tributaries at the saphenous trunk complemented by multiple stab avulsions (see chapter 10). The preoperative value assessed after ten tip-toe exercise was $50.13 \pm 6.56$ mmHg; it passed to $28.82 \pm 7.14$ mmHg six months postoperatively. The difference between pre and postoperative measurements was statistically significant using both Student 's t and Wilcoxon' s tests ($p<0.001$) [270].

## 3. LRR (Light Reflection Reography)

The same group of 73 patients underwent to LRR evaluation preoperatively and 6 months postoperatively. LRR and PPG are both non -invasive methods capable to give a rough estimation of the calf muscular pump based on the slope of the curve obtained with tip-toe exercise. More precisely both methods can assess refilling time non-invasively (Figure 11.1) [19,214]. Refilling time measured preoperatively was $10.12 \pm 2.6$ seconds. After CHIVA I procedure was prolonged to $19.80 \pm 4.91$seconds, confirming the finding measured by the means of EVT (Figure 11.2). The difference between pre and postoperative measurements was statistically significant using both Student 's t and Wilcoxon' s tests ($p<0.001$) [270].

## 4. APG (Air Plethysmography)

APG permits to extrapolate four parameters which investigate several aspect of venous function [19,58,59]. Total Volume (TV), which is the amount of blood to be found in the venous reservoir, and measures the change in volume (in ml air) produced by the passage from the supine position with the leg raised at 45° to the standing position.

Venous Filling Index (VFI), the volume variation produced in a limb in a defined time by the passage from the supine to the standing position. VFI is related to the severity of the reflux and is expressed in ml air/sec.

Ejected Fraction (EF) which is the rate of the reduction of TV after a single tip toe movement. It reflects the calf muscular systole.

Residual Volume Fraction (RVF), the rate of reduction of TV obtainable after ten tip toe movements. This index is linearly and significantly related to ambulatory venous pressure measurement (Figure 11.3).

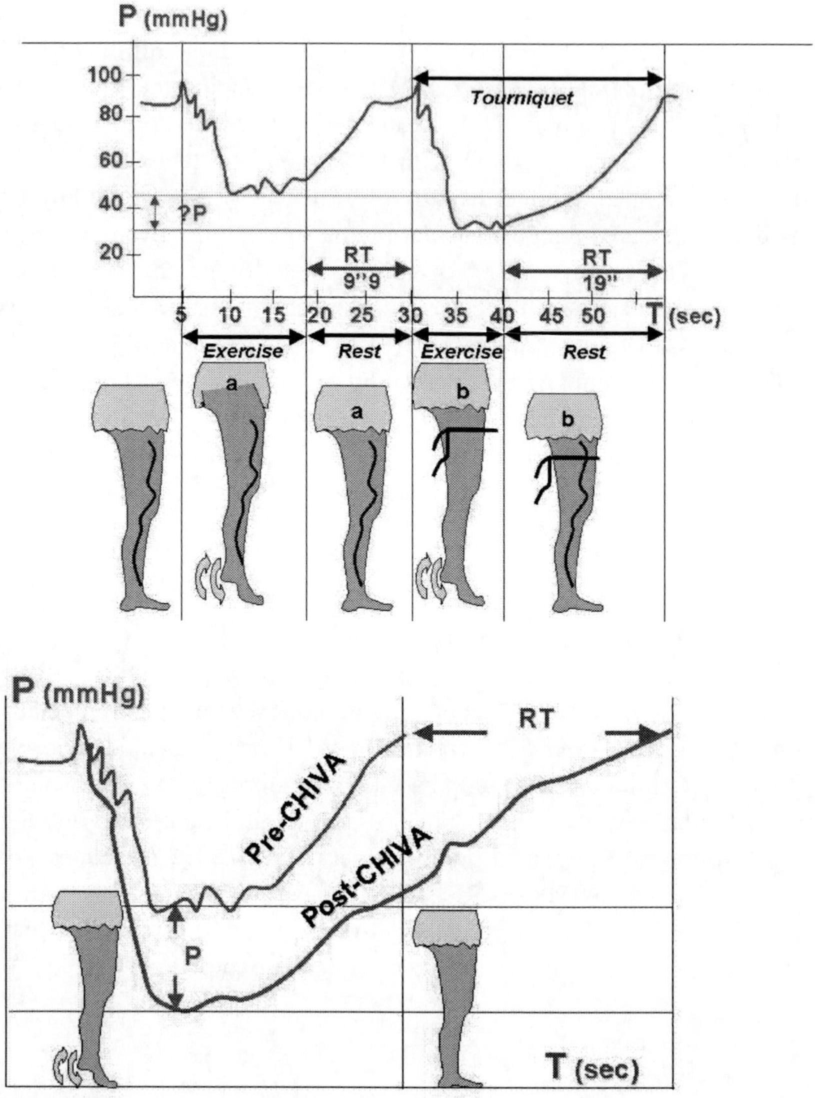


Figure 11.2. Ambulatory Venous Pressure. Top panel: Normal Values P:Pressure. PAE: P after exercise < 30mmHg , ΔP: PEA variation between a and b conditions. RT: refilling time after exercise , i.e. the time necessary to return to the resting pressure, > 18 sec. Normal PAE drop and RT are due to normal haemodynamics which allows the valvulomuscular pump to achieve the dynamic fractionation of the hydrostatic pressure (DFHP). a:In the case( a) the spontaneous PAE is to high > 30 mmHg and RT too short. b: A tourniquet at the proximal thigh corrects the values up to normal. Why? Because the tourniquet closure of the superficial at the thigh restores the DFHP, pressing and so disconnecting a superficial closed shunt probably due to a great saphenous reflux in that case. Bottom panel: The preoperative value assessed after ten tip-toe exercise was $50.13 \pm 6.56$ mmHg, passed to $28.82 \pm 7.14$ mmHg six months postoperatively. Refilling time measured preoperatively was $10.12 \pm 2.6$ seconds. After CHIVA I procedure was prolonged to $19.80 \pm 4.91$secondsThe difference between pre and postoperative measurements was statistically significant using both Student 's t and Wilcoxon' s tests ($p<0.001$).

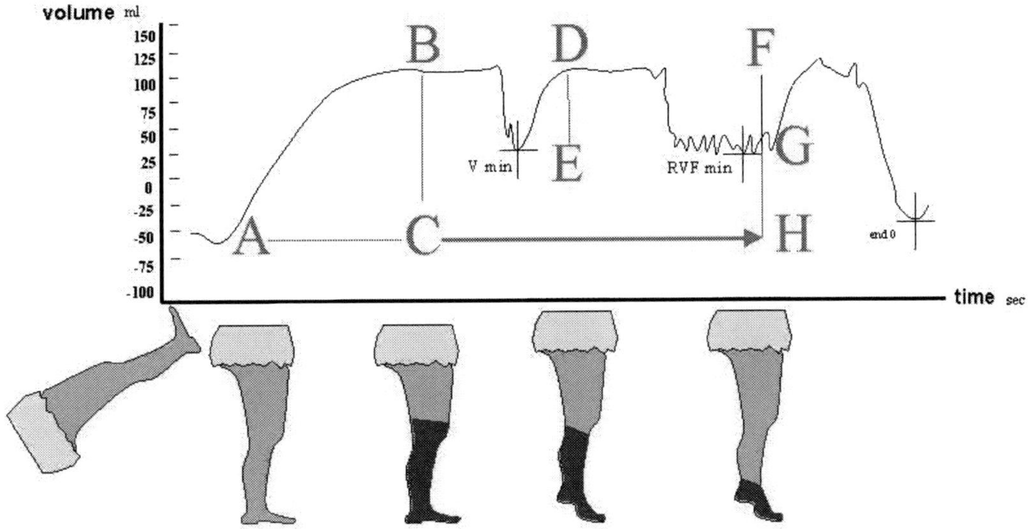


Figure 11.3. APG Trace. TV n.v. < 130ml; total volume of blood in the venous reservoir of the leg = segment BC. VFI n.v. < 2 ml/sec; time for refilling of blood the leg passing from leg elevation to the standing posture = BC/AC. EF n.v. > 55%TV; expelled volume with just one tip-toe exercise, systolic ejection fraction of the calf pump = DE/BC %. RVF n.v. < 30%TV; residual volume in the venous reservoir of the leg = GH/BC%.

APG examination was performed in all cases between 8 and 10 a.m. at the same temperature (23C°), just before CHIVA was performed for correction of chronic venous insufficiency.

Interestingly, APG were measured after simple disconnection of varicose tributaries from the main saphenous trunk, the so called first step of CHIVA II procedure (see chapter 10) [252].

All air-gas plethysmographic parameters, with the exception of Ejection Fraction (EF), significantly improved: Venous Volume (VV) changed from 150 ml ± 9 to 119 ± 6 and 114 ml ± 7 after 1 and 6 months, respectively ($p < 0.0001$), Venous Filling Index (VFI) from 4.9 ml/sec ± 0.5 to 2.3 ±0.2 both after 1 and 6 months, respectively ($p < 0.0001$), and Residual Volume Fraction (RVF) from 42 ml ± 3 to 29.8 ± 2 and 30.2 ± 2 after 1 and 6 months, respectively ($p < 0.0001$).

In the graphics of Figure 11.4 and Figure 11.5 the improvement of VFI and RVF is well apparent, so demonstrating that reflux in the GSV is firmly suppressed by the disconnection of the TV containing the re-entry PV, just eliminating the gradient between the reflux point (i.e. the SFJ) and the re-entry point in the deep veins.

Reflux doesn't exist more until the reappearance of the gradient. Reflux did recur in 15% of the patients in which a re-entry perforating vein newly developed. This time opening of the perforator was found on the main GSV trunk.

Reflux elimination achieved by the elimination of the gradient determines significant improvement in venous function, as assessed by means of APG, and it is not related to a false finding measured by diplex scanning.

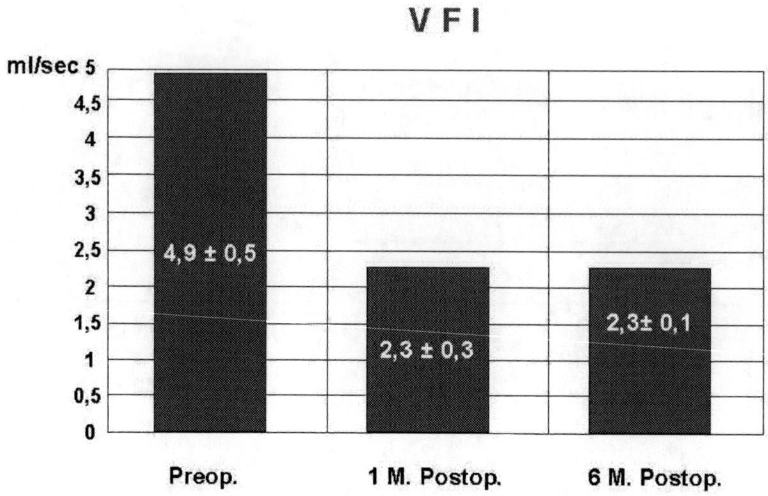


Figure 11.4. VFI changes after 1st step CHIVA 2 PROCEDURE Eur. J. Vasc. Endovasc. Surg. 2001.

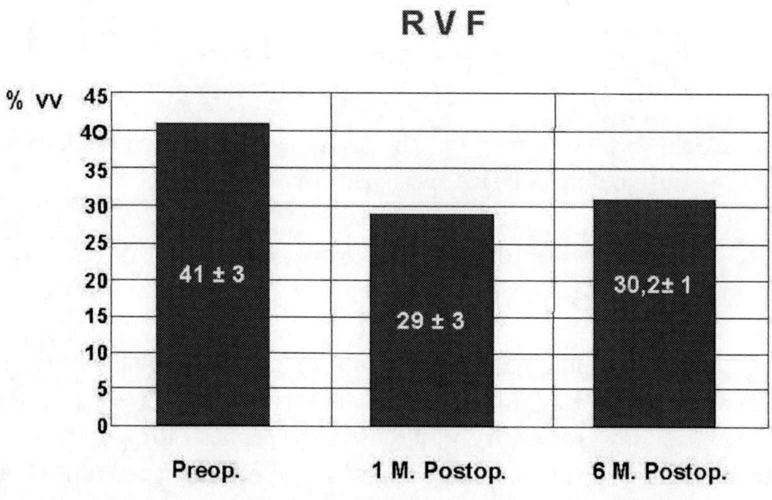


Figure 11.5. RVF changes after 1st step CHIVA 2 PROCEDURE Eur. J. Vasc. Endovasc. Surg. 2001.

## 5. Long Term APG Assesment

Non invasive air gas plethysmography was used for assessment of changes in venous function in a randomized study comparing CHIVA (CHIVA I and CHIVA I +II) to compression in course of active primary ulcers.

Parameters were assessed at the time of randomization and repeated six months and three years later, respectively (Table I).

In the haemodynamic CHIVA group, all four parameters, with the exception of the ejection fraction, significantly improved 6 months after the operation. However, after three years, only Residual Volume Fraction was found to be consistently corrected and significantly improved. However, this is the more important parameter since correlates with AVP and represents the net-volume of blood which remains stowed in the hold of the leg veins after exercise [251].

Interestingly, RVF was found in pathological values only if SF recurrence occurred.

**Table I. Pre and postoperative APG parameters assessed in the surgical group. Grey cells describes postoperative parameters significantly different as compared to preoperative assessment (p < 0.001)**

| *APG assessment* | **TV** | **VFI** | **EF** | **RVF** |
|---|---|---|---|---|
| **Preoperative** | 170 ± 54.6 | 6.7 ± 3.4 | 48 ± 12.5 | 40 ± 15.7 |
| **6 m. after surgery** | **134 ± 44.1 (-25%)** | **3.0 ± 51 (-44%)** | 57.0 ± 18.1 | **29 ± 15.1 -31%** |
| **3 y. after surgery** | 141 ± 42.5 (-16%) | 5.35 ± 2.03 (-5.92%) | 54.0 ± 14.3 (+12%) | **22.5 ± 14.7 -35%** |
| **Ulcer recurrence** | 136.5 ± 6.3 (+2%) | 7.9 ± 4.0 (+21%) | 40.0 ± 14.1 (-24.5%*) | **65.5 ± 6.3 +14%** |

## B. Clinical Results

Clinical results were evaluated in several prospective long term studies, including a meta-analysis which compared haemodynamic CHIVA to stripping [47,56]. More specifically, the results for both stripping and CHIVA homogeneous data available in perspective studies, have been classified by the same examiner into three groups, using Hobbs classification as follows:

1. "Healed" – complete absence of visible varices. Results: stripping = 46%, CHIVA = 60%.
2. "Improved" – residual or newly formed varices visible, but of slight clinical importance. Results: stripping = 45%, CHIVA = 39%.
3. "Unchanged" – complete recurrence of varicosities. Results: stripping = 9%, CHIVA = 1%.

After statistical analysis, using the Pearson test with Bonferroni's modification, the results of CHIVA therapy at the 3-year follow-up point were better than those obtained from the stripping procedure at the same follow-up point (P <0.001).

Clinical results are usually evaluated by the means of Hobbs score. The assessment in CHIVA evaluation was performed by an independent assessor who had not been involved in previous surgical decision making and operative procedure. Hobbs score is measured according to the following criteria [47,56,131,132,140]:

### Objective Assessment:

-class A: no visible and palpable varicose veins

-class B: a few visible and palpable varicose veins with diameter < 5 mm

-class C: remaining or newly formed varicose veins with diameter > 5 mm

-class D: insufficient main trunks and perforator

In addition, functional and cosmetic results were self-assessed by the patients, at the time of the last examination in Hospital, using a simple analogue scale well explained by the indipendent assessor to the patients theirselves:

## Subjective Assessment:

-class A: no inconvenience

-class B: slight functional or cosmetic imperfection, but satisfaction with the result

-class C: appreciable functional or cosmetical failure; improvement but dissatisfaction with the result

-class D: unaltered or increased inconvenience

The four classes, both subjectively and objectively assessed, were divided in accord with the preoperative hemodynamic pattern (Shunt I or III) and tested for significance by chi squared test.

Hobbs score was measured in 186 consecutive haemodynamic correction CHIVA I procedure with 72 months of mean follow-up. CHIVA I procedure was applied in all cases irrespectively of the type of shunt.

Overall saphenous vein patency recorded was 94%, with a mean diameter measured at mid thigh of 4.6 mm as compared to 6.2 mm recorded preoperatively. When patency was demonstrated the saphenous flow was reversed and with low velocity.

Total recurrences/residual varicose veins registered were 11%, 8% for Shunt I and 16 % for Shunt III, respectively.

Symptoms improved in 97% of cases, no-ulcer recurrences were observed in the outcome of the 19 patients in pre-operative clinical class 5 or 6.

Hobbs score: These results are also summarized in Table II. Better results obtained with this technique in patients with Type I Shunt as compared to those objectively and subjectively assessed in Type III Shunt are statistically significant (chi squared=22.144, $p<0.0001$). However, overall evaluation of the technique demonstrated 84% of patients in class A, 11% in class B, 4% in class C and 1% in D (chi squared $p<0.0001$).

This study was really important since demonstrated successful the application of CHIVA I procedure mainly in patients with the out-let of the re-entry perforator on the GSV (Shunt I) (Table II): 92% of disappearance of varicose veins, 99% of saphenous vein patency and when the functional and cosmetic result were subjectively and objectively assessed, we registered excellent and good results (Class A and B of the scale) in 98% and 94% of the cases, respectively.

This finding is not surprising and previous clinical reports of CHIVA technique showed satisfactory results for Type I Shunt but deluding cosmetic results for persistent or recurrent varicose veins in the Type III Shunt, the Achille's heel of the CHIVA theory prior of the introduction of CHIVA in two steps.

Such a results analysis led to consider alternative haemodynamic procedure for type III shunt, which was investigated in a further tailored study.

**Table II. Results in chiva 1 group; Mean follow-up 72 months**

| | **Type I SHUNT** | **Type III SHUNT with re-entry** | **Type III SHUNT without re-entry** | **Type III SHUNT "short or deep"** | **TOTAL** |
|---|---|---|---|---|---|
| VARICOSE VEINS DISAPPEARANCE | 172/186 92% | 16/27 59% | 81/92 87% | 32/35 91% | **89%** |
| VARICOSE VEINS REDUCTION WITH EXERCISE | 9/186 5% | 8/27 30% | 4/92 4% | 2/35 6% | **7%** |
| REFLUX SITE: | | | | | |
| Sapheno-Femoral | 2/186 1% | 1/27 4% | 3/92 3% | 1/35 3% | **2%** |
| Perforators | 6/186 3% | 1/27 4% | 6/92 7% | 1/35 3% | **4%** |
| Sapheno/Tributar | 6/186 3% | 27/27 100% | 2/92 2% | 3/35 9% | **11%** |
| SAPHENOUS VEIN PATENCY | 184/186 99% | 27/27 100% | 74/92 80% | 35/35 100% | **94%** |
| SAPHENOUS VEIN THROMBOSIS | 2/186 1% | 0/27 0% | 18/92 20% | 0/35 0% | **6%** |
| SYMPTOMS IMPROVEMENT | 183/186 98% | 27/27 100% | 84/92 91% | 35/35 100% | **97%** |
| SUBJECT.EVAL* | | | | | |
| Class A | 162/186 87% | 8/27 30% | 74/92 80% | 30/35 86% | **81%** |
| Class B | 21/186 11% | 16/27 59% | 14/92 15% | 3/35 9% | **16%** |
| Class C | 2/186 1% | 2/27 7% | 3/92 3% | 2/35 6% | **3%** |
| Class D | 1/186 1% | 1/27 4% | 2/92 2% | 0/35 0% | **1%** |
| OBJECT. EVAL.* | | | | | |
| Class A | 172/186 92% | 16/27 59% | 81/92 87% | 32/35 91% | **89%** |
| Class B | 4/186 2% | 3/27 11% | 5/92 1% | 4/35 11% | **5%** |
| Class C | 6/186 3% | 7/27 26% | 3/92 1% | 1/35 3% | **4%** |
| Class D | 2/186 1% | 1/27 4% | 3/92 1% | 0/35 0% | **2%** |

**Table III. Hobbs score after first step CHIVA II procedure at 18 months F-up**

| SUBJECTIVE EVALUATION | |
|---|---|
| Class A | 35 pts 87.5% |
| Class B | 5 pts 12.5% |
| Class C | 0 pts 0% |
| Class D | 0 pts 0% |
| OBJECTIVE EVALUATION | |
| Class A | 35 pts 87.5% |
| Class B | 5 pts 12.5% |
| Class C | 0 pts 0% |
| Class D | 0 pts 0% |

## CLINICAL RESULTS OF CHIVA IN TWO STEPS PROCEDURE

40 limbs in 40 patients (26 female, 14 male mean age 52 y.o.) with demonstrated duplex incompetence both of the sapheno-femoral junction (SFJ) and the main GSV trunk with the re-entry perforator located on a tributary [252].

A preoperative skin map was obtained by duplex in order to identify the point where the superficial tributary had to be interrupted. This point correponds to the origin of the varicose TV from the GSV (see chapter 9-10).

All operations were performed under local anaesthesia and consisted in the disconnection of the origin of the TV containing the "re-entry" PV from the main trunk of the GSV. It is mandatory to perform a technically perfect flush ligation on the GSV trunk in order to firmly transform the refluent GSV into a GSV with a forward flow during muscular contraction, but no Doppler-detectable reverse flow during muscular relaxation. The proximal tract of the dilated TV was avulsed through multiple mini-incision technique, sparing the segment immediately above the re-entry PV opening.

Patients were discharged hours after surgery with elastic stockings exerting 20-30 mmHg of pressure at the ankle.

Objective and subjective assessment by using the Hobbs score of the surgical results through the records of the independent assessor are showed in table III.

In all cases after 1 month from the operation duplex investigation demonstrated a GSV with a forward flow during muscular contraction, but no reflux during muscular relaxation. Neither insufficient TV nor PV along the GSV were found.

After 6 months 34 patients maintained such a result. In contrast, six patients (15%) presented with an asymptomatic reflux in the GSV. In these 6 patients, at duplex scanning, the main difference, as compared to the pre-operative examination was the presence of a re-entry PV on the main GSV trunk. No insufficient TV were found in all cases.

# CLINICAL RESULTS OF CHIVA IN PRIMARY VENOUS ULCERS

Haemodynamic CHIVA procedure was further evaluated in a randomized study comparing CHIVA to compression in the treatment of primary venous ulcers [251].

Surgery, in local anaesthesia, consisted in high-ligation complemented by proximal avulsion of the insufficient tributaries (Type I presentation), or in flush ligation and division from the GSV of the insufficient tributaries (Type III presentation).

Patients began to walk 1 hour after the procedure with the ulcer covered by advanced dressing and wearing an elastic stocking exerting 20-30 mmHg of ankle pressure. Patients were discharged within 3 hours and were seen twice a week the first week, and subsequently weekly till the ulcer was healed. Patient follow-up examination occurred every six months along a period of 3 years [24,25].

The difference in ulcer area between the conservative and the CHIVA group, 11 cm2 (3-12) and 10 cm2 (2,6-11,8), respectively, was not significant.

The healing rate was 96% in a period of 63 days (21-180) in the compression group as compared to 100% in 31 days (17-53) recorded in the CHIVA group. No significant difference was demonstrated concerning the rate of healing. However, there was a highly significant ($p<0.005$) difference in the healing time between the two groups.

Finally, ulcer did recur in 9 cases in the compression group along the follow-up (38%) and in 2 cases in the surgical group (9%). The difference is statistically significant ($p < 0.05$). Recurrence analysis by the survivor function of the Kaplan-Meyer estimation is given in Figure 11.6; a significantly better out-come has been demonstrated in the surgical group: $p<0.02$.

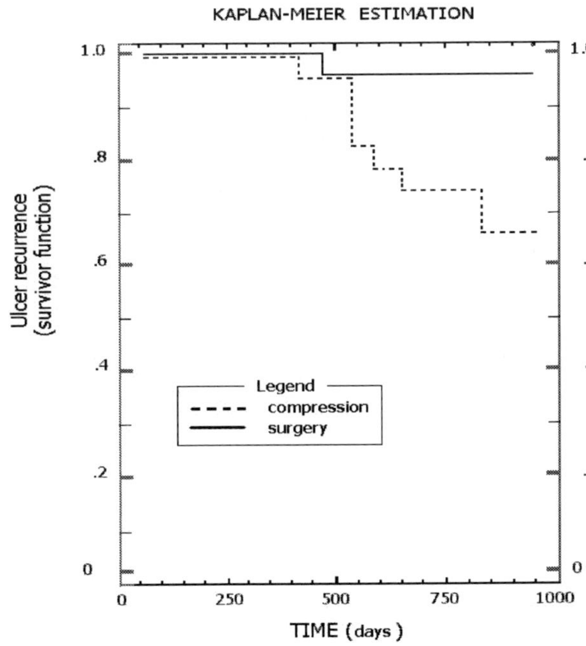


Figure 11.6. Survivor function illustrating ulcer recurrence according to treatment. The better outcome of patients who underwent CHIVA surgery is well apparent.

Ulcer recurrences occurred in two cases as above described. The first case was related to sapheno-femoral recurrence, whereas the second one to further development of a sapheno-popliteal reflux.

Two patients (29%) showed a saphenous reflux after 6 and 30 months, respectively, following the first step procedures for type III hemodynamic presentation: the occurrence of the development of a new re-entry perforator located on the GSV is well established, as above reported. In these two cases we performed the second surgical step, represented by high ligation.

## Quality of Life Assesment

In the same study, SF36 quality of life questionnaire was evaluated. Before interventions no significant differences were found out in the score of the SF-36 questionnaire between the CHIVA and the compression [251].

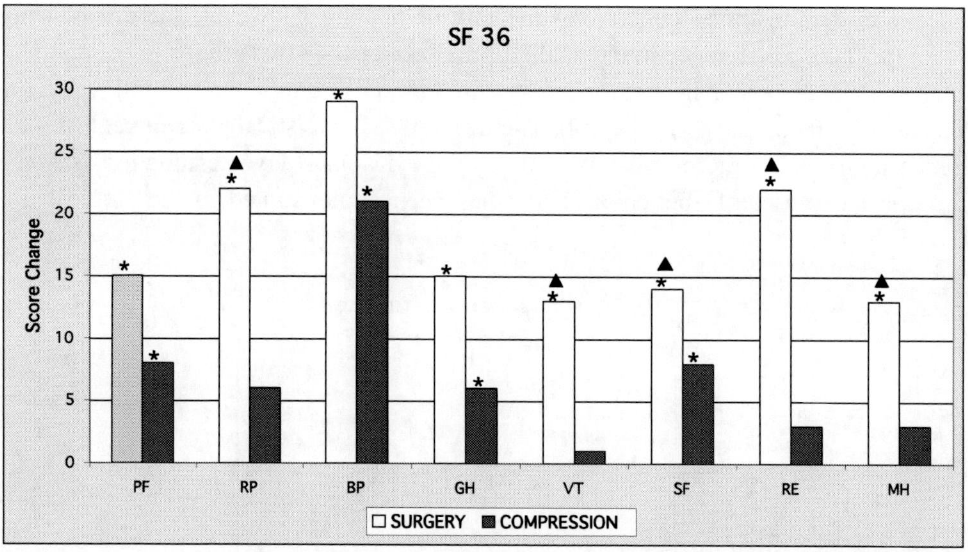


Figure 11.7. Median score differences (end of observation-baseline) are shown for the 8 domains explored by the SF 36 questionnaire. *P<0.05 comparing baseline to end of treatment values, △ P<0.05 comparing surgery vs compression. PF= Physical functioning, RP= Role-physical limitation, BP= Bodily pain, GH= General health, VT= Vitality, SF= Social functioning, RE= Role-emotional limitation, MH= Mental health.

## Randomized Controlled Trials

Stripping procedure is the gold standard in CVD treatment since demonstrated in several RCT to be superior to either sclerotherapy, or high ligation alone, whereas there were no randomised studies assessing in a long-term period the value of conventional stripping versus other surgical procedures [56].

For such a reason, 150 patients affected by CVI, CEAP clinical class 2-6, were randomised to stripping or to CHIVA, preceded by pre-operative Duplex mapping. End-points were: objective and subjective results assessed by the means of the Hobbs score (Hobbs score ranges from 1 to 4,with 4 representing the worst result), either by an independent assessor or by the patients at their own control, respectively; rate of recurrences assessed both by physical and duplex examinations in both groups.

Mean follow-up lasted 10 years, 26 patients were lost, resulting in 54 patients (32 females, and 22 males) in the stripping group, and in 70 patients (59 females, and 11 males) in the CHIVA one. Subjective Hobbs score was not statistically different in both groups. On the contrary, objective assessment resulted significantly better in the CHIVA group (1.94 ±0.09 vs 2.24±0.12, P<0.038). Varicose veins recurrence rate was significantly higher in the stripping group as compared to CHIVA (18% and 35%, respectively, P<0.04), without significant differences in the rate of recurrences from the sapheno-femoral junction.

This study demonstrates that varicose veins more easily recur along time in the Stripping group. Since, no significant differences were found in recurrences from the sapheno-femoral junction, such result could be speculatively related to the presence of a draining saphenous system in the CHIVA group.

At 3 years follow-up the differences above reported were not significant in this and in other RCT, comparing the 2 techniques (Figure 11.8).

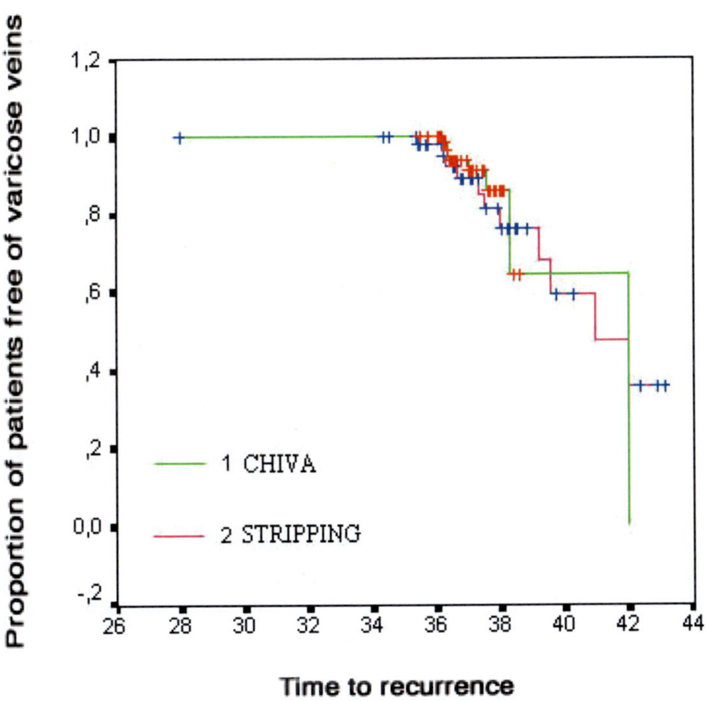


Figure 11.8. This figure shows the survival curve of recurrences at 3.y No significant differences were found between the two techniques at 3 years. In the stripping group the recurrences were caused by pattern # 1,2,3. To the contrary, in the CHIVA group were caused by pattern # 1 and 4 (see Fig.11.10).

In contrast, along the period 3-10 years the different recurrence rate in the two groups becomes well apparent and significant, Mantel test P= 0.004, Tarone test P=0.007, and Breslow test P=0.014. It is noteworthy that, between 3-10 years, in the stripping group the recurrences were caused exclusively by pattern # 5, whereas in the CHIVA patients they were attributable to pattern # 4 (Figure 11.9).

The varicose veins recurrence rate was significantly higher in the stripping group (CHIVA 18%; stripping 35%, P<0.04), without significant differences in the rate of recurrences from the sapheno-femoral junction. The associated risk of recurrence at ten years is increased of more than two times in the stripping group (OR 2.2, 95% CI 1-5, P=0.04).

This RCT demonstrates that varicose veins more easily recur along time in the stripping group. Since, no significant differences were found in recurrences from the sapheno-femoral junction, such result could be speculatively related to the presence of a draining saphenous system in the CHIVA group.

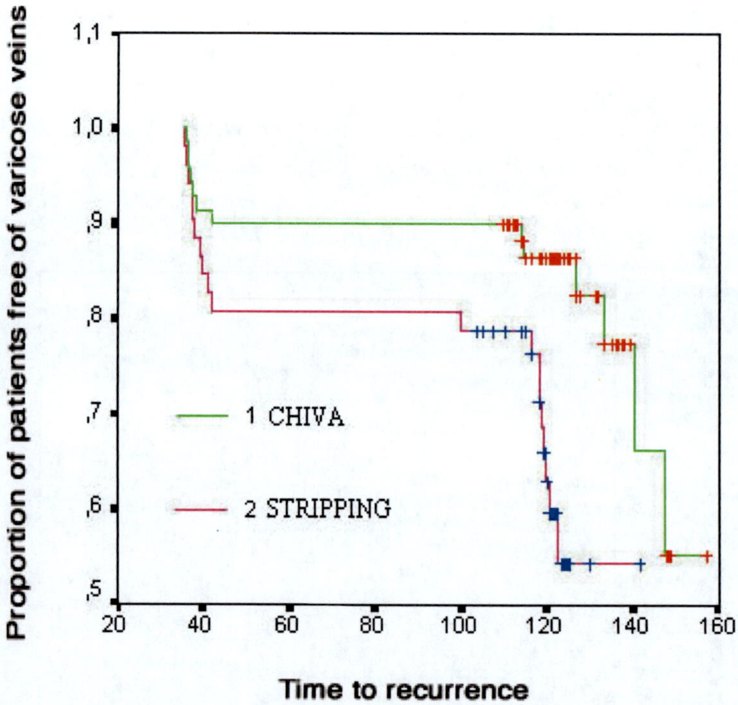


Figure 11.9. Along the period 3-10 years the different recurrence rate in the two groups becomes more and more evident and significant. It is noteworthy that, between 3-10 years, in the stripping group the recurrences were caused exclusively by pattern # 5, whereas in the CHIVA patients they were referred again to new pattern # 4 (see Fig 11.10).

Duplex analysis of the pattern of recurrence is particularly interesting (Figure 11.10). We identified five different haemodynamic patterns of recurrences, differently distributed in the two treatment groups. The presence of combined patterns was the rule in the stripping group, while in the CHIVA group a single pattern of recurrence was more common.

1) ***Type 1 recurrence*** consists of sapheno-femoral recurrence. We found 2 patients out of 70 corresponding to 2.9% in the CHIVA group, and 3 patients out of 54, corresponding to 5.5 % in the stripping group (NS Student's t test).
2) ***Type 2 recurrence:*** consists of reflux coming from the pelvis, through a venous pathway located or in the groin or the perineum, with no associated sapheno-femoral reflux (21). This was present in 1/70 pts, 1.4 % in the CHIVA group vs 2/54 pts, 3.7 % in the Stripping group, NS (Student's t test).
3) ***Type 3 recurrence:*** consists of duplex ultrasound evidence of incompetent thigh perforators not present at the time of the first procedure. This development was not found after ten years in the CHIVA patients (0/70 pts, 0%); while in the Stripping group we have seen 4 patients out of 54 with this pattern (P value NS, Student's t test).
4) ***Type 4 recurrence:*** comprises reflux from the proximal saphenous vein (thigh section) to a varicose tributary. This was only found in the CHIVA group and it is typical of the saphenous vein sparing surgery (13/70 pts., 18.5 % in the CHIVA group vs 0/54 pts, 0% in the stripping group with P value <0.01, Student's t test).
5) ***Type 5 recurrence:*** consists of recurrences from varicose veins greater than 5 mm without any demonstrable escape points or change of compartments. This haemodynamic pattern, in contrast to the previous 4 patterns, is exclusive to the stripping patients and not found in the CHIVA group (0/70 pts, 0% in the CHIVA group vs 12/54 pts, 22% in the stripping group; P<0.01, Student's t test). All the

Duplex results with pattern of reflux in each group are given in figure 11.10.

The main difference between the two groups after 10 years, is the 22% of newly formed varicose veins found in the stripping group, without any detectable reflux point. We believe that this type of recurrence is attributable to the lack of a draining saphenous system [66]. The maintenance of drainage seems to be a decisive factor in avoiding neo-angiogenesis after varicose vein surgery. This observation is confirmed when CHIVA treatment is not correctly performed leading to post-operative GSV thrombosis and occlusion. A non-draining GSV, despite conservative surgery, increases the number of recurrences in comparison to draining GSV systems [45,47,55,270].

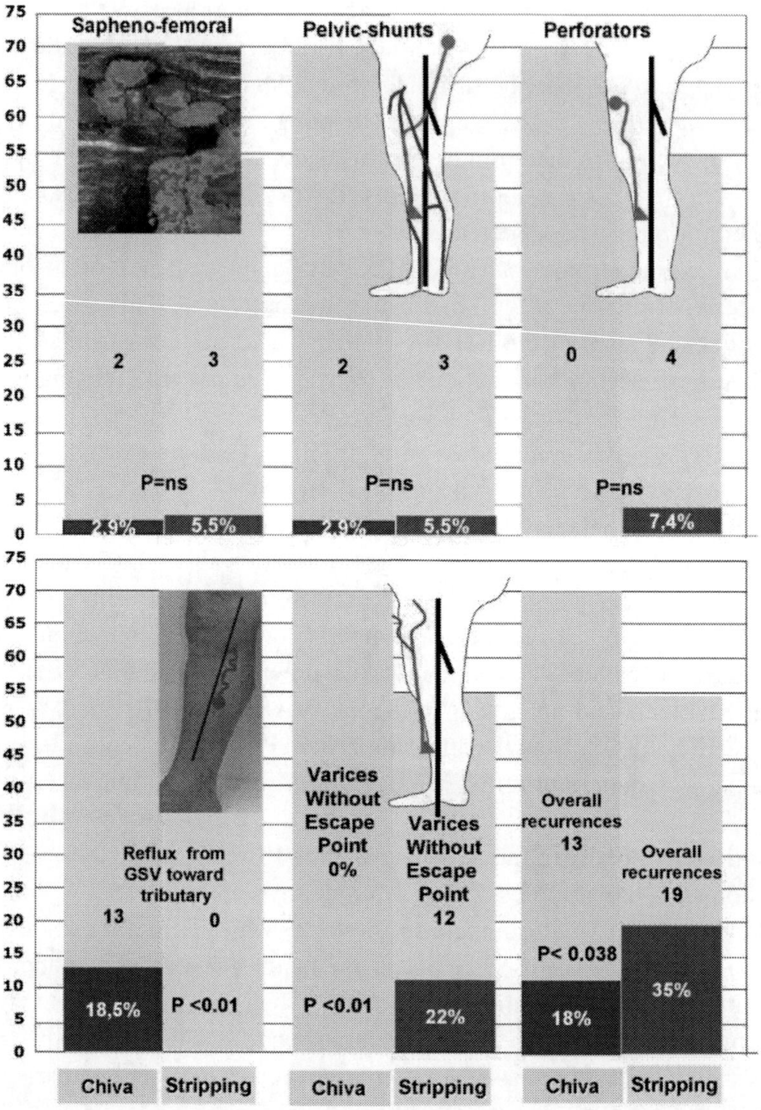


Figure 11.10. Pattern of recurrences after 10 years. Patterns of recurrences find respectively in the CHIVA and stripping group; number of cases and relative rate are reported. Type 1 compares SF recurrences; type 2 recurrences feed by pelvic reflux; type 3 recurrences from perforators. Type 4 reports recurrences due to reflux from the GSV toward a varicose tributary; type 5 varicose veins greater than 0.5 cm in the absence of any detectable reflux point. The last section of the figure summarized total number of patients with recurrences, and the relative rate in both groups.

*Chapter 12*

# THE FALSE PROBLEM OF PERFORATORS

***Paolo Zamboni***
University of Ferrara, Italy.

Perforators in primary CVD are widely considered as an enemy to fight. The original sin is probably due to the general misinterpretation of the classic article written by Frank Cockett on The Lancet [60]. Such hypothesis was that venous hypertension, transmitted to the cutaneous tissue by perforators, in turn causes venous ulcers. The “blow-out” hypothesis was mainly referred to the post-thrombotic legs. In such a condition, outward flow during muscular diastole may occur in the distal leg perforators determining the microcirculatory overload which, in turn, leads to the cascade of events typical of secondary CVD. However, most surgeons were fascinated by the Cockett vision and, despite the fact that it was not supported by relevant scientific data, the era of perforator veins surgery began.

Every severe case of CVD was referred to as the ankle “blow-out” syndrome without any distinction being drawn between a primary and a secondary aetiology in perforating veins incompetence, characterized by opposite patho-physiology, yet.

Previous as well as further scientific data were completely forgotten: the former was simply the Perthes test, a fantastic live-demonstration that, by eliminating superficial reflux, the blood flows down-ward and therefore in-ward to the competent deep veins through the perforators (Figure 12.1).

The latter was the studies of Bjordal, who used electromagnetic flow-metry, and demonstrated that in-ward flow occurred in the distal perforators during exercise in patients with primary CVD (Figure 12.2) [26-30].

The Cockett theory spread by several surgical schools was applied to both primary and post-thrombotic CVD, and, on the basis of my personal discussion with colleagues around the world, I can report that the majority of SEPS surgeons have never read the article in question.

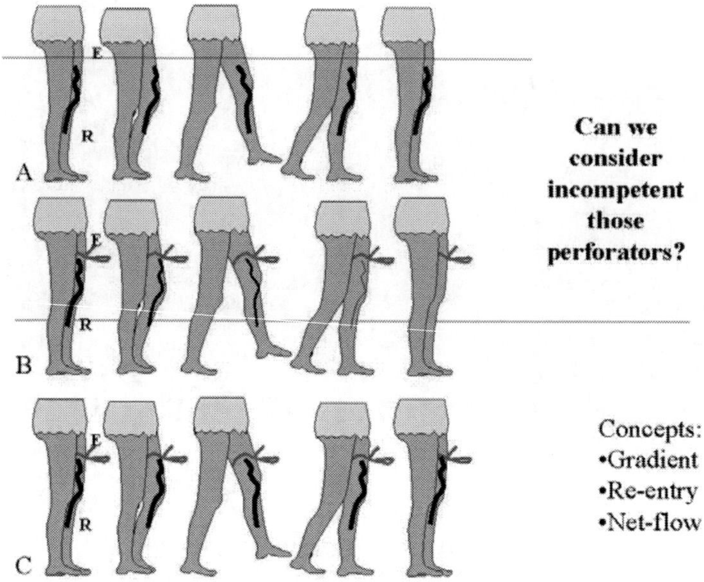


Figure 12.1. Perthes test is a reproducible demonstration of the haemodynamic dependence of distal perforators from superficial reflux. Here is an example of varicose superficial vein related to a closed shunt where E is the refluxing escape point through which the deep blood flows out, then downwards through the superficial incompetent varicose vein, then inward through the re-entry perforator R and then turns back into the deep network. This event occurs only during the valvulo-muscular pump (VMP) diastole because of the valve incompetence (escape point, shunting vein) associated with diastolic reversion of the gradient of pressure. So a flow reversion needs necessarily a valve incompetence AND pressure gradient reversion. When the re-entry perforator is incompetent, retrograde flow can occur only in case of reverse pressure gradient. The Net-flow concept is related to the rate of in-flow and out-flow in bi-directional perforator during stress tests. A: Despite its good condition, the valvulo-muscular pump activated by walk is not powerful enough to narrow the dilate vein of the refluxes the deep blood reclosed shunt. The cause is not into the deep veins through the re-entry perforator R because it is overloaded by thigher pressure to the lower (diastolic reflux fed by the deep veins through the escape point E. B: When the tourniquet presses at the escape point , the diastolic reflux is eliminated and so, the valvulo-muscullar pump power can empty the varicose vein anymore in closed shunt . C: When VMP is impaired and so unable to reverse enough the diastolic pressure gradient (deep venous incompetence or obstacle or muscular inefficiency) the varicose vein doesn't narrow because the net-flow is unfavourable.

During the eighties, Kevin Burnand reported poor results of perforating vein ablation in post thrombotic limbs with ulceration, but the majority of surgeons still continued think them as an enemy. The recent development of SEPS technological and minimal invasive surgery increased perforating ablation throughout the world [115,138,235].

It has been demonstrated by Elfstrom [89] that ablative surgery of the perforating veins significantly reduces the venous drainage of the leg. Illig, unintentionally, demonstrated the same by the means of PPG after SEPS procedures (Figure 12.3) [138,256].

However, despite his poor clinical and PPG results, he stated that PPG is not the best way of assessing SEPS haemodynamic results. The fact that he fails to discuss the poor results of the SEPS procedure and criticizes instead the methodology for assessing the operation indicates the great and unshakable faith of most surgeons in perforating ablation.

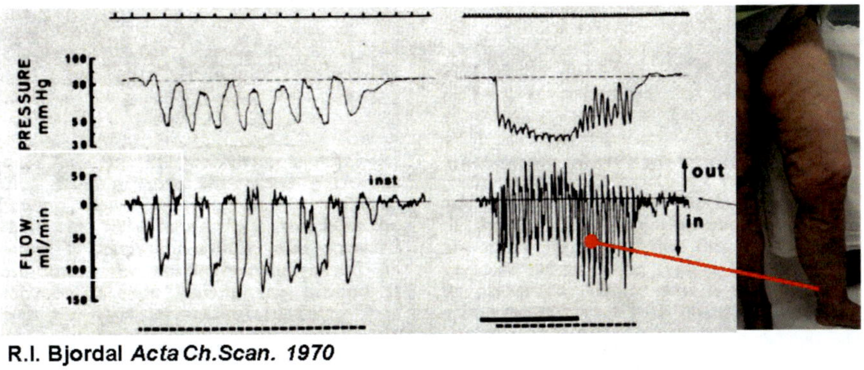


Figure 12.2. Objective measurement of positive NET FLOW in distal perforators by the means of electromagnetic flow-metry [282]. The prevalence of in-ward flow during muscular diastole determines the fall of ambulatory venous pressure (modified from Bjordal).

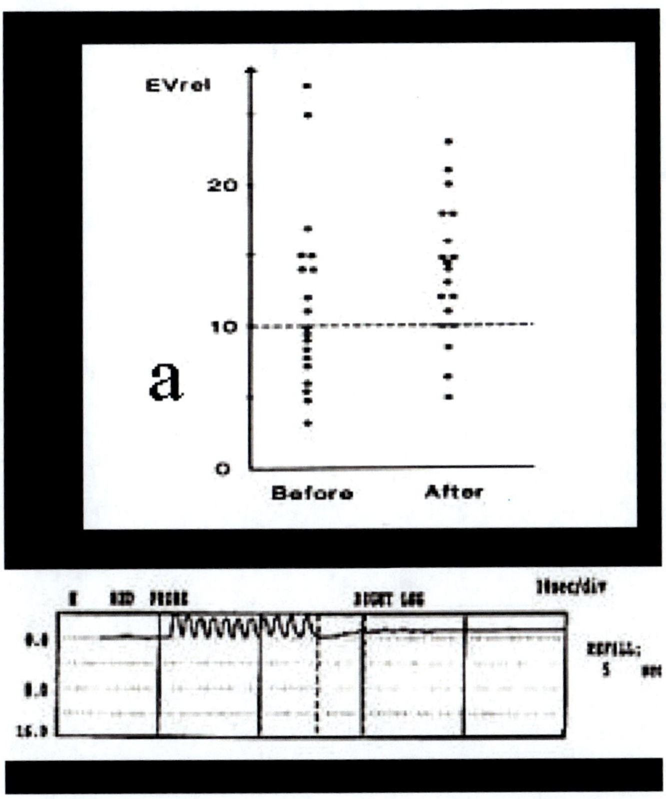


Figure 12.3. Haemodynamic results of indiscriminate avulsion of terminal perforators demonstrate worsening of venous drainage: In the top panel, by the unchanged expelled volume (EV) after the operation (mod. From Elfstrom), and in the bottom panel by the flat curve of PPG (mod. from Illig).

And yet, every day in our vascular lab, Duplex scanning in primary cases demonstrates a bi-directional flow in the Cockett veins with a permanent in-ward flow during muscular diastole! (Figure 12.4).

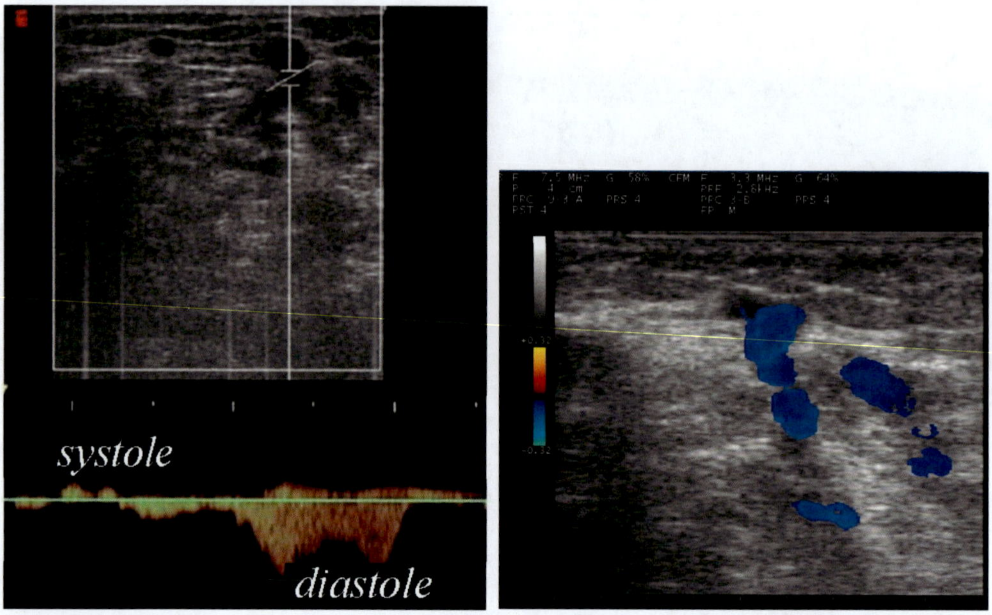


Figure 12.4. The great misunderstanding is the equivalence of perforating veins exhibiting a bi-directional flow with insufficient perforating veins. In primary cases, bi-directional distal perforators show an in-ward flow in muscular diastole with a positive net-flow. A) Duplex trace of a Cockett perforator with the in ward direction at muscular relaxation; B) Blue colour of re-entry at muscular relaxation in a bi-trunk Shermann perforator with the opening on the saphenous vein.

Surprisingly, this finding is considered pathological by many investigators, despite the "net profit" proven both by the Perthes test and electromagnetic flow-metry. In my opinion, it is incorrect to consider insufficient those perforator veins that exhibit bi-directional flow without a critical evaluation of their haemodynamic significance in the context of an insufficient saphenous system. No distinction is made between perforating veins with regards to the flow direction during calf muscular contraction or relaxation [70].

Coleridge Smith has reported that bi-directional flow is commonly found in the distal perforators of normal subjects and therefore cannot be considered diagnostic of insufficiency [212].

The bi-directional criterion creates many limitations, doubts and probably errors both in investigating and in operating.

Furthermore, the standards adopted for duplex assessment of perforator reflux does not permit the identification of re-entry perforators and/or perforators with prevalent in-ward flow, even if bi-directional. These vessels in certain limbs are useful for drainage and cannot be more considered pathological perforating veins. This is the reason of the reduction of venous drainage after perforating veins surgery (Figure 12.4). Careful assessment by colour Doppler of in ward flow during muscular diastole could identify useful pathways for the venous drainage from the lower extremities.

In my opinion, the third element of misconception of the role of perforating veins are studies showing that incompetent perforating veins are associated with recurrent varicose veins.

Such a finding is certainly not surprising. Ablative surgery causes removal of the natural basin of superficial blood collection (saphenous vein) and of its drainage pathways. Residual veins need to drain blood and a gradient guides the flow inward through perforating veins. Thus, the increased number of perforating veins are not a cause but instead a consequence of the new hemodynamic and pathophysiologic scene. This occurs some years after a stripping procedure, even when it is technically correct (see long term results after stripping chapter 11).

Finally, an important element of the perforating veins misconception in primary cases can be brought back to the use of phlebography in clinical practice, of course widely utilized in the pre-ultrasounds medical era. Unfortunately, phlebography doesn't provide any information about blood flow direction in the perforating veins during muscular contraction/relaxation, but just static, sometimes impressive, images of the vein system. In static conditions the valves are open and the blood distribution in the veins regularly occurs by reason of the principle of communicating vessels.

## 1. Incompetent Perforators: Terminal, Non-Terminal and Terminalized

Within the field of 'private circulations', or venous shunt in primary cases, by the means of duplex we can detect perforators exhibiting a bi-directional flow, usually considered insufficient.

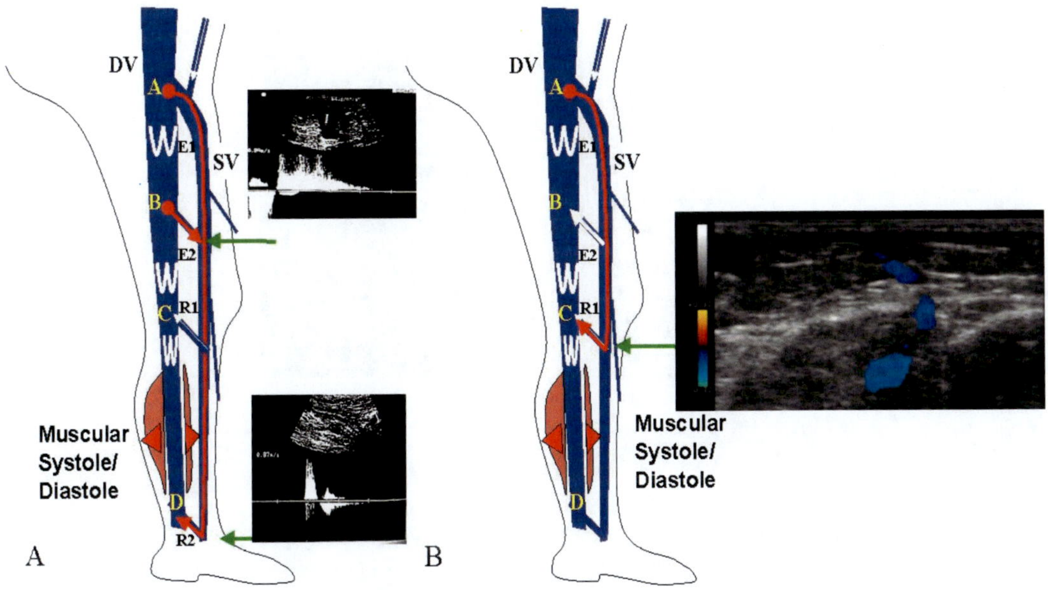


Figure 12.5. Proximal perforators are more likely to show out-ward flow in muscular diastole, and are usually defined non-terminal perforators (panel A, top trace). In contrast, in primary cases, distal or terminal perforators demonstrate out- ward flow in systole and in-ward flow in diastole (panel A, bottom trace), or just in-ward flow (panel B).

Further analysis of flow direction in muscular systole and diastole, allows distinction in two categories [49]:

a) **"Terminal"** incompetent perforators or those in the **"terminal zone,"** that is, located in the most distal part of the 'private circulation' and representing natural re-entry points (Figure 12.5);
b) **"Non-terminal"** incompetent perforators or those located along the pathway of the 'private circulation' (Figure 12.5);

During muscle contraction the majority of the incompetent perforators aspirates blood from the superficial circulation to the deep circulation (Figure 12.6), while a minority produces systolic reflux; this however can be observed mainly in the terminal zone, due to sudden acceleration applied distally to the deep veins by the calf contraction (Figure 12.5 panel A, bottom). During muscle relaxation the incompetent perforators in the terminal zone aspirate blood from the superficial circulation to the deep circulation. It is important to note, however, that perforators producing a systolic reflux (those in the terminal zone) are "compensating for" primary varices since the bias between rates of systolic reflux and diastolic re-entry is weighted in favour of the re-entry rate, as Bjordal has shown. Such perforators therefore are incompetent but "**sufficient**," i.e., functionally compensatory.

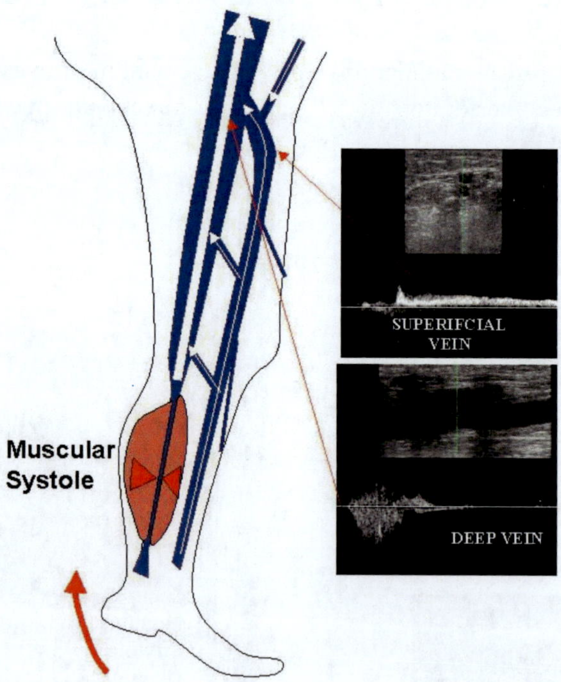


Figure 12.6. Muscular contraction applies more energy to deep veins as compared to superficial one resulting in increased Doppler flow velocity. According to Bernoulli law and Venturi effect (see Pitot's tubes) this contributes to the aspiration of blood from the superficial to-ward the deep veins in proximal perforators and/or junction level during muscular contraction. The consequent drop in lateral pressure in the deep veins determines an in-ward flow at muscular contraction (Bernoulli Law).

We found this pattern in the vast majority of perforating veins investigated by duplex. In primary cases, exactly 2200/2337 (94,1%) perforators demonstrated an in-ward flow in muscular diastole, and were prevalently located in the Cockett and paratibial groups.

Non-terminal incompetent perforators, on the other hand, may demonstrate diastolic reflux from the deep circulation to the superficial circulation as one progresses from the terminal zone; this is promoted by a pressure gradient from deep level to surface level. This gradient is evidently related to the increased diastolic velocity of the superficial reflux and the consequent drop in lateral pressure on the superficial side by reason of the Bernouilli principle and Venturi effect. The diastolic reflux from the non-terminal perforator supplies the secondary reflux from the incompetent perforator. In our survey we found this pattern in 137/2337 (5.9%) perforators with an out-ward flow in muscular diastole, prevalently located in at the thigh.

Compression below the non-terminal perforator interrupts the secondary 'private circulation' and causes the diastolic reflux to disappear. This procedure also helps to demonstrate the flow inversion in diastole from surface level to deep level, just as with the terminal perforators.

This phenomenon has been called **"terminalization"** of the perforating veins. From a physics perspective, it is the result of reduced diastolic velocity of the primary reflux and of decreased compliance, which in turn is due to the reduced rate of output from the system. The result of both of these events is an increase in superficial lateral pressure, which inverts the gradient that favors aspiration of blood toward the deep circulation (see chapter 1).

Since the perforator terminalization phenomenon reduces the height of the hydrostatic column as well as the compliance of the system, while increases the superficial lateral pressure. Such change of haemodynamic forces automatically limits the degree of systolic reflux and restores balance to the flow of blood between the two systems (Figure 12.7).

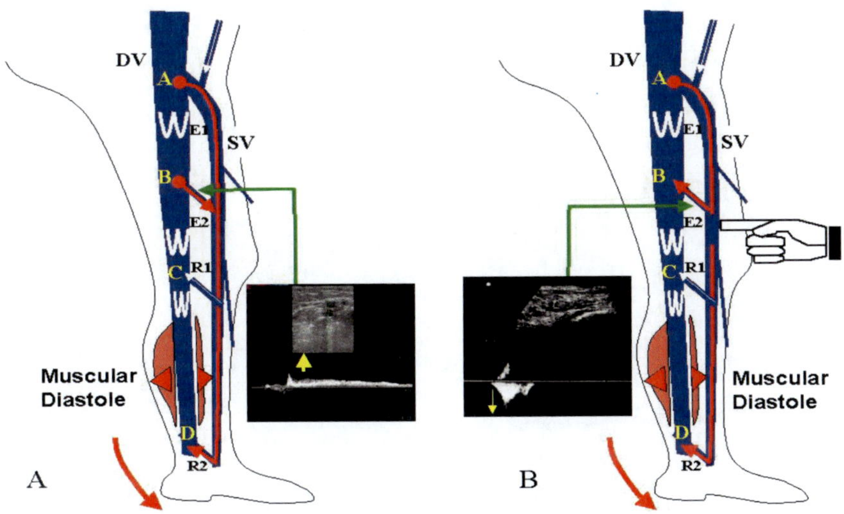


Figure 12.7. Terminalization Phenomenon of an incompetent Hunter perforator, with evident reflux in E2. In b, finger compression below the superficial outlet, by modifying the haemodynamic forces, determines in-ward flow in diastole.

It is important to note that some non-terminal perforators stop refluxing in diastole (at least at a velocity that is detectable on Doppler) simply by reduction of the velocity of the retrograde flow on the surface; this happens when a primary reflux point (for example at the sapheno-femoral junction) is closed and the system is transformed from a refluxing system to an outflow system. Evidence of this may be found by observing the hemodynamics of a perforator after application of manual pressure to the primary reflux point (generally assumed to be the saphenofemoral junction) or by compressing a refluxing saphenous trunk.

A terminal or terminalized perforator should be considered as a hemodynamically valid re-entry whenever drainage of the system through the perforator is detected during the relaxation stage.

From the diagnostic perspective, emptying may be obtained either by a compression-release procedure or by a sway test with the patient standing. Achievement of drainage can be verified either directly by placing the pulsed Doppler sample volume within the perforator or indirectly by detecting a retrograde flow in the vessel longitudinally connected directly or indirectly to the perforator. In this latter case, of course, incompetent tributaries located above the targeted perforator should be excluded by finger compression in order to avoid the effects of other re-entry's upon the retrograde flow in the vessel in question.

# REFERENCES

[1] Abbott W.M., Megerman J., Hasson J.E., L'Italien G.J., Warnock D.F. "Effect of compliance mismatch on vascular graft patency" *J. Vasc. Surg.* 1987;5:376-82

[2] Agus GB, Mancini S, Magi G; IEWG. The first 1000 cases of Italian Endovenous-laser Working Group (IEWG).Rationale, and long-term outcomes for the 1999-2003 period. *Int Angiol.* 2006 Jun;25(2):209-15.

[3] Allegra C, Antignani PL, Bergan JJ, Carpentier PH, Coleridge-Smith P,Cornu-Thenard A, Eklof B, Partsch H, Rabe E, Uhl JF, Widmer MT; "International Union of Phlebology Working Group. The "C" of CEAP: suggested definitions and refinements: an International Union of Phlebology conference of experts." *J Vasc Surg.* 2003 Jan;37(1):129-31. No abstract available.

[4] Allegra C, Bergan J."Update on fundamental causes and management of chronic venous insufficiency. Executive summary" *Angiology.* 2003 Jul-Aug;54 Suppl 1:S1-

[5] Arbeille P, Kerbeci P, Greaves D, Schneider S, Hargens A, Hughson R. Arterial and venous response to Tilt with LBNP test after a 60 day HDT bedrest(WISE study). *J Gravit Physiol.* 2007 Jul;14(1):P47-8

[6] Bahnini A, Bailly M, Chiche L, Franceschi C. [Ambulatory conservative hemodynamic correction of venous insufficiency. Technique, results] *Ann Chir.* 1997;51(7):749-60.

[7] Bailly M. [Ambulatory and hemodynamic treatment of venous insufficiency (CHIVA cure).Report of an atypical case] *J Mal Vasc.* 1992;17(3):241-9.

[8] Bailly M. "Cartographie CHIVA. In: *Encyclopédie Médico-Chirurgicale*" Paris, 43-161-B, p. 1-4

[9] Bailly M. "Résultats de la Cure C.H.I.V.A. In: *Techniques et stratégie en Chirurgie Vasculaire*" Jubilé de J.M. Cormier. Edition A.E.R.C.V., Paris,1992: 255-71

[10] Baird R.N., Abbott W.M. "Elasticity and compliance of canine femoral and jugular vein segments" *Am. J. Physiol.*1977;233(1):H15-21

[11] Baird R.N., Abbott W.M. "Pulsatile blood flow in arterial graft" *Lancet* 1976;1976:948-50

[12] Baird R.N., Kidson I.G., L'Italien G.J., Abbott W.M. "Dynamic compliance of arterial graft" *Am. J. Physiol.* 1977;233(5):H568-72

[13] Bartolo M, Nicosia PM, Antignani PL, Raffi S, Ricci S, Marchetti M, Pittorino L. Noninvasive venous pressure measurements in different venous diseases. A new case collection. *Angiology*. 1983 Nov;34(11):717-23.

[14] Bassi G. "La fisiopatologia delle varici safeniche essenziali. In *"Compendio di terapia flebologica"* Ed. Minerva Medica, pp 23-30

[15] Bassi G. "Les mecanismes et les effects des recidives apres traitments actifs de veines perforantes insuffisantes" *Phlebologie* 1987; 40:743-752

[16] Bassi G. "Zur chirurgischen Behandlung der insuffizienten Perforanten des Beines" *Vasa* 1975; 5:252

[17] Bassi G.l. "*Le varici degli arti inferiori*" Minerva Medica, 1962

[18] Bastide. G, Lefebvre D. The "rete venosum plantare" (the plantar venous network or Lejars' venous sole of the foot. *Phlebologie*. 1993 Apr-Jun;46(2):169-71.

[19] Belcaro G., Christopoulos D., Nicolaides A.N. "Basic data related to normal and abnormal lower extremity hemodynamics" *Ann Vasc Surg* 1991; 5:306

[20] Bergan J, Pascarella L, Mekenas L."Venous disorders: treatment with sclerosant foam" *J Cardiovasc Surg (Torino)*. 2006 Feb;47(1):9-18.

[21] Bergan JJ, Pascarella L. "Severe chronic venous insufficiency: primary treatment with sclerofoam" *Semin Vasc Surg*. 2005 Mar;18(1):49-56.

[22] Bergan JJ, Rattner Z."Endovenous therapy"—2005 *Acta Chir Belg*. 2005 Feb;105(1):12-5.

[23] Bergan JJ, Schmid-Schonbein GW, Smith PD, Nicolaides AN, Boisseau MR, Eklof B. Chronic venous disease. *N Engl J Med*. 2006 Aug 3;355(5):488-98.

[24] Bicknell C, Cheshire NJ. The role of superficial venous operations for leg ulceration. *Br J Hosp Med* (Lond). 2006 Jun;67(6):305-8.

[25] Bishop C.C.R., Jarrett P.E.M. "Outpatient varicose vein surgery under local anesthesia" *Br J Surg* 1986; 73:821-822

[26] Bjordal R. "Simultaneous pressure and flow recordings in varicose veins of the lower extremity" *Acta Chir Scand* 1970; 136:309-317

[27] Bjordal R.I. "Circulation patterns in incompetent perforating veins in the calf and in the saphenous system in primary varicose veins" *Acta Chir. Scand*. 1972; 138:251

[28] Bjordal R.I. "Pressure patterns in the saphenous system in patients with venous leg ulcers" *Acta Chir Scand* 1971; 137:495-501

[29] Bjordal R.I. "The clinical implications and therapeutical consequences of the observed hemodynamic patterns" In: *Perforating veins*. Urban & Schwarzenberg, Munchen, 1981

[30] Bjordal R.J. *"Blood Circulation in varicose veins of the lower extremities"* Universitetsforlaget. Oslo 1972

[31] Blanchmaison P., Griton P., Hugentobler J.P., et al "Les valvules ostiales du sujet variqueux. Examen endoscopique" *Phlebologie 44*:615-622, 1991

[32] Boersma W. "Quelques remarques sur l'origine périphérique des veins communicantes de la jambe" *Phlébologie, 20*: 437-443, 1967

[33] Browse NL, Burnand KG.. The cause of venous ulceration. *Lancet*. 1982 Jul 31;2(8292):243-5.

[34] Burton A. *"Fisiologia e Biofisica della circolazione"* Il Pensiero Scientifico Editore, Roma, 1969

[35] Caggiati A, Bergan JJ, Gloviczki P, Eklof B, Allegra C, Partsch H;"International Interdisciplinary Consensus Committee on Venous Anatomical Terminology. Nomenclature of the veins of the lower limb: extensions, refinements, and

[36] Caggiati A, Bergan JJ. The saphenous vein: derivation of its name and its relevant anatomy. *J Vasc Surg* 2002 Jan;35(1):172-5

[37] Caggiati A, Ricci S. The caliber of the human long saphenous vein and its congenital variations. *Ann Anat*. 2000 Mar;182(2):195-201.

[38] Caggiati A, Ricci S. The long saphenous vein compartment. *Phlebology*. 1997;12:107–111.

[39] Caggiati A. Fascial relations and structure of the tributaries of the saphenous veins. *Surg Radiol Anat* 2000;22(3-4):191-6

[40] Caggiati A. Fascial relationships of the short saphenous vein. *J Vasc Surg* 2001 Aug;34(2):241-6

[41] Caggiati A. The saphenous venous compartments. *Surg Radiol Anat* 1999;21(1):29-34

[42] Camilli S., Guarnera G. "*L' insufficienza venosa primaria e le possibilità della chirurgia ricostruttiva*" Padova: Piccin, 1993

[43] Campanello M., Hammarsten J., Forsberg C., Bernland P., Henrikson O., Jensen J. Standard Stripping Versus Long Saphenous Vein-Saving surgery for primary varicose veins: a prospective, randomised study with the patients as their own controls. *Phlebology* 1996; 11:45-9.

[44] Campbell W.A. "Sapheno-femoral reconnection in recurrent varicose veins" *J. Derm. Surg. Onc*. 1994;20:67-68

[45] Cappelli M, Lova RM, Ermini S, Turchi A, Bono G, Bahnini A, Franceschi C. Ambulatory conservative hemodynamic management of varicose veins: critical analysis of results at 3 years. *Ann Vasc Surg*. 2000 Jul;14(4):376-84.

[46] Cappelli M, Molino Lova R, Ermini S, Giangrandi I, Giannelli F, Zamboni P. Haemodynamics of the sapheno-femoral complex: an operational diagnosis of proximal femoral valve function. *Int Angiol*. 2006 Dec;25(4):356-60.

[47] Cappelli M, Molino Lova R, Ermini S, Turchi A, Bono G, Franceschi C. Comparison between the CHIVA cure and stripping in the treatment of varicose veins of the legs: follow-up of 3 years. *J Mal Vasc*. 1996;21(1):40-6.

[48] Cappelli M, Molino Lova R, Ermini S, Zamboni P."Hemodynamics of the sapheno-femoral junction. Patterns of reflux and their clinical implications." *Int Angiol*. 2004 Mar;23(1):25-8.

[49] Cappelli M., Ermini S., Turchi A., Bono G. "Considérations hémodynamiques sur les perforantes" *Phlébologie* 1994, 47, 4: 389-393.

[50] Cappelli M., Ermini S., Turchi A., Bono G. "La sclerose échoguidée" Abstracts XI° Congrès mondial de l'Union internationale de phlébologie Montreal 1992

[51] Cappelli M., Ermini S., Turchi A., Bono G. "Les reflux d'origine pelvienne" Abstracts XI° Congrès mondial de l'Union internationale de phlébologie Montreal 1992

[52] Cappelli M., Ermini S., Turchi A., Bono G. “Perchè conservare le safene” Atti XI° congresso nazionale della Società Italiana di Flebologia Clinica e Sperimentale. Torino 1994

[53] Cappelli M., Ermini S., Turchi A., Bono G., Molino Lova R. “Considérations hémodynamiques sur la vidange saphénienne” *Phlébologie* 1995, 48, 4: 491-498

[54] Cappelli M., Ermini S., Turchi A., Bono G., Molino Lova R. “Réflexions sur quelques aspects généraux d'hydrodynamique et d'hydrostatique” *Phlébologie* 1995, 48, 3: 367-370

[55] Cappelli M., Molino Lova R., Ermini S., Turchi A., Bono G., Bahanini A., Franceschi C.I. “La Cure C.H.I.V.A. dans le traitement de la Maladie Variqueuse : analyse critique des résultats après trois ans” *Ann. Chir. Vasc.* 2000; 14 : 376-84.

[56] Carandina S, Mari C, De Palma M, Marcellino MG, Cisno C, Legnaro A, Liboni A,Zamboni P. Varicose vein stripping vs haemodynamic correction (CHIVA): a long term randomised trial. *Eur J Vasc Endovasc Surg.* 2008 Feb;35(2):230-7. Epub 2007 Oct 26.

[57] Cavezzi A, Labropoulos N, Partsch H, Ricci S, Caggiati A, Myers K, Nicolaides A, Smith PC. Duplex ultrasound investigation of the veins in chronic venous disease of the lower limbs--UIP consensus document. Part II. Anatomy. *Eur J Vasc Endovasc Surg.* 2006 Mar;31(3):288-99.

[58] Christopoulos D., et al. “Venous reflux: quantification and correlation with the clinical severity of chronic venous disease” *Br. J. Surg.* 1988; 75:352

[59] Christopoulos D., Nicolaides A.N., Szendro G., Irvine A.T., Bull M.T., Eastcott H.G. “Air-plethysmography and the effect of elastic compression on venous hemodynamics of the leg” *J Vasc Surg* 1987; 5:148

[60] Cockett FB, Jones DE The ankle blow-out syndrome. *Lancet 1*; 17, 1953

[61] Coleridge-Smith P, Labropoulos N, Partsch H, Myers K, Nicolaides A, Cavezzi A. Duplex ultrasound investigation of the veins in chronic venous disease of the lower limbs--UIP consensus document. Part I. Basic principles. *Eur J Vasc Endovasc Surg.* 2006 Jan;31(1):83-92

[62] Consiglio L., Giorgi G “ Terapia di exeresi o conservativa?” *Minerva Ang.* 1991;16, sup.1: 442-3.

[63] Corcos L, Dini S, De Anna D, Marangoni O, Ferlaino E, Procacci T, Spina T,Dini M. The immediate effects of endovenous diode 808-nm laser in the greater saphenous vein: morphologic study and clinical implications. *J Vasc Surg.* 2005 Jun;41(6):1018-24; discussion 1025.

[64] Cox S.J., Wellwood J.M., Martin A. “Saphenous nerve injury caused by stripping the long saphenous vein” *Br. Med. Journal* 1974; 286:415-7 8

[65] Creton D. 125 reinterventions for recurrent popliteal varicose veins after excision of the short saphenous vein. Anatomical and physiological hypoteses of the mechanism of recurrence. *J Mal Vasc* 1999 Feb; 24(1):30-6

[66] Creton D. A nondraining saphenous system is a factor of poor prognosis for long-term results in surgery of Great Saphenous vein recurrences. *Dermatol. Surg.* 2004; 30:5:May.

[67] Creton D.: *Recidive variquese poplitée après chirurgie du reflux saphène externe 56 rèinterventions poplitées*, Phlebologie, 1996, 49: 205-212

[68] Cromer A.H. *"Physics for the Life Sciences"* New York, Mc Graw Hill, 1977, pp136-45

[69] Crotty T.P. "An investigation of radial reflux in an isolated peripheral canine vein segment" *Phlebology 10*: 115-121, 1995

[70] Danielsson G, Eklof B, Kistner RL. Association of venous volume and diameter of incompetent perforator veins in the lower limb--implications for perforator vein surgery. *Eur J Vasc Endovasc Surg*. 2005 Dec;30(6):670-3.

[71] Darke S.G.: "The morphology of recurrent varicose veins" *Eur. J. Vasc. Surg.* 1992;512-7. 8

[72] Dauzat M. *"Ultrasonographie vasculaire diagnostique"* Vigot, Paris, 1991

[73] Davies A.H., Magee T.R., Baird R.N., Sheffield E., Horrocks M. "Pre-bypass morphological changes in vein grafts" *Eur J Vasc Surg* 1993; 7:642-647

[74] Davies A.H., Magee T.R., Baird R.N., Sheffield E., Horrocks M. "Vein compliance: a preoperative indicator of vein morphology and of veins at risk of vascular graft stenosis" *Br. J. Surg.* 1992;79:1019-21

[75] Davies A.H., Magee T.R., Hayward J., Harris R., Baird R.N., Horrocks M. "Non-invasive methods of measuring venous compliance" *Phlebology* 1992;7:78-81

[76] De Palma M, S.Carandina, P.Mazza, P. Fortini, A. Legnaro, A. Palazzo, A. Liboni, P. Zamboni. Perforator of the popliteal fossa and short saphenous vein insufficiency. *Phlebology*, 2005,20:170-174

[77] De Simone J.G. "Etude de la valvule ostiale de la crosse de la saphene interne et de la parietale de la veine femorale" *Phlebologie 44*:427-459, 1991

[78] DeCamp P.T., Ward J.A., Ochsner A. "Ambulatory venous pressure studies in postphlebitic and other disease states" *Surgery* 1951; 29:365-380

[79] Delis KT, Husmann M, Kalodiki E, Wolfe JH, Nicolaides AN. In situ hemodynamics of perforating veins in chronic venous insufficiency. *J Vasc Surg*. 2001 Apr;33(4):773-82.

[80] Delis KT, Knaggs AL, Khodabakhsh P. Prevalence, anatomic patterns, valvular competence, and clinical significance of the Giacomini vein. *J Vasc Surg*. 2004 Dec;40(6):1174-83.

[81] Della Corte M. *"Manuale di fisica medica"* Società Editrice Universo 1988

[82] Disselhoff BC, der Kinderen DJ, Moll FL. Is there recanalization of the great saphenous vein 2 years after endovenous laser treatment? *J Endovasc Ther*. 2005 Dec;12(6):731-8.

[83] Dodd H.: the varicose tributaries of the popliteal vein, *Brit. J. Surg*, 1965, vol 52, n° 5 May 350-354

[84] Dunn CW, Kabnick LS, Merchant RF, Owens R, Weiss RA. Endovascular Radiofrequency Obliteration Using 90 degrees C for Treatment of Great Saphenous Vein. *Ann Vasc Surg*. 2006 Jul 25;

[85] Edwards J.E., Edwards E.A. "The saphenous valves in varicose veins" *Am. Heart J. 19*:338-351, 1940

[86] Einarsson E., Eklof B., Neglén P. "Sclerotherapy or Surgery as Treatment for Varicose Veins: a Prospective Randomized Study" *Phlebology* 1993; 8: 22-26

[87] Eklof B, Rutherford RB, Bergan JJ, Carpentier PH, Gloviczki P, Kistner RL,Meissner MH, Moneta GL, Myers K, Padberg FT, Perrin M, Ruckley CV, Smith PC,Wakefield TW; "American Venous Forum International Ad Hoc Committee for Revisionof the CEAP Classification. Revision of the CEAP classification for chronic venous disorders: consensus Statement" *J Vasc Surg*. 2004 Dec;40(6):1248-52.

[88] Eklof B. "Modern Treatment of Varicose Veins" *Br. J. Surg*. 1988; 75: 297-98

[89] Elfstrom J, In: Tesi M, Dormandy JA (eds): *Superficial and deep venous disease of the lower limbs*. Edizioni Minerva Medica, Torino 1984 pp 258-60.

[90] Escribano JM, Juan J, Bofill R, Maeso J, Rodriguez-Mori A, Matas M. Durability of reflux-elimination by a minimal invasive CHIVA procedure on patients with varicose veins. A 3-year prospective case study. *Eur J Vasc Endovasc Surg*. 2003 Feb;25(2):159-63.

[91] Escribano JM, Juan J, Bofill R, Rodriguez-Mori A, Maeso J, Fuentes JM, Matas M. Haemodynamic strategy for treatment of diastolic anterograde giacomini varicose veins. *Eur J Vasc Endovasc S*urg. 2005 Jul;30(1):96-101.

[92] Escribano JM."Regarding "Optimal therapy for advanced chronic venous insufficiency" *J Vasc Surg*. 2003 Aug;38(2):411; author reply 411

[93] Evans R.L., Pelley J.W., Quenemoen L. "Some simple geometric and mechanical characteristics of mammalian blood vessels" *Am. J. Physiol*. 1960;199:1150-6

[94] Fegan W.G. "Varicose veins: the "Bob-sleigh" theory" *Phlebology 8*: 142-144, 1993

[95] Fegan W.G., Kline L. "The cause of varicosity in superficial veins of the lower limb" *Br. J. Surg. 59*: 798-801, 1972

[96] Fichelle JM, Carbone P, Franceschi C. [Results of ambulatory and hemodynamic treatment of venous insufficiency (CHIVA cure)]*J Mal Vasc*. 1992;17(3):224-8.

[97] Fischer R., Linde N., Duff C., Jeanneret C., Chandler JG., Seeber P. Late recurrent saphenofemoral junction reflux after ligation and stripping of a greater saphenous vein. *J. Vasc. Surg*. 2001; 34:236-40.

[98] Fligelstone L. , Salaman R., Oshodi T., Wright I., Pugh N., Shandall A., Lane I. Flush saphenofemoral ligation and multiple stab phlebectomy preserve a useful greater saphenous vein four years after surgery. *J. Vascular Surg*. 1995 ;22 :588-92.

[99] Fligelstone L., Carolan G., Pugh N., Shandall A., Lane I. "An assessment of the long saphenous vein for potential use as a vascular conduit after varicose vein surgery" *J. Vasc. Surg*. 1993; 18:836-40 8

[100] Franceschi C. [Ambulatory and hemodynamic treatment of venous insufficiency (CHIVA cure)] *J Mal Vasc*. 1992;17(4):291-300.

[101] Franceschi C. [Conservative hemodynamic ambulatory treatment of venous insufficiency]*Soins Chir*. 1992 Mar;(133):29-31.

[102] Franceschi C. [Measures and interpretation of venous flow in stress tests. Manual compression and Parana manoeuver. Dynamic reflux index and Pstakis index] *J Mal Vasc*. 1997 May;22(2):91-5.

[103] Franceschi C. [The conservative and hemodynamic treatment of ambulatory venous insufficiency] *Phlebologie*. 1989 Nov-Dec;42(4):567-8.

[104] Franceschi C. "La cure CHIVA et la critique: 14 responses et 1 conclusion" *STV* 1993; 5:491-497

[105] Franceschi C.l. *"Théorie et Pratique de la Cure Conservatrice et Hémodynamique de l' Insuffisance Veineuse en Ambulatiore"* Précy-sous-Thil: Editions de l' Armançon, 1988

[106] Francheschi C, Bahnini A. Treatment of lower extremity venous insufficiency due to pelvic leak points in women. *Ann Vasc Surg*. 2005 Mar;19(2):284-8

[107] Franco G. "Exploration ècho-Doppler des veines perforantes des membres inférieurs" *Actualités Vasculaires Internationales*, nov. 1992 n° 6

[108] Franco G. "La Cure Hémodynamique de l' Insuffisance Veineuse en Ambulatiore (CHIVA). Révolution ou régression" *J. Mal. Vasc*. 1992; 17; 301-307

[109] Franco G. Ultrasonographic exploration for recurrent varicose veins in the popliteal fossa after surgery. *J Mal Vasc*. 1997 Dec ; 22(5) : 336-42

[110] Frings N, Nelle A, Tran P, Fischer R, Krug W. Reduction of neoreflux after correctly performed ligation of the saphenofemoral junction. A randomized trial. *Eur J Vasc Endovasc Surg*. 2004 Sep;28(3):246-52.

[111] Georgiev M, Myers KA, Belcaro G. The thigh extension of the lesser saphenous vein: from Giacomini's observations to ultrasound scan imaging. *J Vasc Surg*. 2003 Mar;37(3):558-63.

[112] Georgiev M. "The femoro-popliteal vein: Ultrasound anatomy, diagnosis and office surgery" *Dermatol Surg*. 1996 22: 57-62

[113] Gillot C.l. "Les veines perforantes internes de la jambe, de la cheville et du pied" *Phlébologie* 1994 47, n°1, 76-104

[114] Glass G.M. "Neovascularisation in recurrence of the varicose great saphenous vein following transection" *Phlebology* 1987; 2:81-92

[115] Gloviczki P, Bergen JJ, Rhodes JM, Canton LG, Harmsen S, Ilstrup D. Mid-term results of endoscopic perforator vein interruption for chronic venous insufficiency: lessons learned from the North American Subfascial Endoscopic Perforator Surgery registry. *J Vasc Surg* 1999;29:489-502.

[116] Goren G., Tellin A.E. "Ambulatory stab evulsion phlebectomy for truncal varicose veins" *Am. J. Surg*. 1991; 162:166-74

[117] Gorny P. "Les excés de la "Philosophie" conservatrice dans la chirurgie des varices" *Phlébologie* 1995, 48, 3: 303-305

[118] Gorny Ph., Blanchemaison Ph., Chahine D., Hutinel B., Chanvallon C., Payen B., Reinharez D. "Chirurgie Conservatrice et Ambulatiore: étude comparative entre CHIVA et Crossectomie chez 321 patients opérés de la saphène interne. Discussion" *Phlébologie* 1995, 48, 2: 255-259

[119] Gorny Ph., Chahine D., Payen B., Hutinel B., Blanchemaison Ph., Renaudin J.M., Tran-Duy S. "Crossectomie, éveinage court ou long? Une étude comparative chez 703 patients opérés de la veine saphène interne. Analyse des résultas" *Phlébologie* 1995, 48, 4: 487-490

[120] Gorny Ph., Reinharez D., Hutinel B., Radier P., Blanchemaison Ph., Payen B., Tran-Duy S. "Chirurgie post-stripping en ambulatoire" *Phlébologie* 1994, 47, 3: 265-273

[121] Goulbourne I.A., Ruckley C.V. "Operations for hernia and varicose vein in a day-bed unit" *Br. Med. J*. 1979; 2:712-714

[122] Green G.E., Hutchinson J.E., Mc Cord C. "Choice of saphenous vein segments for aortocoronary grafts" *Surgery* 1971; 69:924-7

[123] Guarnera G., Furgiuele S., Di Paola F.M., Camilli S. "Recurrent varicose veins and primary deep venous insufficiency: relationship and therapeutic implications" *Phlebology* 1995; 10:98-102

[124] Guex J.J., Hiltbrand B., Bayron J.M., Henri F., Allaert F.A., Perrin M. "Anatomical patterns in varicose vein disease: a duplex scanning study" *Phlebology* 1995; 10:94-97

[125] Haeger K. "Five year results of Radical Surgery for Superficial Varices with or without Coexistent Perforator Insufficiency" *Acta Chir. Scand.* 1966; 131: 38-49

[126] Hammarsten J., Bernland P., Campanello M., Falkenberg M., Henrikson O., Jensen J. A study of the mechanisms by which haemodynamic function improves following Long Saphenous vein-saving surgery. . *Phlebology* 1996; 11: 102-5.

[127] Hammarsten J., Campanello M., Pederson P. "Long saphenous vein sparing surgery for varicose veins. Correspondence" *Eur. J. Vasc. Surg.* 1993;7:763-4. 8

[128] Hammarsten J., Pedersen P., Cederlund C.G., Campanello M. "Long saphenous vein sparing surgery for varicose veins. A long term follow-up" *Eur. J. Vasc. Surg.* 1990; 4:361-4. 8

[129] Harada RN, Katz ML, Comerota A: A non invasive screening test to detect critical deep venous reflux" *J Vasc Surg* 1995, 22: 532-37

[130] Hartmann K, Klode J, Pfister R, Toussaint M, Weingart I, Waldermann F,Hartmann M. Recurrent varicose veins: sonography-based re-examination of 210 patients 14 years after ligation and saphenous vein stripping. *Vasa.* 2006 Feb;35(1):21-6.

[131] Hobbs J.T . Surgery or slerotherapy for varicose veins: 10year results of a random trial. *Lancet* 1978; 27;1(8074):1149.

[132] Hobbs J.T. "Surgery and Sclerotherapy in the treatment of Varicose Veins" *Arch. Surg.* 1974; 109: 793-96

[133] Hobbs JT The enigma of the gastrocnemius vein *Phlebology* 1988;3:8-12

[134] Hobbs JT. Varicose veins arising from the pelvis due to ovarian vein incompetence. *Int J Clin Pract.* 2005 Oct;59(10):1195-203.

[135] Hojensgard I.C., Sturup H. "Venous pressure in primary and postthrombotic varicose veins. A study of the statics and dynamics of the venous system of the lower extremity under pathological conditions" I. *Acta Chir. Scand.* 1949; 99:133-153

[136] Hugentobler J.P., Blanchmaison P. "CHIVA cure. Etude de 96 patients opres de juin 1988 a juin 1990" *J. Mal. Vasc.* 1992;17:218-23

[137] Ibegbuna V, Delis KT, Nicolaides AN. Haemodynamic and clinical impact of superficial, deep and perforator vein incompetence. *Eur J Vasc Endovasc Surg.* 2006 May;31(5):535-41.

[138] Illig GK "Photoplethysmography and calf muscle pump function after subfascial endoscopic perforator ligation" *J Vasc Surg* 1999; 30: 1067-76

[139] International Consensus Committee. "Classification and grading of chronic venous disease in the lower limbs: A Consensus Statement" *Phlebology* 1995;10:42-5

[140] Jakobsen B.H. "The value of different forms of treatment for varicose veins" *Br. J. Surg.* 1979;66:182-84

[141] Kakkos SK, Bountouroglou DG, Azzam M, Kalodiki E, Daskalopoulos M, Geroulakos G. Effectiveness and safety of ultrasound-guided foam sclerotherapy for recurrent varicose veins: immediate results. *J Endovasc Ther*. 2006 Jun;13(3):357-64.

[142] Kistner RL, Eklof B, Masuda EM. Deep venous valve reconstruction. *Cardiovasc Surg*. 1995 Apr;3(2):129-40.

[143] Kistner R.L., Ferris E.B., Randhaw G., Kamida C. "A method of performing descending venography" *J. Vasc. Surg*. 1986; 4:464-468

[144] Koyano K, Sakaguchi S. Selective stripping operation based on Doppler ultrasonic findings for primary varicose veins of the lower extremities. *Surgery* 1988; 103:615-9

[145] Kupinsky A.M., Evans S.M., Khan, Zorn T.J. "Ultrasonic characterization of the saphenous vein" *Cardiovasc. Surg*. 1993 1:513-7

[146] Labropoulos N, Leon L, Engelhorn CA, Amaral SI, Rodriguez H, Kang SS, Mansour AM, Littooy FN. Sapheno-femoral junction reflux in patients with a normal saphenous trunk. *Eur J Vasc Endovasc Surg*. 2004 Dec;28(6):595-9.

[147] Labropoulos N, Leon L, Kwon S, Tassiopoulos A, Gonzalez-Fajardo JA, Kang SS, Mansour MA, Littooy FN. Study of the venous reflux progression. *J Vasc Surg*. 2005 Feb;41(2):291-5.

[148] Labropoulos N, Leon LR Jr. Duplex evaluation of venous insufficiency. *Semin Vasc Surg*. 2005 Mar;18(1):5-9.

[149] Labropoulos N, Manalo D, Patel NP, Tiongson J, Pryor L, Giannoukas AD."Uncommon leg ulcers in the lower extremity" *J Vasc Surg*. 2007 Mar;45(3):568-573. Epub 2007 Jan 25.

[150] Labropoulos N, Tassiopoulos AK, Bhatti AF, Leon L. Development of reflux in the perforator veins in limbs with primary venous disease. *J Vasc Surg*. 2006 Mar;43(3):558-62.

[151] Labropoulos N, Tiongson J, Pryor L, Tassiopoulos AK, Kang SS, AshrafMansour M, Baker WH. Definition of venous reflux in lower-extremity veins. *J Vasc Surg*. 2003 Oct;38(4):793-8.

[152] Labropoulos N, Tiongson J, Pryor L, Tassiopoulos AK, Kang SS, Mansour MA,Baker WH. Nonsaphenous superficial vein reflux. *J Vasc Surg*. 2001 Nov;34(5):872-7.

[153] Large J. "A conflict in vascular surgery" *Aust. N. Z. J. Surg*. 1985; 55:373-6

[154] Large J. "Surgical treatment of saphenous varices with preservation of the main great saphenous trunk" *J. Vasc. Surg*. 1985; 2:886-91 8

[155] Larson R.H., Lofgren E.P., Myers T.T., Lofgren K.A. "Long-term Results After Vein Surgery" *Mayo Clin. Proc*. 1974; 49: 114-17

[156] Laurikka J., Sisto T., Salenius J.P., Tarkka M., Auvinen O. "Long Saphenous Vein Stripping in the Treatment of Varicose Veins: Self- and Surgeon-Assessed Results After 10 Years" *Phebology* 1994; 9: 13-16

[157] Lemaire R. "Les structures motrices responsables de l'écoulement veineux" *Journal des maladies vasculaires Tome* 14 n° 2 1989 95-99

[158] Lemasle Ph, Uhl Jf, Lefebvre-Vilarderbo M, Baud JM. Proposition d'une definition echographique de la grande saphene et des saphenes accessories a l'etage crural. *Phlébologie* 1996; 49:279-86.

[159] Lewis J.D., Parsons D.C.S., Needham T.N., Douglas J.N., Hobbs J.T., Nicolaides A.N. "The use of venous pressure measurements and directional Doppler recording in distinguishing between superficial and deep valvular incompetence in patients with venous insufficiency" *Br. J. Surg.* 1973;60:312-8

[160] Li AKC "A technique for re-exploration of the s-f junction" *Br.J. Surg* 1975 62; 745-46

[161] Liddle AD, Davies AH. Pelvic congestion syndrome: chronic pelvic pain caused by ovarian and internal iliac varices. *Phlebology*. 2007;22(3):100-4.

[162] Lin JC, Iafrati MD, O'Donnell TF Jr, Estes JM, Mackey WC. Correlation of duplex ultrasound scanning-derived valve closure time and clinical classification in patients with small saphenous vein reflux: Is lesser saphenous vein truly lesser? *J Vasc Surg.* 2004 May;39(5):1053-8.

[163] Lofgren E.P. and Lofgren K.A. "Recurrence of Varicose Veins After the Stripping Operation" *Arch. Surg.* 1971; 102: 111-14

[164] Lofgren K.A., Ribisi A.P., Myers T.T."An evaluation of stripping versus ligation for varicose veins" *Arch. Surg.* 1958; 76:310-316 8

[165] Lurie F, Creton D, Eklof B, Kabnick LS, Kistner RL, Pichot O, Sessa C, Schuller-Petrovic S. Prospective randomised study of endovenous radiofrequency obliteration(closure) versus ligation and vein stripping (EVOLVeS): two-year follow-up. *Eur J Vasc Endovasc Surg.* 2005 Jan;29(1):67-73.

[166] Lye C.R., Sumner D.S., Strandness D.E. "The transcutaneous measurement of the elastic properties of the human saphenous vein femoro-popliteal bypass graft" *Surg. Gynaecol. Obst.* 1975;141:891-5

[167] Maeso J, Juan J, Escribano J, Allegue NM, Di Matteo A, Gonzalez E, Matas M. Comparison of clinical outcome of stripping and CHIVA for treatment of varicose veins in the lower extremities. *Ann Vasc Surg.* 2001 Nov;15(6):661-5.

[168] Maleti O, Lugli M. Neovalve construction in postthrombotic syndrome. *J Vasc Surg.* 2006 Apr;43(4):794-9.

[169] Mandolesi S. e Coll. *"Etude orthodynamique par Doppler cw du réseau veineux superficiel dans les syndromes par obstacle de décharge des membres inférieures"* XI° Congres Mondial de l'Union Internationale de Phlébologie Montreal 1992

[170] Marongiu G.M. "In quali casi e' indicata la crossectomia isolata nel trattamento della malattia varicosa essenziale? E infine se ne puo' intravedere una indicazione a scopo profilattico?" *Atti Giornate Flebologiche Algheresi*, pag. 43-46, 1989

[171] Mashiah A., Rose S.S., Hod I. "The scanning electronic microscope in the pathology of varicose veins" *Israel J. Med. Sci.* 27:202-206, 1991

[172] Masuda E.M., Kistner R.L., Eklof B. "Prospective study of duplex scanning for venous reflux: comparison of Valsalva and pneumatic cuff techniques in the reverse Trendelemburg and standing positions" *J.Vasc. Surg.* 1994; 20: 711-20

[173] May R. "Nomenclature of the surgically most important connecting veins. In: *Perforating veins*" Urban & Schwarzenberg, Munchen, 1981

[174] Mc Farlane R., Godwin R.J., Barabas A.P. "Are varicose veins and coronary bypass surgery incompatible?" *Lancet* 1985; ii:859

[175] McMullin G.M., Coleridge-Smith P.D., Scurr J.H. "Objective assesment of high ligation without stripping the long saphenous vein" *Br. J. Surg.* 1991; 78:1139-42 8

[176] Meissner MH, Gloviczki P, Bergan J, Kistner RL, Morrison N, Pannier F, Pappas PJ, Rabe E, Raju S, Villavicencio JL. Primary chronic venous disorders. *J Vasc Surg*. 2007;46:54-67.

[177] Mellman J. Wupperman Th. "Morphometric properties of incompetent perforaiting veins in the phlebogram" In May R. *Perforating Veins. Urban unt Schwarzenberg*. Munchen, Wien Baltimore, 1981

[178] Mendes RR, Marston WA, Farber MA, Keagy BA. Treatment of superficial and perforator venous incompetence without deep venous insufficiency: is routine perforator ligation necessary? *J Vasc Surg*. 2003;38:891-5.

[179] Mendoza E. *Duplexsonographie der oberflachlichen beinvenen*. Steinkopff-Verlag, Darmstadt 2007.

[180] Munn S.R., Morton J.B., Mac Berth W.A.A.G., Mac Leish A.R. "To strip or not to strip the long saphenous vein? A varicose veins trial" *Br. J. Surg*. 1981; 68: 426-8

[181] Navarro TP, Delis KT, Ribeiro AP. Clinical and hemodynamic significance of the greater saphenous vein diameter in chronic venous insufficiency. *Arch Surg* 2002; 137:1233-1237;

[182] Negus D. "Should the incompetent saphenous vein be stripped to the ankle?" *Phlebology* 1986;1:33-6. 8

[183] Nicolaides A.N., Zukowski A.J. "The value of dynamic venous pressure measurements" *World J. Surg*. 1986; 10:919-924

[184] Nicolaides AN, The International Consensus Group" The investigation of chronic venous insufficiency. A Consensus Statement". *Circulation* 2000, 102 (20):e126

[185] Nicolaides AN; Cardiovascular Disease Educational and Research Trust; European Society of Vascular Surgery; The International Angiology Scientific Activity Congress Organization; International Union of Angiology; Union Internationale de Phlebologie at the Abbaye des Vaux de Cernay. Investigation of chronic venous insufficiency: A consensus statement (France,March 5-9, 1997).*Circulation*. 2000 Nov 14;102(20):E126-63.

[186] Norgren L, Thulesius O, Gjöres JE, Söderlundh S. Foot-volumetry and simultaneous venous pressure measurements for evaluation of venous insufficiency. *Vasa*. 1974;3(2):140-7.

[187] Patel D.J., Greenfield J.C. Jr., Fry D.L. "In vivo pressure-length-radius relationship of certain blood vessel in man and dog" In: Ahinger EO ed. *Pulsatile blood flow*. New York: Mc Graw Hill, 1964:293-305

[188] Payne S.P.K., London N.J.M., Jagger C., et al. "Clinical significance of venous reflux detected by duplex scanning" *Br. J. Surg*. 1994; 81:39-41

[189] Perrin M, Allaert FA. Intra- and Inter-observer Reproducibility of the Recurrent Varicose Veins after Surgery (REVAS) Classification. *Eur J Vasc Endovasc Surg*. 2006 Sep;32(3):326-32.

[190] Perrin M, Guidicelli H, Rastel D. Surgical techniques used for the treatment of varicose veins: survey of practice in France *J Mal Vasc*. 2003;28;277-86

[191] Perrin MR.,Labropoulos N., Leon LR. Jr. Presentation of the patient with recurrent varices after surgery (REVAS). *J. Vasc. Surg*. 2006; 43:327-34.

[192] Phifer TJ, Gerlock AJ Jr, Rich NM, McDonald JC. Long-term patency of venous repairs demonstrated by venography. *J Trauma*. 1985 Apr;25(4):342-6.

[193] Pollack A.A., Wood E.H. "Venous pressure in the saphenous vein at the ankle in man during exercise and changes in posture" *J. Appl. Phys*. 1949; 1:649-662

[194] Pozzi L. *"Elementi di emodinamica"*La Medicina Internazionale, 1972 n° 15

[195] Rabe E. "The classification of insufficient perforating veins by color duplex sonography" *Phlebology* 1994; 23:146-148

[196] Raju S., Fredericks R. "Valve reconstruction procedures for nonobstructive venous insufficiency: rationale, techniques and results in 107 procedures with two-to eight-year follow-up" *J. Vasc. Surg*. 1988; 7:301-310

[197] Raju S, Neglen P. High prevalence of nonthrombotic iliac vein lesions in chronic venous disease: a permissive role in pathogenicity. *J Vasc Surg*. 2006 Jul;44(1):136-43; discussion 144.

[198] Rettori R. Postoperative recurrence of varicosities at the level of the popliteal fossa. Anatomic data guiding the ultrasonographic exploration and surgical sequelae. *J Mal Vasc*. 1998 Feb ; 23 (1) : 54-60

[199] Ricci S, Georgiev M, Jawien A, Zamboni P. Sciatic nerve varices. *Eur J Vasc Endovasc Surg*. 2005 Jan;29(1):83-7.

[200] Ricci S., Caggiati A., Echoanatomical Patterns of the Long Saphenous Vein in Patients with Primary Varices and in Healty Subjects. *Phlebology Volume 14*, Issue 2, pp 54-58.

[201] Ricci S., Georgiev M., Goldman M. *"Ambulatory Phlebectomy"* Mosby Y. B., New York 1995

[202] Rich NM. Complications of vascular injury management. *Surg Clin North Am*. 2002 Feb;82(1):143-74.

[203] Rich NM. Management of venous trauma. *Surg Clin North Am*. 1988 Aug;68(4):809-21.

[204] Rivlin S. "The surgical cure of primary varicose veins" *Br. J. Surg*. 1975; 62: 913-17

[205] Rizzi A, Quaglio D, Vasquez G, Mascoli F, Amadesi S, Calo G, Regoli D, ZamboniP. Effects of vasoactive agents in healthy and diseased human saphenous veins. *J Vasc Surg*. 1998 Nov;28(5):855-61.

[206] Rose S.S., Ahmed A "Some thoughts on the etiology of varicose veins" *J. Cardiovasc. Surg*. 27:534-543, 1986

[207] Ruckley CV, Evans CJ, Allan PL, Lee AJ, Fowkes FG. Chronic venous insufficiency: clinical and duplex correlations. The Edinburgh Vein Study of venous disorders in the general population. *J Vasc Surg*. 2002 Sep;36(3):520-5.

[208] Rutheford R.B., Sawyer J.D., Jones D.N. "The fate of residual saphenous vein after partial removal or ligation" *J. Vasc. Surg*. 1990;12:422-26

[209] Rutherford EE, Kianifard B, Cook SJ, Holdstock JM, Whiteley MS Incompetent perforating veins are associated with recurrent varicose veins *Eur J Vasc Endovasc Surg* 2001;75:458.

[210] Sales CM, Bilof ML, Petrillo KA, Luka NL. Correction of lower extremity deep venous incompetence by ablation of superficial venous reflux. *Ann Vasc Surg* 1996; 10: 186–189.

[211] Sarin S., Scurr J.H., Coleridge Smith P.D. "Saphenofemoral junction recurrence after surgical ligation" *J. Derm. Surg. Onc.* 1994;20:70

[212] Sarin S., Scurr J.H., Smith Coleridge P.D., Medial calf perforators in venous disease: the significance of outward flow, *J Vasc Surg* 1992;16:40-6.

[213] Sarin S., Shields D.A., Farrah J., Scurr J.H., Coleridge-Smith P.D. "Does venous function deteriorate in patients waiting for varicose surgery?" *J. R. Soc. Med.* 1993; 86:21-23

[214] Sarin S., Shields D.A., Scurr J.H., et al "Photopletismography: A valuable non invasive tool in the assessment of venous dysfunction" *J. Vasc. Surg.* 16:154-162, 1992

[215] Sarin S., Sommerville K., Farah J., Scurr J.H., Coleridge Smith P.D. "Duplex ultrasonography for assessment of venous valvular function of the lower limb" *Br. J. Surg.* 1994; 81:1591-5 8

[216] Shah D.M, Chang BB, Leopold PW, Corson JD, Leather RP, Karmody AM. The anatomy of the greater saphenous venous system" *J. Vasc. Surg.* 1987; 6:107-13 12

[217] Sharif MA, Soong CV, Lau LL, Corvan R, Lee B, Hannon RJ. Endovenous laser treatment for long saphenous vein incompetence. *Br J Surg*. 2006 Jul;93(7):831-5.

[218] Stacey MC, Burnand KG, Layer GT, Pattison M. Calf pump function in patients with healed venous ulcers is not improved by surgery to the communicating veins or by elastic stockings. *Br J Surg* 1988; 75:436-9.

[219] Stegall F.H. "Muscle Pumping in the Dependente Leg" *Circulation Reserch*. July 1966 Vol. XIX

[220] Stiegler H., Rotter G., Standl R., et al. "The value of color-coded duplex sonography in the diagnosis of perforating vein insufficiency: a prospective study in 94 patients" *VASA* 1994; 23:109-113

[221] Stolic "Terminology, division and systematic anatomy of communicating veins" In: *Perforating Veins*, May R. et al., Urban Schwarzenberg, Munchen Wien Baltimore, 1981

[222] Sturup H., Hojensgard I.C. "Venous pressure in varicose veins in patients with incompetent communicating veins. A study of the statics and dynamics of the venous system of the lower extremity under pathological conditions" *Acta Chir. Scand.* 1949; 99:518-525

[223] Sullivan E.D., Peter D.J., Cranley J.J. "Realtime B-mode venous ultrasound" *J. Vasc. Surg.* 1984;1:465-71

[224] Szendro G., Nicolaides A.N., Zukowski A. et al "Duplex scanning in the assessment of deep venous incompetence" *J. Vasc. Surg.* 1986; 4:237

[225] Talbot S.R. *"B-mode evaluation of peripheral veins"* Semin. Ultrasound CT MR 1988;9:295-319

[226] Taulaniemi E. "On the treatm0ent of varices"*Acta Chir. Scand.* 1963, 125: 429-432

[227] Tessari L. "Messa a punto sul metodo emodinamico della malattia varicosa"Atti Giornate Flebologiche Algheresi, pag. 521-24 1989

[228] Thiery L.: Anatomie chirurgicale de la fosse poplitée, *Phlebologie*, 1986, 39 (1), 57-66

[229] Thiery L.: Le problème des perforantes, *Phlebologie*, 1988, 41 (1), 215-228

[230] Thomson H. The surgical anatomy of the superficial and perforating veins of the lower limb. *Ann R Coll Surg Engl*. 1979;61:198–205.

[231] Thulesius O. "Vein wall characteristics and valvular function in chronic venous insufficiency" *Phlebology* 1993; 8:94-98

[232] Thulesius O, Norgren L, Gjöres JE. Foot-volumetry, a new method for objective assessment of edema and venous function. *Vasa*. 1973;2(4):325-9.

[233] Thulesius O., Ugaily-Thulesius L., Neglen P., Shuhaiber H. "The role of the endoteluim in the control of venous tone: studies on isolate,d human veins" *Clin Physiol* 1988; 8:359-366

[234] Tibbs J. D. Fletcher E. W. L. "Direction of flow in superficial veins as a guide to venous disorders in lower limbs" *Surgery*, 1983; 93; 6; pp. 758-767

[235] Ting AC, Cheng SW, Ho P, Poon JT, Wu LL, Cheung GC. Reduction in deep vein reflux after concomitant subfascial endoscopic perforating vein surgery and superficial vein ablation in advanced primary chronic venous insufficiency. *J Vasc Surg*. 2006 Mar;43(3):546-50.

[236] Ting AC, Cheng SW, Wu LL, Cheung GC. Changes in venous hemodynamics after superficial vein surgery for mixed superficial and deep venous insufficiency. *World J Surg*. 2001 Feb;25(2):122-5.

[237] Traissac B, Sagardoy G. [Role of elastic containment with calibrated biflex bandages in the treatment of venous insufficiency in athletes and in vascular rehabilitation] *Phlebologie*. 1986 Jan-Mar;39(1):173-82.

[238] Trendelenburg F. "Ueber die Unterbindung der Saphena magna bei Unterschenkelvaricen" *Beitr Klin. Chir*. 1981; 7:195

[239] Tretbar L.L. "Ambulatory venous blood flow in the long saphenous vein before and after clipping the sapheno-femoral junction" *J. Surg. Derm. Onc*. 1994;20: 69-70

[240] Umeh H.N., Faber R.G., Reece-Smith H., Galland R.B. "Impact of a waiting list initiative on a general surgical waiting list" *Ann. R. Coll. Surg*. Engl. (Suppl) 1994; 39:103-105

[241] Van Bemmelen PS, Beach K, Bedford G, Strandness DE Jr. The mechanism of venous valve closure. Its relationship to the velocity of reverse flow. *Arch Surg*. 1990 May;125(5):617-9.

[242] Van Cleef J.F. "Modèl dynamique de la pompe musculaire du mollet dans l'insuffisance veineus Profonde" *Phlébologie*, 1992, 45, n° 3, pp. 259-263

[243] Van Cleef J.F., Hugentobler J.P., Desnaux P., et al "Quelques aspects endoscopiques de valvules chez la variqueux" *Phlebologie 44*:623-627, 1991

[244] Varty K., Jones L., Porter E., Bell P.R.F., London N.J.M.L. "A quantitative study of long saphenous vein morphology in patients undergoing arterial surgery" *Phlebology* 1995; 10:90-93

[245] Villaviciencio L. "The anatomic basis for the unreliability of the Doppler examination under Valsalva manouver" *Phlebologie-Phlebology 92*, vol. 2, ed. by Martimbeau P.R., Prescott R., Zummo M. Paris: Libbey, 1992, 2:9

[246] Vin F, Chleir F, Ultrasonography of postoperatively recurrent varicose vein in the area of the short saphenous vein. *Ann chir* 2001 May; 126(4):320-4

[247] Walsh JC, Bergan JJ, Beeman S, Comer T: Femoral venous reflux abolished by greater saphenous vein stripping; *Ann.Vasc Surg* 1994, 8, 566-70

[248] Winterborn RJ, Foy C, Earnshaw JJ. Causes of varicose vein recurrence: late results of a randomized controlled trial of stripping the long saphenous vein. *J Vasc Surg*. 2004 Oct;40(4):634-9.

[249] Winterborn RJ, Jones L, Earnshaw JJ. Response to: The lateral accessory saphenous vein--a common cause of recurrent varicose veins. *Ann R Coll Surg* Engl. 2004 Nov;86(6):490.

[250] Woodyer A.B., Dormandy J.A. “Is it necessary to strip the long saphenous vein?” *Phlebology* 1986;1:221-4. 8

[251] Zamboni P, Cisno C, Marchetti F, Mazza P, Fogato L, Carandina S, De Palma M, Liboni A. Minimally invasive surgical management of primary venous ulcers vs. compression treatment: a randomized clinical trial. *Eur J Vasc Endovasc Surg*. 2003 Apr;25(4):313-8.

[252] Zamboni P, Cisno C, Marchetti F, Quaglio D, Mazza P, Liboni A. Reflux elimination without any ablation or disconnection of the saphenous vein. A haemodynamic model for venous surgery. *Eur J Vasc Endovasc Surg*. 2001 Apr;21(4):361-9.

[253] Zamboni P, De Palma M, Carandina S, Fogato L, Fortini P, Legnaro A, Mazza P, Ricci S. The "T" vein of the leg. *Dermatol Surg*. 2004 May;30(5):750-2

[254] Zamboni P, Escribano JM. Regarding 'Reflux Elimination Without any Ablation or Disconnection of the Saphenous Vein. A Haemodynamic Model for Venous Surgery' and 'Durability of Reflux-elimination by a Minimal Invasive CHIVA Procedure on Patients with Varicose Veins. A 3-year Prospective Case Study'. *Eur J Vasc Endovasc Surg*. 2004 Nov;28(5):567.

[255] Zamboni P, Marcellino MG, Cappelli M, Feo CV, Bresadola V, Vasquez G, Liboni A. Saphenous vein sparing surgery: principles, techniques and results. *J Cardiovasc Surg* (Torino). 1998 Apr;39(2):151-62.

[256] Zamboni P. Regarding Photoplethysmography and calf muscle pump function after subfascial endoscopic perforator ligation *J Vasc Surg* 2000; 32: 1039-40

[257] Zamboni P. La chirurgia conservativa del sistema venoso superficiale. Faenza: Gruppo Editoriale Faenza Editrice, 1996:3-9.

[258] Zamboni P., D. Quaglio, C. Cisno, F. Marchetti, M. Giacometti, M.G. Marcellino: “Evaluation ultrasonique de la pression veineuse ambulatoire dans l’insuffisance veineuse primaire”. *Phlebologie* 1999;52; 2.

[259] Zamboni P., D. Quaglio, C. Cisno, F. Marchetti, S. Lanzara, P. Mazza The relationship between diameter and pressure in the insufficient saphenous vein *Journal of Phlebology*, 2002;vol 2, num1, 19-23.

[260] Zamboni P., D.Quaglio, F.Marchetti, C.Cisno, P.Mazza, L.Fogato.The value of the ultrasonic perthes test in predicting the outcome of saphenous vein sparing surgery . *Int. Angiology* 2001 vol. 20, June, Suppl. 1 to issue n° 2, 142

[261] Zamboni P., F. Portaluppi, M.G Marcellino, D.Quaglio, R.Manfredini, A. Liboni , RJ Stoney: “In vitro > in vivo assessment of vein wall properties”. *Ann Vasc Surg* 1998;12:324-329.

[262] Zamboni P., F. Portaluppi, M.G. Marcellino, L.Pisano, R. Manfredini, A.Liboni: “Ultrasonographic assessment of ambulatory venous pressure in superficial venous incompetence”. *J. Vasc. Surg*. 1997,26: 796-803.

[263] Zamboni P., Feo C., Marcellino M.G., Manfredini R., Vettorello G.F., De Anna D. "Angiovideoassisted hemodynamic correction of varicose vein" *Int. Angiology* 1995; 14:202-208

[264] Zamboni P, Gemmati D. Clinical implications of gene polymorphisms in venous leg ulcer: a model in tissue injury and reparative process. *Thromb Haemost*. 2007 Jul;98(1):131-7.

[265] Zamboni P., Gasbarro V., Marcellino M.G. "Exetrnal valvuloplasty of the sapheno-femoral junction" *Vasc.Surg. 28*: 327-36, 1994

[266] Zamboni P., Gasbarro V., Pozza E., De Anna D., Murgia A.P., Donini A., et al. "External valvuloplasty of the sapheno-femoral junction and tributaries preservation" In: *Phlebologie 92*, Paris: John Libbey Eurotext, 1992:1252:1254

[267] Zamboni P., Liboni A. "External valvuloplasty of the sapheno-femoral junction using perforated prosthesis" *Phlebology* 1991, 6:141-147

[268] Zamboni P., M. Cappelli, MG Marcellino, AP Murgia, L.Pisano, P.Fabi: "Does a saphenous varicose vein exist?" *Phlebology* 1997;12: 74-77.

[269] Zamboni P., M.G. Marcellino, L. Pisano, D. Quaglio, V.Gasbarro, D.De Anna, A. Liboni: A new hook-dissector for ambulatory phlebectomy. *Abstract Annual Congress North American Society*

[270] Zamboni P., M.G. Marcellino, L.Pisano, M. Cappelli, V. Bresadola, G. Vasquez, A. Liboni: Saphenous vein sparing surgery: indications, techniques and results. *J Cardiovasc Surg* 1998;39: 151-162.

[271] Zamboni P., Marcellino M.G., Feo C., Berta R., Vasquez G., Pansini G.C. "When CHIVA treatment could be video guided" *Dermatol. Surg*. 1995; 21:621-625

[272] Zamboni, Serena Lanzara, Francesco Mascoli, Alberto Caggiati*, Alberto Liboni Inflammation in venous disease. *Review. Int. Ang*. 2008, in press

[273] Zamboni P., Marcellino M.G., Feo C., Pisano L., Vasquez G., Bertasi M., Liboni A. "Alternative saphenous vein sparing surgery for future grafting" *Pan. Min. Med 37*: 190-97, 1996.

[274] Zamboni P., Marcellino M.G., Gasbarro V., Viaggi R., R. Manfredini, Liboni A., Donini I. "Primary varices hemodynamic correction with intraoperative angioscopy" *J. Dermatol. Surg. Oncol*. 1994, 20:69

[275] Zamboni P., Marcellino M.G., Portaluppi F., Manfredini R., Quaglio D., Liboni A. "The probability of lower saphenous vein compliance in advanced varicose vein disease" World Congress of Phlebology 1995, Abstract book.

[276] Zamboni P., Marcellino M.G., Portaluppi F., Manfredini R., Quaglio D., Liboni A. "The relationship between in vitro and in vivo venous compliance measurement" *Int. Angiology 2*: 17-18;1996.

[277] Zamboni P., Marcellino M.G., Quaglio D., Vasquez G., Murgia A.P., Pisano L., Feo C. "A reliable non invasive methods for venous compliance measurements" *Phlebology* 1995;10 suppl.1:277-9

[278] Zamboni P.. Pathophysiology of Perforators in Primary Chronic Venous Insufficiency *World Journal of Surgery*, 2005;29;1:115-8

[279] Zamboni P, Izzo M, Tognazzo S, Carandina S, De Palma M, Catozzi L, Caggiati A, Scapoli G, Gemmati D. The overlapping of local iron overload and HFE mutation in

venous leg ulcer pathogenesis. *Free Radic Biol Med.* 2006 May 15;40(10):1869-73. Epub 2006 Feb 14.Comment in: *Free Radic Biol Med.* 2006 May 15;40(10):1700-1.

[280] Zamboni P.MD, Caterina Cisno MD, Federica Marchetti MD, Paolo Mazza MD, Luisella Fogato MD, Sergio Carandina MD, Massimiliano De Palma MD, and Alberto Liboni MD Haemodynamic CHIVA correction surgery vs compression for primary venous ulcers: first year results **Phlebology*, 2004,19(1): 28-34.

[281] Zamboni P.MD, Marcello Izzo MD, Fogato Luisella MD, Carandina Sergio MD, and Vincenzo Lanzara PhD Urine haemosiderin: a novel marker to assess the severity of chronic venous disease. *J. Vasc. Surg.*, 2003;37:132-6

[282] Zamboni P.Regarding: Treatment of superficial and perforator venous incompetence without deep venous insufficiency: is routine perforator ligation necessary? *J. Vasc. Surg.*, 2004; 39(5):1144-1145

[283] Zamboni P, Gianesini S. Response to Letter to Editor re: Varicose Vein Stripping vs Haemodynamic Correction (CHIVA): a Long Term Randomised Trial, by S. Carandina, C. Mari, M. De Palma, M.G. Marcellino, C. Cisno, A. Legnaro, A. Liboni, P. Zamboni, in Eur J Vasc Endovasc Surg 2008;35(2):230-237. *Eur J Vasc Endovasc Surg.* 2008 Apr 5 [Epub ahead of print]

[284] Zamboni P, D Quaglio, C Cisno, F Marchetti, L Cisno, MG Marcellino, The relationship between ultrasonic ambulatory venous pressure and residual volume fraction. *Phlebology* 1999. 14:146-150.

## About The Authors

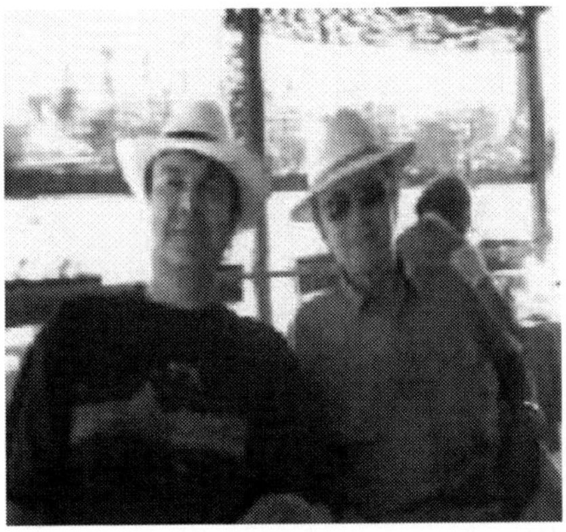

Claude Franceschi MD, Director of the Vascular Laboratories of Hospitals Saint Joseph and Pitié-Salpétrière in Paris, France. In 1977, published the first text book about Doppler Vascular Diagnosis at the early appearance of non invasive diagnosis in clinical Medicine. In 1988 published Theory and Practice of the Cure CHIVA, an innovative text of venous haemodynamics which deeply influenced the practice of Phlebology, especially in Europe.

Paolo Zamboni, Professor of Surgery and Director of the Vascular Diseases Center of University of Ferrara, Italy. He created a multi-disciplinary research group involved in the study of venous diseases. The staff includes experts both in basic and in clinical sciences, who collaborate back to back in common and innovative research programs.

### Contributing Authors

Massimiliano De Palma, MD
Sergio Carandina, MD
Sergio Gianesini, MD
Erica Menegatti, RVT

Department of Surgery, Vascular Diseases Center, University of Ferrara, Italy.

# INDEX

## A



## B

## Q



## R



## S

## T

## U



## V



## W